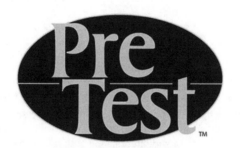

# Physiology

PreTest™ Self-Assessment and Review

T0204794

## Notice

Medicine is an ever-changing science. As new research and clinical experience broaden our knowledge, changes in treatment and drug therapy are required. The authors and the publisher of this work have checked with sources believed to be reliable in their efforts to provide information that is complete and generally in accord with the standards accepted at the time of publication. However, in view of the possibility of human error or changes in medical sciences, neither the authors nor the publisher nor any other party who has been involved in the preparation or publication of this work warrants that the information contained herein is in every respect accurate or complete, and they disclaim all responsibility for any errors or omissions or for the results obtained from use of the information contained in this work. Readers are encouraged to confirm the information contained herein with other sources. For example and in particular, readers are advised to check the product information sheet included in the package of each drug they plan to administer to be certain that the information contained in this work is accurate and that changes have not been made in the recommended dose or in the contraindications for administration. This recommendation is of particular importance in connection with new or infrequently used drugs.

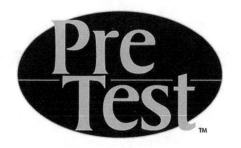

# Physiology
## PreTest™ Self-Assessment and Review
### Thirteenth Edition

**Patricia J. Metting, PhD**
Professor, Departments of Physiology & Pharmacology and Medicine
Vice Provost and Associate Dean for Student Affairs
The University of Toledo College of Medicine
Toledo, Ohio

**James F. Kleshinski, MD**
Associate Professor, Department of Medicine
Associate Dean for Admissions
The University of Toledo College of Medicine
Toledo, Ohio

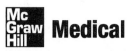 **Medical**

New York   Chicago   San Francisco   Lisbon   London   Madrid   Mexico City
Milan   New Delhi   San Juan   Seoul   Singapore   Sydney   Toronto

**The McGraw·Hill Companies**

**Physiology: PreTest™ Self-Assessment and Review, Thirteenth Edition**

1 2 3 4 5 6 7 8 9 0    DOC/DOC    14 13 12 11 10

ISBN 978-0-07-162350-6
MHID 0-07-162350-7

This book was set in Berkeley by Glyph International Limited.
The editors were Kirsten Funk and Cindy Yoo.
The production supervisor was Sherri Souffrance.
Project management was provided by Madhu Bhardwaj, Glyph International Limited.
The cover designer was Maria Scharf.
RR Donnelley was printer and binder.

**Library of Congress Cataloging-in-Publication Data**

Metting, Patricia J.
    Physiology: PreTest self-assessment and review.—13th ed. / Patricia J. Metting,
    James F. Kleshinski.
       p.; cm.
    Rev. ed. of: Physiology. 12th ed. / [edited by] Patricia J. Metting.
    c2007.
    Includes bibliographical references and index.
    ISBN 978-0-07-162350-6 (pbk.)
    1. Human physiology—Examinations, questions, etc.   I. Kleshinski, James F.
    II. Physiology. III. Title.
    [DNLM: 1. Physiological Phenomena—Examination Questions.
    2. Physiology—Examination Questions. QT 18.2 M595p 2010]
    QP40.P47    2010
    612.0076—dc22                                        2009054281

To my husband, Mike Metting, and our children,
Megan and Patrick Metting,
and
To my wife, Olga Kleshinski, and our children,
Jimmy and Olivia Kleshinski,
For your unconditional love and encouragement and the sacrifices you have made over the years in deference to our professional activities and responsibilities. We hope that somehow you know that there has never been anything more important in our lives than all of you.

PM and JK

# Student Reviewers

**Maxx Gallegos**
University of Kansas School of Medicine
Class of 2011

**Russel Kahmke**
SUNY Upstate Medical University
Class of 2010

**Daniel Marcovici**
Sackler School of Medicine
Tel Aviv University
Class of 2011

**S. Kendall Smith**
MD/PhD Candidate
University of Kansas School of Medicine
Class of 2012

**Sheree Perron**
Eastern Virginia Medical School
Class of 2010

# Contents

# Introduction

Each *PreTest™ Self-Assessment and Review* is designed to allow allopathic and osteopathic medical students, as well as international medical graduates, a comprehensive and convenient way to assess and review their knowledge of a particular medical science, in this instance, physiology. The 500 questions have been organized to parallel the Content Outline for the United States Medical Licensing Examination (USMLE™) Step 1 (http://www.usmle.org/Examinations/step1/step1_content.html). By familiarizing yourself with the Step 1 Content Outline, you will get a more accurate idea of the subject areas covered in each section. For example, acid-base balance and high-altitude physiology are topics covered under General Principles: Multisystem Processes and oxygen and carbon dioxide transport are covered in the chapter on the Physiology of the Hematopoietic and Lymphoreticular Systems, rather than under Respiratory or Renal Physiology, where you likely learned them during your medical school education. The value of organizing the questions this way is that the Step 1 Content Outline is used by the National Board of Medical Examiners (NBME) in the score reports that go to each examinee to provide them with their relative performance in each of the various areas tested by the USMLE Step 1. Thus, when you eventually find out how you performed in each category, you will have a more accurate understanding of your areas of strength and weakness.

*Physiology: PreTest™* has been updated to incorporate a clinical vignette and/or graphic interpretation in every question. In this way, the questions in *Physiology: PreTest™* more closely parallel the length and the degree of difficulty of the questions that you should expect to find on the USMLE Step 1.

*Physiology: PreTest™* will also be a valuable resource for osteopathic medical students studying for the Comprehensive Osteopathic Medical Licensing Examination (COMLEX)-USA. Similar to Step 1 of the USMLE, Level 1 of the COMLEX-USA, administered by the National Board of Osteopathic Medical Examiners, Inc., emphasizes an understanding of the basic science mechanisms underlying health and disease, and is constructed with clinical presentations in the context of medical problem solving (http://www.nbome.org).

Each question in *Physiology: PreTest™* is followed by multiple answer options. For each question, select the *one best* answer from the choices given. Each question is also accompanied by the correct answer and its explanation. The explanation provides the reason why the correct answer is correct and, in most cases, the reasons why the wrong answers are wrong.

The explanations also provide additional information relevant to the clinical vignette and the basic science topic the question is intended to test. The references accompanying each question are from popular and excellent physiology, pathophysiology, and internal medicine textbooks. Step 1 is the first of three exams required for medical licensure in the United States. Although it is a test that examines knowledge of the basic sciences, the expectation is that you can apply the basic knowledge in clinical problem solving. By using clinical vignettes and clinical reference texts, our hope is that your preparation for the USMLE Step 1 (and/or COMLEX-USA Level 1) will also serve to enhance your ability to function competently in the clinical environment. The material in the referenced pages will provide a more expansive description of the subject matter covered by the question.

One effective way to use the *PreTest*™ is to use it as a review for each topic area. Start by reading the High-Yield Facts on a selected topic found at the beginning of the book. The High-Yield Facts are not meant to be a complete list of all of the important facts, concepts, and equations necessary for understanding physiology. Those that are included, however, offer a solid foundation and should be included in your review of physiology in preparation for a class test or for the USMLE Step 1. Once you've completed your reading on a topic, answer the questions for that chapter. As you check your answers, be sure to read the explanations, as they are designed to reinforce and expand on the material covered by the questions. If you are still unsure of why the correct answer is correct, you should also read the referenced text pages.

*PreTest*™ can also be used as a practice testing session. Set aside two-and-a-half hours, and answer 150 of the questions, writing the answers on a separate sheet of paper. Once you have completed all 150, then you can go back and compare your answers to the ones provided in the book. This exercise will help you assess your level of competence and confidence prior to taking the USMLE Step 1. Whichever way you use *PreTest*™, an important part of your review can be found in the explanations.

Good luck on your exam and best wishes for your clinical training. Keep in mind that there is a *PreTest*™ available for the other basic sciences, as well as in each of the required clinical disciplines, so we encourage you to make the *PreTest*™ series your review books of choice throughout the preclinical and clinical portions of the medical school curriculum, as well as during your preparation for Step 1 and Step 2 Clinical Knowledge (CK) of the USMLE or for the COMLEX-USA Level 1 and Level 2-Cognitive Evaluation (CE).

# Acknowledgments

We are indebted to all of The University of Toledo College of Medicine medical students past and present, who have challenged us to be vigilant in correlating the basic and clinical sciences. We wish to thank Jeffrey P. Gold, MD, Provost and Executive Vice President for Health Affairs and Dean of the College of Medicine at The University of Toledo, Joseph I. Shapiro, MD, Mercy Heath Partners Education Professor and Chairman, Department of Medicine, The University of Toledo, and all of our faculty colleagues for their support and encouragement.

The contributions of the authors of all previous editions of this book are gratefully acknowledged. In addition, the input of the medical student reviewers was valuable for enhancing the quality of this latest edition. We would also like to thank Kirsten Funk, Editor, Medical Publishing Division, McGraw-Hill Professional, for her editorial assistance and guidance throughout the preparation of this text, Cindy Yoo, Project Development Editor, and Sherri Souffrance, Production Supervisor, McGraw-Hill Professional, for their assistance in the production phase, and Madhu Bhardwaj, Glyph International limited, for her involvement in the typesetting and revisions.

# High-Yield Facts in Physiology

## GENERAL PRINCIPLES: CELLULAR PHYSIOLOGY

*(References: Ganong, pp 1-49. Widmaier et al, pp 43-54, 96-136.)*

### Membrane Transport Mechanisms

The transport of ions, gases, nutrients, and waste products through biological membranes is essential for many cellular processes. Membrane transport mechanisms can be classified as *passive* (do not require energy input, as with simple diffusion or facilitated diffusion) and *active transport* (requires energy input). Membrane transport mechanisms can also be classified as either *simple diffusion* (does not require a membrane transporter, eg, diffusion through the lipid bilayer or diffusion through ion channels) or *mediated transport* (requiring an integral membrane protein transporter, as with facilitated diffusion or active transport).

*Diffusion* is defined as the net flux of a substance from an area of higher concentration to an area of lower concentration from movement solely by random thermal motion, which does not require energy input.

*Facilitated diffusion* is a type of mediated transport, but is a passive process in which carrier proteins move substances in the direction of their electrochemical gradients (eg, glucose transport in adipose tissue and muscle).

*Active transport* is a carrier-mediated transport process that requires energy to transport substances against their electrochemical gradients. The most important primary active transporter in mammalian cells is the $Na^+$-$K^+$ pump, which generates energy from the hydrolysis of ATP. Secondary active transport processes derive their energy from ion gradients. One example is the glucose transporter, which uses energy derived from the $Na^+$ electrochemical gradient.

Table 1 summarizes the major characteristics of the various membrane transport processes. Note that nonpolar substances, such as oxygen, carbon dioxide, and fatty acids, are transported by simple diffusion through the lipid bilayer of biological membranes. Ions and hydrophilic solutes, which do not readily cross the lipid bilayer, utilize an integral membrane protein to cross the membrane either via diffusion through a protein channel or via a carrier-mediated transport process.

## TABLE I. MAJOR CHARACTERISTICS OF MEMBRANE TRANSPORT MECHANISMS

| | Diffusion Through Lipid Bilayer | Diffusion Through Ion Channel | Facilitated Diffusion | Primary Active Transport | Secondary Active Transport |
|---|---|---|---|---|---|
| Direction of net flux | High to low concentration | High to low concentration | High to low concentration | Low to high concentration | Low to high concentration |
| Use of energy and source | No, passive | No, passive | No, passive | Yes, ATP | Yes, ion gradient |
| Equilibrium or steady state | $C_o = C_i$ | $C_o = C_i^a$ | $C_o = C_i$ | $C_o \neq C_i$ | $C_o \neq C_i$ |
| Uses integral membrane protein | No | Yes | Yes | Yes | Yes |
| Exhibits saturation kinetics | No | No | Yes, mediated transport | Yes, mediated transport | Yes, mediated transport |
| Chemical specificity | No | Yes | Yes | Yes | Yes |
| Typical molecules using pathway | Nonpolar: $O_2$, $CO_2$, fatty acids | Ions: $Na^+$, $K^+$, $Ca^{2+}$ | Polar: glucose | Ions: $Na^+$, $K^+$, $Ca^{2+}$, $H^+$ | Polar: amino acids, glucose, some ions |

[a]In the presence of a membrane potential, the intracellular and extracellular ion concentrations will not be equal at equilibrium.
(Modified, with permission, from Widmaier EP, Raff H, Strang KT. *Vander's Human Physiology: The Mechanisms of Body Function*. 11th ed. New York, NY: McGraw-Hill; 2008: 108.)

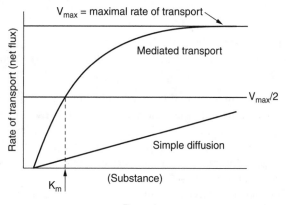

Figure I

The kinetics of diffusion versus carrier-mediated transport processes vary, as depicted in Figure 1.

Simple diffusion of a substance is described by the Fick equation, as follows:

$$\text{Net flux} = A \times ([S1] - [S2]) \times D/d$$

where

A is area available for diffusion,

[S1] − [S2] is concentration gradient of the substance across the membrane,

d is distance for diffusion,

D is diffusion coefficient of the substance,

= solubility coefficient/$\sqrt{\text{gram molecular weight}}$ of the substance.

According to the Fick equation, substances will diffuse more rapidly if the substance has a smaller mass, if the surface area for diffusion is increased, and if the concentration of the substance in one region greatly exceeds the concentration in the other region. For diffusion across membranes, the magnitude of the net flux is also directly proportional to the membrane permeability coefficient for the molecule.

*Mediated transport* exhibits saturation kinetics described by the Michaelis-Menten equation, as follows:

$$\text{Net flux} = V_{max} \times [S]/K_m + [S],$$

where
  $V_{max}$ is the maximal rate of transport.
  [S] is the concentration of the transported substance.
  $K_m$ is the concentration required for half-maximal transport of the
  substance.

Osmosis is a term given to the passive diffusion of water across a semi-permeable membrane from a compartment in which the solute concentration is lower (chemical potential of water is higher) to a compartment in which the solute concentration is higher (chemical potential of water is lower), as depicted in Figure 2. A semipermeable membrane is permeable to water but impermeable to solutes.

The flow of water through membranes by osmosis is described by the osmotic flow equation:

$$Flow = \sigma \times L \times (\pi_1 - \pi_2),$$

where
  $\sigma$ is reflection coefficient.
  $L$ is hydraulic conductivity.
  $\pi_1 - \pi_2$ is osmotic pressure difference across membrane.

The reflection coefficient ($\sigma$) is an index of the membrane's permeability to a solute and varies between 0 and 1. Particles that are impermeable

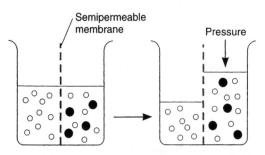

**Figure 2**
Diagrammatic representation of osmosis. Water molecules are the open circles and solute molecules are the closed circles. Osmosis is the passive flow of water molecules across a semipermeable membrane from a compartment in which the chemical potential of water is higher (solute concentration is lower) to a compartment in which the chemical potential of water is lower (solute concentration is higher). *(Reproduced, with permission, from Ganong WF. Review of Medical Physiology. 22nd ed. New York, NY: McGraw-Hill;2005: 5.)*

to the membrane have a reflection coefficient of 1. Particles that are freely permeable to the membrane have a reflection coefficient of 0.

The *osmotic pressure* ($\pi$) of a solution is the pressure necessary to prevent solute migration. The osmotic pressure (in units of mm Hg) is calculated with the van't Hoff equation:

$$\pi = R\,T\,(\varphi ic),$$

where

R is the ideal gas constant.
T is absolute temperature.
$\varphi$ is the osmotic coefficient.
i is the number of ions formed by the dissociation of a molecule.
c is the molar concentration of solute.
($\varphi ic$) is the osmolarity of the solution.

The value of i is 1 for nonionic substances such as glucose and urea, 2 for substances such as HCl, NaCl, KCl, $NH_4Cl$, $NaHCO_3$, and $MgSO_4$, and 3 for compounds such as $CaCl_2$ and $MgCl_2$.

A value of 1 is often used as an approximate value of $\varphi$. Thus, the osmolarity and osmotic pressure of 1 M $CaCl_2$ > 1 M NaCl > 1 M glucose.

Similarly, a 1 M solution of glucose has approximately the same osmolarity and osmotic pressure as 0.5 M $NaHCO_3$ or 0.33 M $MgCl_2$.

One osmol is equal to 1 mol of solute particles. The osmolarity is the number of osmoles per liter of solution, whereas the osmolality is the number of osmoles per kilogram of solvent. In the body, osmolal concentrations are expressed as osmoles per kilogram of water.

The term tonicity is used to describe the osmolality of a solution relative to plasma. Solutions that have the same osmolality as plasma (~300 mOsm/L) are isotonic; those with greater osmolality are hypertonic; and those with lesser osmolality are hypotonic.

The plasma membranes of most cells are relatively impermeable to many of the solutes of the extracellular fluid but are highly permeable to water. Thus the movement of water by osmosis leads to swelling or shrinking of cells. As shown in Figure 3, cells shrink when placed in hypertonic solutions and swell when placed in hypotonic solutions.

The steady-state volume of a cell can be calculated as:

$$\pi_{initial} \times V_{initial} = \pi_{final} \times V_{final}$$

Isotonic solutions are commonly used for intravenous fluid administration and as drug diluents because administration of an isotonic solution

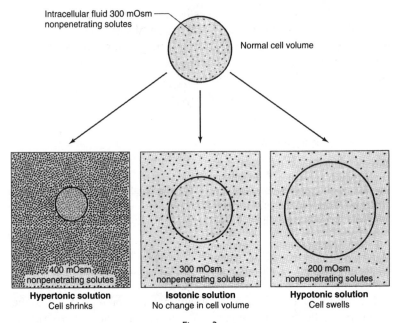

Figure 3
Cell volume changes with hypertonic, isotonic, and hypotonic solutions. *(Reproduced, with permission, from Widmaier EP, Raff H, Strang KT. Vander's Human Physiology: The Mechanisms of Body Function. 11th ed. New York, NY: McGraw-Hill;2008: 111.)*

does not produce changes in cell volume, that is, no net water movement. Isotonic saline has a concentration of 154 mM NaCl, containing $154 \times 2$ or 308 mM of osmotically active particles. An isotonic solution of glucose is a 5% dextrose solution.

## Intercellular Connections and Communication

Two types of connections form between the cells comprising a tissue. One type of junction serves to fasten the cells to one another and to surrounding tissues. Examples of fastening junctions that lend strength and stability to tissues include tight junctions or zona occludens, desmosomes, zona adherins, hemidesmosomes, and focal adhesions. The other type of connection between cells serves the purpose of transferring ions and other molecules from cell to cell. This type of junction is called a gap junction, though transport of ions across epithelial cells can occur via tight junctions.

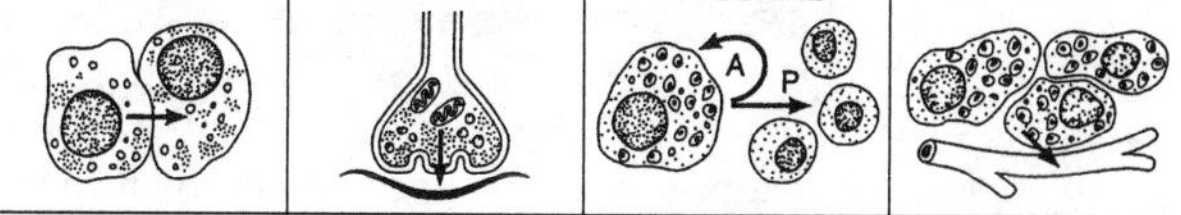

| | GAP JUNCTIONS | SYNAPTIC | PARACRINE AND AUTOCRINE | ENDOCRINE |
|---|---|---|---|---|
| Message transmission | Directly from cell to cell | Across synaptic cleft | By diffusion in interstitial fluid | By circulating body fluids |
| Local or general | Local | Local | Locally diffuse | General |
| Specificity depends on | Anatomic location | Anatomic location and receptors | Receptors | Receptors |

**Figure 4**

*Types of intercellular connections and communication. (Reproduced, with permission, from Ganong WF. Review of Medical Physiology. 22nd ed. New York, NY: McGraw-Hill;2005:36.)*

In addition to the direct cell-to-cell communication via gap junctions, cells communicate with each other via chemical messengers in the extracellular fluid by a number of processes, including neural, endocrine, and paracrine communication (Figure 4).

In the case of intercellular communication mediated by chemical messengers in the extracellular fluid, there are generally "first messengers," which constitute the extracellular ligands that bind to receptors in the cell membrane, and "second messengers," which are the intracellular mediators that bring about the changes in cell function produced by binding of the "first messenger." The principal mechanisms by which chemical messengers exert their intracellular effects are summarized in Table 2.

## GENERAL PRINCIPLES: MULTISYSTEM PROCESSES

*(Fauci et al, pp 274-295. Ganong, pp 1-4, 240-247, 713-738. Levitzky, pp 163-188. Stead et al, pp 221-237. Widmaier et al, pp 2-17, 78-92, 477, 500-527.)*

### Body Fluid Compartments

Water is the most abundant constituent in the body. The percentage of water in the body is a function of body fat. The greater the percentage of body fat, the lower the percentage of body water.

- *Total body water* (TBW) is approximately 60% of lean body mass.
- *Intracellular fluid* (ICF) comprises about two-thirds of TBW (40% of body mass).

| TABLE 2. PRINCIPAL MECHANISMS FOR INTRACELLULAR EFFECTS OF CHEMICAL MESSENGERS | |
| --- | --- |
| Mechanism | Examples |
| Open or close ion channels in cell membrane | Acetylcholine on nicotinic cholinergic receptor<br>Norepinephrine on $K^+$ channel in the heart |
| Act via cytoplasmic or nuclear receptors to increase transcription of selected mRNAs | Thyroid hormones, retinoic acid, steroid hormones |
| Activate phospholipase C with intracellular production of diacylglycerol (DAG) and inositol triphosphate ($IP_3$), which activates protein kinase C | Angiotensin II<br>Norepinephrine via $\alpha_1$-adrenergic receptor<br>Vasopressin via $V_1$ receptor |
| Activate or inhibit adenylyl cyclase, causing increased or decreased intracellular production of cyclic AMP with corresponding activation or inactivation of protein kinase A | Norepinephrine via $\beta_1$-adrenergic receptor (increased cAMP and PK-A)<br>Norepinephrine via $\alpha_2$-adrenergic receptor (decreased cAMP and PK-A) |
| Increase cyclic GMP in cell, which activates cGMP-dependent protein kinase | Atrial natriuretic peptide<br>Nitric oxide |
| Increase tyrosine kinase activity of cytoplasmic portions of transmembrane receptors | Insulin<br>Growth factors (EGF, PDGF)<br>Macrophage colony-stimulating factor |
| Increase serine or threonine kinase activity | TGF-$\beta$<br>MAP kinases |

(Modified, with permission, from Ganong WF. *Review of Medical Physiology*. 22nd ed. New York, NY:McGraw-Hill; 2005: 38.)

*Extracellular fluid* (ECF) is one-third of TBW (20% of body mass). The ECF water is further divided into:

- *Intravascular (plasma) water*, which comprises approximately one-fourth of ECF or one-twelfth TBW
- *Extravascular (interstitial) water*, which comprises approximately three-fourths of ECF or one-fourth TBW

The solute or particle concentration of a fluid is its osmolality. Water shifts between the ECF and ICF in order to maintain osmotic equilibrium between the two compartments.

- The normal range of plasma osmolality is 280 to 300 mOsm/kg.

- Plasma osmolality can be estimated as:

$$2\ [Na^+] + \frac{[Glucose]}{18} + \frac{[BUN]}{2.8}$$

The composition of the extracellular and intracellular fluids is shown in Table 3. The distribution of substances between the intracellular and extracellular fluid is unequal due to the membrane potential and the presence of various transporters and ion channels in the plasma membrane.

**TABLE 3. ECF AND ICF COMPOSITION**

|  | Extracellular Concentration, mM | Intracellular Concentration, mM[a] |
|---|---|---|
| $Na^+$ | 150 | 15 |
| $K^+$ | 5 | 150 |
| $Ca^{2+}$ | 1 | 0.0001 |
| $Mg^{2+}$ | 1.5 | 12 |
| $Cl^-$ | 110 | 7 |
| $HCO_3^-$ | 24 | 10 |
| $P_i$ | 2 | 40 |
| Amino acids | 2 | 8 |
| Glucose | 5.6 | 1 |
| ATP | 0 | 4 |
| Protein | 0.2 | 4 |

[a]The intracellular concentrations differ slightly from one tissue to another, but the concentrations shown above are typical of most cells. For $Ca^{2+}$, values represent free concentrations. Total calcium levels, including the portion sequestered by proteins or in organelles, approach 2.5 mM (extracellular) and 1.5 mM (intracellular). (Reproduced, with permission, from Widmaier EP, Raff H, Strang KT. *Vander's Human Physiology: The Mechanisms of Body Function.* 11th ed. New York, NY: McGraw-Hill;2008: 107.)

## Fluid and Electrolyte Balance and Disorders

The extracellular osmolarity is controlled by antidiuretic hormone (ADH), also known as vasopressin. Increases in osmolarity stimulate the release of ADH from the posterior pituitary gland. ADH returns osmolarity toward normal by decreasing the amount of water excreted by the kidney. When osmolarity is decreased, ADH release is decreased and osmolarity is returned toward normal by increased water excretion. ADH is also secreted in response to low blood pressure. Under these conditions, reabsorption of water by the kidneys can make the extracellular fluid hypotonic.

Plasma osmolality is elevated in:

- Dehydration
- Hypernatremia

- Diabetes insipidus
- Uremia
- Hyperglycemia
- Mannitol therapy
- Hypercalcemia
- Toxin ingestion (ethanol, methanol, ethylene glycol)

Plasma osmolality is decreased in:

- Syndrome of inappropriate antidiuretic hormone (SIADH)
- Hyponatremia
- Overhydration
- Addison disease
- Hypothyroidism

The extracellular volume is controlled by the NaCl content of the extracellular fluid. Hypovolemia, or volume depletion, generally refers to a state of combined salt and water loss exceeding intake, leading to ECF volume contraction. The loss of $Na^+$ may be renal or extrarenal (Table 4.)

---

### TABLE 4. CAUSES OF HYPOVOLEMIA

I. ECF volume contracted
   A. Extrarenal $Na^+$ loss
      1. Gastrointestinal (vomiting, nasogastric suction, drainage, fistula, diarrhea)
      2. Skin/respiratory (insensible losses, sweat, burns)
      3. Hemorrhage
   B. Renal $Na^+$ and water loss
      1. Diuretics
      2. Osmotic diuresis
      3. Hypoaldosteronism
      4. Salt-wasting nephropathies
   C. Renal water loss
      1. Diabetes insipidus (central or nephrogenic)
II. ECF volume normal or expanded
   A. Decreased cardiac output
      1. Myocardial, valvular, or pericardial disease
   B. Redistribution
      1. Hypoalbuminemia (hepatic cirrhosis, nephrotic syndrome)
      2. Capillary leak (acute pancreatitis, ischemic bowel, rhabdomyolysis)
   C. Increased venous capacitance
      1. Sepsis

---

(Reproduced, with permission, from Fauci AS, Braunwald E, Kasper DL, et al. *Harrison's Principles of Internal Medicine,* 17th ed. New York: McGraw-Hill, 2008:276).

NaCl content is controlled by aldosterone and atrial natriuretic peptide (ANP). Extracellular volume is monitored by low-pressure baroreceptors within the thoracic venous vessels and the atria and by pressure receptors within the afferent arteriole of the kidneys. ANP release is controlled directly by stretch receptors within the right atrium.

Aldosterone secretion is controlled by the renin-angiotensin system. Renin is released from the juxtaglomerular cells (JG cells) of the kidney in response to:

- Decreased perfusion pressure within the afferent arteriole
- Sympathetic stimulation of the JG cells
- Decreased Cl⁻ concentration in fluid bathing the macula densa

Renin catalyzes the conversion of angiotensinogen to angiotensin I. Angiotensin I is converted to angiotensin II (AII) by angiotensin-converting enzyme (ACE) located within the lung. AII stimulates aldosterone secretion from the adrenal cortex gland.

*Hyponatremia* is defined as a serum sodium concentration < 134 mEq/L. The causes of hyponatremia are subdivided into three categories based on the coexisting serum osmolarity and fluid status as shown in Table 5.

| TABLE 5. CAUSES OF HYPONATREMIA | | Urine Osm | Urine Sodium |
|---|---|---|---|
| **Hypovolemic** | Extrarenal: GI losses, skin losses, lung losses, third-spacing (fistula, burns, vomiting, diarrhea, GI suction, edema, pancreatitis) | ↑ | ↓ |
| | Renal: Diuretics, intrinsic renal damage (including acute tubular necrosis), partial urinary tract obstruction | ↑ | ↑ |
| | Adrenal insufficiency (Addison) | ↑ | ↑ |
| **Isovolemic** | Water intoxication | ↓ | ↓ |
| | SIADH | ↑ | ↑ |
| **Hypervolemic** | CHF, liver cirrhosis, and the nephrotic syndrome | ↑ | ↓ |

↓ = decreased; ↑ = increased.
(Reproduced, with permission, from Stead LG, Stead SM, Kaufman MS, et al. *First Aid for the Medicine Clerkship*. 2nd ed. New York, NY: McGraw-Hill;2006:228.)

| TABLE 6. CAUSES OF HYPERNATREMIA | | Urine Osm | Urine Sodium |
|---|---|---|---|
| Hypovolemic | Renal loss: Osmotic diuresis (glycosuria, urea), acute/ chronic renal failure, partial obstruction | N/↓ | ↑ |
| | Extrarenal loss: Hyperpnea, excessive sweating | ↑ | ↑ |
| | Extrarenal loss: Diarrhea, burns, moderate sweating | ↑ | ↓ |
| | Iatrogenic (bicarbonate, dialysis, salt tablets) | ↑ | ↑ |
| Isovolemic | Diabetes insipidus (from any cause) | ↓ | ↓ |
| Hypervolemic | Mineralocorticoid excess (e.g., Conn's syndrome) | N/↓ | N/↓ |

↓ = decreased; ↑ = increased; N = normal.
(Reproduced, with permission, from Stead LG, Stead SM, Kaufman MS, et al. *First Aid for the Medicine Clerkship*. 2nd ed. New York, NY: McGraw-Hill;2006:229.)

*Hypernatremia* is defined as a serum sodium concentration greater than 145 mEq/L. The causes of hypernatremia are subdivided into three categories based on the coexisting fluid status as shown in Table 6.

Potassium is the major intracellular cation. The normal plasma $K^+$ concentration is 3.5-5 mmol/L, whereas the normal intracellular concentration is approximately 150 mmol/L (Table 3). The ratio of intracellular to extracellular $K^+$ (normally 38:1) is the principal result of the resting membrane potential and is essential for normal neuromuscular function. Virtually all regulation of renal $K^+$ excretion and total body $K^+$ balance occurs in the distal nephron. Potassium secretion is regulated by aldosterone. Aldosterone is secreted by the zona glomerulosa cells of the adrenal cortex in response to increases in extracellular $K^+$ or angiotensin II, causing $K^+$ secretion to increase. $K^+$ transport into cells is increased by epinephrine and insulin.

The causes of *hypokalemia*, defined as a plasma $K^+$ concentration less than 3.5 mEq/L, are shown in Table 7. The causes of *hyperkalemia*, defined as a plasma $K^+$ concentration greater than 5 mEq/L, are shown in Table 8.

## TABLE 7. CAUSES OF HYPOKALEMIA

I. Decreased intake
  A. Starvation
  B. Clay ingestion
II. Redistribution into cells
  A. Acid-base
    1. Metabolic alkalosis
  B. Hormonal
    1. Insulin
    2. $\beta_2$-Adrenergic agonists (endogenous or exogenous)
    3. $\alpha$-Adrenergic antagonists
  C. Anabolic state
    1. Vitamin $B_{12}$ or folic acid (red blood cell production)
    2. Granulocyte-macrophage colony stimulating factor (white blood cell production)
    3. Total parenteral nutrition
  D. Other
    1. Pseudohypokalemia
    2. Hypothermia
    3. Hypokalemic periodic paralysis
    4. Barium toxicity
III. Increased loss
  A. Nonrenal
    1. Gastrointestinal loss (diarrhea)
    2. Integumentary loss (sweat)
  B. Renal
    1. Increased distal flow: diuretics, osmotic diuresis, salt-wasting nephropathies
    2. Increased secretion of potassium
      a. Mineralocorticoid excess: primary hyperaldosteronism, secondary hyperaldosteronism (malignant hypertension, renin-secreting tumors, renal artery stenosis, hypovolemia), apparent mineralocorticoid excess (licorice, chewing tobacco, carbenoxolone), congenital adrenal hyperplasia, Cushing's syndrome, Bartter's syndrome
      b. Distal delivery of non-reabsorbed anions: vomiting, nasogastric suction, proximal (type 2) renal tubular acidosis, diabetic ketoacidosis, glue-sniffing (toluene abuse), penicillin derivatives
      c. Other: amphotericin B, Liddle's syndrome, hypomagnesemia

(Reproduced, with permission, from Fauci AS, Braunwald E, Kasper DL, et al. *Harrison's Principles of Internal Medicine.* 17th ed. New York, NY: McGraw-Hill;2008: 281.)

| TABLE 8.  CAUSES OF HYPERKALEMIA |
|---|

I. Renal failure
II. Decreased distal flow (i.e., decreased effective circulating arterial volume)
III. Decreased K⁺ secretion
    A. Impaired Na⁺ reabsorption
       1. Primary hypoaldosteronism: adrenal insufficiency, adrenal enzyme deficiency (21-hydroxylase, 3β-hydroxysteroid dehydrogenase, corticosterone methyl oxidase)
       2. Secondary hypoaldosteronism: hyporeninemia, drugs (ACE inhibitors, NSAIDs, heparin)
       3. Resistance to aldosterone: pseudohypoaldosteronism, tubulointerstitial disease, drugs (K⁺-sparing diuretics, trimethoprim, pentamidine)
    B. Enhanced Cl⁻ reabsorption (chloride shunt)
       1. Gordon's syndrome
       2. Cyclosporine

Note: ACE, angiotensin-converting enzyme; NSAIDs, nonsteroidal anti-inflammatory drugs.
(Reproduced, with permission, from Fauci AS, Braunwald E, Kasper DL, et al. *Harrison's Principles of Internal Medicine*. 17th ed. New York, NY: McGraw-Hill;2008: 283.)

## Acid-Base Balance and Disorders

Each day, approximately 15,000 mmol of volatile acid ($CO_2$) and 50 to 100 mEq of fixed acid (hydrochloric acid, lactic acid, phosphoric acid, sulfuric acid, etc) are produced by metabolism. The pH of the extracellular fluid is maintained by buffering the acid as it is formed and excreting the acid over time. The kidneys require approximately 24 hours to excrete the fixed acids. $CO_2$ is rapidly excreted by the lungs.

When $CO_2$ is added to water, it forms carbonic acid ($H_2CO_3$), a reaction that is catalyzed by the enzyme carbonic anhydrase (CA). Once formed, carbonic acid rapidly dissociates into $H^+$ and $HCO_3^-$

$$CO_2 + H_2O \xrightarrow{CA} H_2CO_3 \longleftrightarrow H^+ + HCO_3^-$$

The *pH of plasma* is calculated with the Henderson-Hasselbalch equation:

$$pH = 6.1 + \log [HCO_3^-]/[\text{dissolved } CO_2]$$
$$= 6.1 + \log [HCO_3^-]/(PCO_2 \text{ in mm Hg} \times 0.03 \text{ mEq/L/mm Hg})$$

**TABLE 9. CHARACTERISTICS OF PRIMARY ACID-BASE DISORDERS**

| Disorder | pH | Primary Disturbance | Compensatory Response |
|---|---|---|---|
| Respiratory acidosis | ↓ | ↑$Pa_{CO_2}$ (alveolar hypoventilation) | ↑$[HCO_3^-]$ (↑ renal $H^+$ excretion) |
| Respiratory alkalosis | ↑ | ↓$Pa_{CO_2}$ (alveolar hyperventilation) | ↓ $[HCO_3^-]$ (↓renal $H^+$ excretion) |
| Metabolic alkalosis | ↑ | ↑$[HCO_3^-]$ (gain of $HCO_3^-$; loss of $H^+$) | ↑$Pa_{CO_2}$ (alveolar hypoventilation) |
| Metabolic acidosis | ↓ | ↓$[HCO_3^-]$ (gain of $H^+$; loss of $HCO_3^-$) | ↓$Pa_{CO_2}$ (alveolar hyperventilation) |

Arterial $PCO_2$ is normally maintained at 40 mm Hg by the lungs and arterial $HCO_3^-$ concentration is normally maintained at 24 mEq/L by the kidneys. Thus, normally,

$$\text{Arterial pH } 6.1 + \log 24/(0.03 \times 40) = 6.1 + \log 20/1 = 7.40.$$

The normal ratio of $[HCO_3^-]/[\text{dissolved } CO_2] = 20/1$. The four primary acid-base disorders result from abnormalities that alter the normal 20/1 ratio of $[HCO_3^-]/[\text{dissolved } CO_2]$, as summarized in Table 9. Compensation for the acid-base disorders involves an attempt by the body to minimize the change in pH caused by the primary disorder by restoring the ratio of $[HCO_3^-]/[\text{dissolved } CO_2]$ toward its normal value. In order to do so, if the primary disorder is a metabolic acid-base disturbance causing a change in the $[HCO_3^-]$, then the appropriate respiratory compensatory response will change the $Pa_{CO_2}$, and thus the $[\text{dissolved } CO_2]$ in the same direction. If the primary disorder is respiratory in origin, causing a change in the denominator of the ratio, then there will be renal compensation geared toward changing the $[HCO_3^-]$ in the same direction as the primary change in $Pa_{CO_2}$. The causes of the four primary acid-base disorders are listed in Tables 10 to 13.

## TABLE 10. CAUSES OF RESPIRATORY ACIDOSIS (ALVEOLAR HYPOVENTILATION)

I. Airway obstruction
  A. Chronic obstructive lung disease
  B. Upper airway obstruction
II. Chest wall restriction
  A. Kyphoscoliosis
  B. Pickwickian syndrome
III. Respiratory center depression
  A. Anesthetics
  B. Sedatives
  C. Opiates
  D. Brain injury or disease
  E. Severe hypercapnia, hypoxia
IV. Neuromuscular disorders
  A. Spinal cord injury
  B. Phrenic nerve injury
  C. Poliomyelitis
  D. Myasthenia gravis
  E. Guillain-Barré syndrome
  F. Administration of curare-like drugs
  G. Respiratory muscle diseases

## TABLE 11. CAUSES OF RESPIRATORY ALKALOSIS (ALVEOLAR HYPERVENTILATION)

I. Respiratory center stimulation
  A. CNS
    1. Anxiety
    2. Hyperventilation syndrome
    3. Inflammation (encephalitis, meningitis)
    4. Stroke
    5. Tumors
  B. Drugs or hormones
    1. Salicylates
    2. Progesterone
    3. Hyperthyroidism
  C. Reflex
    1. Hypoxemia
    2. High altitude
    3. Metabolic acidosis
    4. Sepsis, fever
    5. Pulmonary embolism
    6. Pulmonary edema
    7. Congestive heart failure
    8. Asthma
II. Iatrogenic mechanical overventilation
III. Liver failure

**TABLE 12.  CAUSES OF METABOLIC ALKALOSIS**

I. Loss of hydrogen ions
   A. Vomiting
   B. Nasogastric suction
   C. Gastric fistulas
   D. Diuretic therapy
   E. Severe magnesium or potassium deficiency
   F. Overproduction of mineralocorticoids (Cushing syndrome; primary hyperaldosteronism; renal artery stenosis)
   G. Ingestion of mineralocorticoids (licorice ingestion; chewing tobacco)
   H. Inherited disorders (Bartter syndrome; Liddle syndrome; Gitelman syndrome)
II. Ingestion or administration of excess bicarbonate or other bases
   A. Intravenous bicarbonate
   B. Ingestion of bicarbonate or other bases (eg, antacids)

**TABLE 13.  CAUSES OF METABOLIC ACIDOSIS**

| Normal Anion Gap (Hyperchloremia) | Increased Anion Gap (Normochloremic) |
|---|---|
| I. Gastrointestinal loss of $HCO_3^-$<br>  A. Diarrhea<br>  B. Small bowel or pancreatic drainage or fistula<br>  C. Ureterosigmoidostomy, jejunal loop, ileal loop conduit<br>  D. Drugs<br>II. Renal loss of $HCO_3^-$<br>  A. Carbonic anhydrase inhibitors<br>  B. Renal tubular acidosis (RTA)<br>III. Miscellaneous<br>  A. Dilutional acidosis<br>  B. Hyperalimentation | I. Lactic acidosis<br>II. Ketoacidosis<br>  A. Diabetic<br>  B. Starvation<br>  C. Alcoholic<br>III. Ingestion of toxic substances<br>  A. Salicylate overdose<br>  B. Paraldehyde poisoning<br>  C. Methyl alcohol ingestion<br>  D. Ethylene glycol ingestion<br>IV. Failure of acid excretion<br>  A. Acute renal failure<br>  B. Chronic renal failure |

## PHYSIOLOGY OF THE HEMATOPOIETIC AND LYMPHORETICULAR SYSTEMS

*(Ganong, pp 515-546, 666-670. Levitzky, pp 142-162. Widmaier et al, pp 459-476, 500-507.)*

## Oxygen Transport in the Blood

$O_2$ is transported in the blood in two transport forms: (1) dissolved in plasma and (2) chemically combined with hemoglobin. The concentration of a gas dissolved in a liquid is proportional to its partial pressure and its solubility in the liquid. The solubility coefficient of oxygen in plasma at body temperature and pressure is 0.003 mL $O_2$/100 mL blood/mm Hg. The concentration of $O_2$ combined with hemoglobin is determined by the equation:

$$HbO_2 \text{ (mL/dL blood) [Hb] (g/dL blood)} \times 1.34 \text{ mL } O_2/\text{g Hb} \times \%O_2 \text{ saturation}$$

As shown in Table 14, the total $O_2$ content is the sum of the dissolved oxygen and the oxyhemoglobin content. Over 98% of the oxygen delivered to the blood is bound to hemoglobin (HbO$_2$), an amount 65 times greater than the amount dissolved in the arterial blood. Nonetheless, the dissolved oxygen is critical because it determines the amount of oxygen that combines with hemoglobin, as depicted by the oxyhemoglobin dissociation curve (Figure 5).

Oxygen delivery is the product of the cardiac output and the arterial oxygen content. Oxygen extraction is the difference between the arterial and venous oxygen contents (a-v $O_2$). According to the Fick equation, cardiac output (CO) can be calculated as the ratio of the oxygen consumption ($\dot{V}O_2$) and the oxygen extraction.

$$\text{Cardiac output (CO)} = (\dot{V}O_2)/\text{a-v } O_2$$

## Reaction of Hemoglobin and Oxygen

Hemoglobin is a protein with four subunits, each of which has a heme moiety attached to a polypeptide chain (HbA: two $\alpha$ and two $\beta$ chains). Heme is a

| TABLE 14. TOTAL $O_2$ CONTENT IN ARTERIAL AND VENOUS BLOOD | | | |
|---|---|---|---|
| | Dissolved $O_2$ | HbO$_2$ | Total |
| Arterial blood (100 mm Hg PO$_2$; 97% sat; 15 g/dLHb) | 0.3 mL $O_2$/dL | 19.5 mL $O_2$/dL | 19.8 mL $O_2$/dL |
| Venous blood (40 mm Hg PO$_2$; 75% sat; 15 g/dLHb) | 0.12 mL $O_2$/dL | 15.1 mL $O_2$/dL | 15.2 mL $O_2$/dL |

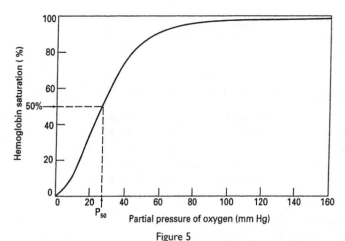

**Figure 5**

Oxyhemoglobin Dissociation Cure. *(Reproduced, with permission, from Levitzky, MG. Pulmonary Physiology, 7th ed. New York: McGraw-Hill, 2007:146.)*

complex consisting of a porphyrin and one atom of a ferrous ($Fe^{2+}$) iron. Each of the four iron atoms can bind reversibly one molecule of $O_2$ ($Hb_4 + O_2 = Hb_4O_2$). The plot of the four reversible reactions of hemoglobin and oxygen is represented by the *oxyhemoglobin dissociation curve*, which shows the relationship between the $PO_2$ of the plasma and the percent of hemoglobin saturated with oxygen.

The oxyhemoglobin dissociation curve has a characteristic sigmoidal shape reflecting the increased affinity of hemoglobin for oxygen as each additional molecule of oxygen binds to the four subunits of hemoglobin (cooperative binding). Conversely, dissociation of oxygen from hemoglobin facilitates additional dissociation. As a result, the slope of the curve decreases as one goes from low to high $PO_2$ values, with a plateau reached when the $PO_2$ is above approximately 80 mm Hg. This is important physiologically because the S-shape facilitates oxygen loading in the pulmonary capillaries, and oxygen unloading at the tissues. Also, there is an important physiological safety factor because a patient with a relatively low arterial $PO_2$ still has a relatively high $O_2$ saturation (eg, 90% $SO_2$ at 60 mm Hg $PO_2$).

A rightward shift of the oxyhemoglobin dissociation curve is indicative of a decrease in $HbO_2$ affinity with less oxygen uptake at the pulmonary capillaries but greater release of oxygen to the tissues. The $P_{50}$, that is, the $PO_2$ at which hemoglobin is 50% saturated with oxygen, is increased above the normal value of approximately 27 mm Hg. Factors that shift the oxy-hemoglobin dissociation curve to the right include:

• Hyperthermia
• Increased $Pco_2$ or decreased pH (known as the Bohr effect)
• Increased [2,3-bisphosphoglycerate (2,3-BPG)] in erythrocytes

A leftward shift of the oxyhemoglobin dissociation curve denotes a higher-than-normal $HbO_2$ affinity with greater oxygen uptake at the pulmonary capillaries delivery but less oxygen released at the tissue level. The $P_{50}$ is lower than normal when affinity is increased. Factors that shift the oxyhemoglobin dissociation curve to the left include:

• Hypothermia
• Alkalosis or decreased $Pco_2$ (Bohr effect)
• Decreased erythrocyte 2,3-BPG (also known as DPG) concentration
• Carbon monoxide

The $Hb-O_2$ curve for fetal Hb (HbF) is shifted to the left of that for normal adult hemoglobin (HbA) because there is poor binding of 2,3-BPG to the γ-chains in HbF compared to the β-chains in HbA. The presence of carbon monoxide in the blood increases the affinity of hemoglobin for any oxygen that is already bound, thereby shifting the curve to the left.

There are hundreds of hemoglobin variants that have been described, most of which result from single-point mutations. Hb variants are often classified as high affinity versus low affinity based on their $P_{50}$ values.

## $CO_2$ Transport in the Blood

Like oxygen, carbon dioxide can be physically dissolved in the plasma or chemically combined with hemoglobin (carbaminohemoglobin). Only approximately 5% of total $CO_2$ is dissolved, and, in contrast to oxygen combined to hemoglobin, carbaminohemoglobin only constitutes approximately 10% of total $CO_2$ in the blood. The majority of $CO_2$ in the blood (80%-90%) is transported as bicarbonate, a product of the dissociation of carbonic acid from the $CO_2$ hydrolysis catalyzed by carbonic anhydrase, as discussed earlier.

There is no carbonic anhydrase in the plasma, so the $CO_2$ hydration equation proceeds very slowly in plasma. In contrast, the presence of carbonic anhydrase in red blood cells results in most $HCO_3^-$ being formed within erythrocytes. However, the $HCO_3^-$ then diffuses down its concentration gradient from RBCs into the plasma in exchange for $Cl^-$, a process called the chloride shift, which is mediated by Band 3, a major membrane protein. Because of the chloride shift, the Cl⁻ content of the red cells in the venous blood is greater than that in the arterial RBCs.

The total $CO_2$ content in blood (~50 mL/dL) is much greater than total arterial $O_2$ content (~20 mL/dL).

## NEUROPHYSIOLOGY

*(Ganong, pp 6-8, 51-64, 85-277. Widmaier et al, pp 151-277, 323-342.)*

### Ionic Equilibria and Membrane Potentials

All cells have membrane potentials. The magnitude of the membrane potential is determined by the membrane permeability and the concentration gradient of the ions that are permeable to the membrane.

In the resting state, the membrane is primarily permeable to K⁺ and, therefore, the resting membrane potential is close to the equilibrium potential for K⁺.

The equilibrium potential (*E*) is calculated with Nernst equation:

$$E_{ion} = 61.5 \log C_{out}/C_{in}.$$

The equilibrium potential for K⁺ is −90 mv, for Na⁺ is +60 mv, and for Cl⁻ is −70 mv.

The resting membrane potential is calculated with the Goldman equation:

$$E_M = -61.5 \times \log \left[ (P_{Na} \times [Na_{in}]) + (P_K \times [K_{in}])/(P_{Na} \times [Na_{out}]) + (P_K \times [K_{out}]) \right]$$

Because neither $E_K$ nor $E_{Na}$ is at the $E_M$ of −70 mv, one would expect the cell to gradually gain Na⁺ and lose K⁺ if only passive electrical and chemical forces were acting on the membrane. In other words, there is more K⁺ and less Na⁺ in the neurons than can be accounted for by electrochemical gradients. This condition is maintained by the electrogenic Na⁺ − K⁺ pump, that is, Na⁺, K⁺-ATPase, which pumps three Na⁺ out of the cell for every two K⁺ it pumps into the cell for each molecule of ATP hydrolyzed.

### Action Potential

If an axon is stimulated and the current has sufficient intensity, an action potential will be produced.

The *action potential* begins with an initial depolarization of about 15 mv (Figure 6).

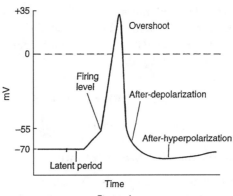

**Figure 6**
**The action potential.**

Once the impulse reaches threshold intensity at about −55 mv, a full action potential is produced as characterized by a rapid upstroke that overshoots the zero potential to approximately +35 mv. After the *overshoot*, the potential reverses and rapidly repolarizes toward the resting level. The sharp rise and fall constitute the *spike potential* of the neuron, which only lasts a millisecond or so. After repolarization is approximately 70% complete, the rate of repolarization decreases for about 4 ms (called *after-depolarization*) and is followed by an overshoot of the resting potential, called the *after-repolarization*, which is only 1 to 2 mv, but lasts about 40 ms. The action potential is said to be *"all or none"* because it will not occur if a stimulus is subthreshold, and if a stimulus is at or above threshold, the action potential occurs with a constant amplitude and forms regardless of the strength of the stimulus.

Action potentials are produced by ionic fluxes controlled by voltage-gated ion channels. Depolarization is produced by activation of voltage-gated $Na^+$ channels, which increases sodium conductance, that is, membrane permeability to $Na^+$. The action potential moves toward the equilibrium potential for $Na^+$ (+60 mv), but does not reach it, primarily because the increase in sodium conductance is brief. Repolarization occurs because (1) the $Na^+$ channels enter a closed or inactivated state before returning to the resting state, and (2) voltage-gated $K^+$ channels open, which increases the membrane conductance to $K^+$, resulting in $K^+$ efflux from the cell. The opening of the $K^+$ channels is slower and more prolonged than the opening of $Na^+$ channels, and the slow return of the $K^+$ channels to the closed state accounts for the after-hyperpolarization, as the membrane approaches the equilibrium potential of $K^+$.

## Functions of Nerves and the Nervous System

Neurons generally have four important functional areas:

(1) A receptor or dendritic zone, where multiple local potentials generated by synaptic connections are integrated

(2) A site where propagated action potentials are generated, which is close to the receptor zone, and includes the initial segment in spinal motor neurons and the initial node of Ranvier in cutaneous sensory neurons

(3) An axonal process that transmits propagated impulses to nerve endings at various rates depending on whether the axons are myelinated or unmyelinated

(4) The nerve endings, where action potentials cause the secretion of synaptic transmitters

Synaptic transmission is used to transmit information from one cell to another. The synaptic transmitter, released from the presynaptic cell by exocytosis, diffuses across a synaptic cleft and binds to a receptor on the postsynaptic cell. The effect produced on the postsynaptic cell depends on both the synaptic transmitter and the receptor. Acetylcholine, which binds to the end plate of skeletal muscle cells, and glutamate and γ-amino butyric acid (GABA), which bind to the postsynaptic membranes of many central nervous system membranes, open ion-selective channels. Norepinephrine and acetylcholine, which bind to the postsynaptic membranes of smooth muscle cells, produce their effect by activating a G protein which, in turn, activates an enzyme-mediated response.

Nerve fiber types are classified into A, B, and C groups based on their various speeds of conduction and fiber diameter (Table 15).

A numerical classification is often used for sensory neurons, as shown in Table 16.

• Sensory receptors (touch, pain, temperature, smell, taste, sound, and sight) are activated by environmental stimuli. The stimulus produces a receptor potential; the magnitude of the receptor potential is proportional to the stimulus. The receptor potential produces a train of action potentials. Tonic receptors fire as long as the stimulus is present and encode intensity. Phasic receptors slow down or stop firing during the presentation of the stimulus and encode velocity.

• The vestibular system provides information about the position and movement of the head, coordinates head and eye movements, and initiates reflexes that keep the head and body erect. Lesions to the vestibular system result in loss of balance and nystagmus.

### TABLE 15. NERVE FIBER TYPES

| Fiber Type | Function | Fiber Diameter (μm) | Conduction Velocity (m/s) | Spike Duration (ms) | Absolute Refractory Period (ms) |
|---|---|---|---|---|---|
| **A** | | | | | |
| α | Proprioception; somatic motor | 12-20 | 70-120 | | |
| β | Touch, pressure, motor | 5-12 | 30-70 | 0.4-0.5 | 0.4-1 |
| γ | Motor to muscle spindles | 3-6 | 15-30 | | |
| δ | Pain, cold, touch | 2-5 | 12-30 | | |
| **B** | Preganglionic autonomic | < 3 | 3-15 | 1.2 | 1.2 |
| **C** | | | | | |
| Dorsal root | Pain, temperature, some mechano-reception, reflex responses | 0.4-1.2 | 0.5-2 | 2 | 2 |
| Sympathetic | Postganglionic sympathetics | 0.3-1.3 | 0.7-2.3 | 2 | 2 |

A and B fibers are myelinated; C fibers are unmyelinated.
(Reproduced, with permission, from Ganong WF. *Review of Medical Physiology*. 22nd ed. New York, NY:McGraw-Hill;2005:61.)

### TABLE 16. CLASSIFICATION OF SENSORY NEURONS

| Number | Origin | Fiber Type |
|---|---|---|
| Ia | Muscle spindle, annulospiral ending | Aα |
| Ib | Golgi tendon organ | Aα |
| II | Muscle spindle, flower-spray ending; touch, pressure | Aβ |
| III | Pain and cold receptors; some touch receptors | Aδ |
| IV | Pain, temperature, and other receptors | Dorsal root C |

(Reproduced, with permission, from Ganong WF. *Review of Medical Physiology*. 22nd ed. New York, NY:McGraw-Hill;2005:61.)

- The cortex is responsible for cognition, language, emotions, and motivation.
- Movement is initiated by the motor cortex. Motor commands reach the spinal cord through the pyramidal system (corticospinal tract) and the nonpyramidal system (corticoreticular and corticovestibular pathways). Lesions to the nonpyramidal system cause spasticity.
- The basal ganglia and cerebellum assist in the control of movement. Lesions to the basal ganglia produce paucity of movement or uncontrolled movements.
- Lesions to the cerebellum produce uncoordinated movements.

Some neurological movement disorders are highlighted in Table 17.

### TABLE 17. EXAMPLES OF MOVEMENT DISORDERS

| Disease | Possible Cause | Clinical Manifestations |
|---|---|---|
| Tardive dyskinesia | Dopamine antagonists used to treat psychotic diseases | Rapid, irregular movements (chorea) or slow, writhing movements (athetosis) of the face, mouth, and limbs |
| Parkinson disease | Degeneration of the substantia nigra dopaminergic neurons | Tremor at rest, bradykinesia, cogwheel rigidity |
| Huntington disease | Degeneration of GABA-ergic neurons with the striatum | Chorea, ataxia, dementia |
| Hemiballism | Lesion of the contralateral subthalamic nucleus | Sudden flinging movements of the proximal limbs |

## Special Senses

### Hearing

Sounds are detected by the hair cells within the organ of Corti of the inner ear. The organ of Corti consists of the hair cells and an overlying membrane called the tectorial membrane to which the cilia of the hair cells are attached. Sounds entering the outer ear cause the tympanic membrane to vibrate. Vibration of the tympanic membrane causes the middle ear bones (malleus, incus, and stapes) to vibrate, which in turn causes the fluid within the inner ear to vibrate.

The inner ear is divided into three chambers (scala vestibuli, scala media, and scala tympani). The scala vestibuli is separated from the scala media by Reissner membrane; the scala media, and the scala tympani are separated by the basilar membrane. The stapes is attached to the membrane of the oval window, which separates the middle ear from the scala vestibuli. The scala tympani is separated from the middle ear by the round window. The organ of Corti sits on the basilar membrane. The fluid within the scala vestibuli and scala tympani (perilymph) is similar to interstitial fluid; the fluid within the scala media (endolymph) resembles intracellular fluid, in that it contains a high concentration of $K^+$ (Figure 7).

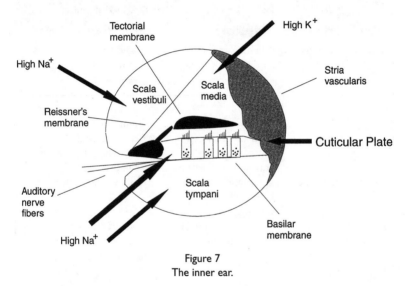

**Figure 7**
The inner ear.

Vibration of the stapes causes the fluid within the scala tympani to vibrate, which in turn causes the basilar membrane to vibrate. Vibration of the basilar membrane causes the cilia to bend back and forth. Bending the stereocilia toward the kinocilium causes $K^+$ channels on the hair cells to open; bending the stereocilia away from kinocilium causes $K^+$ channels to close. Auditory hair cells are unusual because they are depolarized by the flow of $K^+$ into the cell. $K^+$ can flow into the hair cells because the endolymph surrounding the apical portions of the hair cells contains a high $K^+$ concentration (Figure 8).

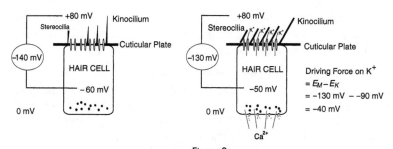

Figure 8
The auditory hair cell and K$^+$ channels.

The basilar membrane is most stiff at the base of the cochlea (near the middle ear) and most compliant at the apex of the cochlea. High-frequency sounds cause a greater vibration of the stiff portion of the cochlea, and, therefore, the hair cells located near the base of the cochlea transmit information about high-frequency sounds to the auditory cortex. Similarly, low-frequency sounds are transmitted to the auditory cortex by the hair cells near the apex of the cochlea, which are located on the more compliant portions of the basilar membrane.

### Sight

Light is detected by the rods and cones contained in the retina of the eye. The retina contains five types of neurons:

- Photoreceptors (rods and cones)
- Bipolar cells
- Ganglion cells
- Horizontal cells
- Amacrine cells

Light rays from distant objects are normally focused on the photoreceptors by the cornea and the relaxed lens. When objects are brought closer to the eye, they are kept focused on the retina by the accommodation reflex, which causes the refractive power of the lens to increase. The photoreceptors contain photopigments, which absorb light. There are four photopigments in the retina: rhodopsin, which is found in the rods, and one in each of the three cone types. Each photopigment contains two components:

(1) Opsin, a group of integral membrane proteins, which is different in each of the four photopigments and determines the wavelength of light absorbed.

(2) A chromophore molecule, retinal, which is a derivative of vitamin A, is the same in each photopigment, and is the actual light-sensitive part of the photopigment that undergoes isomerization by light.

The photoreceptors are unusual because they hyperpolarize when they are stimulated by light. When the rods and cones are not stimulated, they are depolarized by the flow of $Na^+$ into the cell through $Na^+$ channels held in the open state by cGMP. The photoisomerization of retinal from its 11-*cis* form to its all-*trans* form activates rhodopsin and the other photopigments, which in turn activates a G protein called transducin. Activated transducin activates a cGMP phosphodiesterase (PDE). Hydrolysis of cGMP causes $Na^+$ channels on the rod and cone outer segments to close, which produces the membrane hyperpolarization (Figure 9).

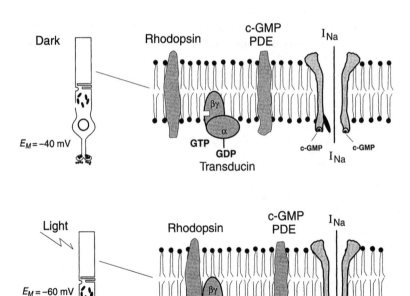

Figure 9
The photoreceptors.

The neurotransmitter keeps the bipolar cells and, therefore, the ganglion cells, in a polarized and relatively quiescent state. Hyperpolarization of the photoreceptors stops the release of an inhibitory neurotransmitter, which in turn causes bipolar cells to depolarize. The bipolar cells stimulate ganglion cells, which in turn convey information about the light stimulus to the visual cortex. The ganglion cells are the only cells in the retina to produce an action potential. Their axons form the optic nerve.

## MUSCULOSKELETAL PHYSIOLOGY

*(Ganong, pp 65-84, 547-549. Widmaier et al, pp 254-295.)*

Three types of skeletal muscle fibers have been identified based upon their maximal shortening velocities and the predominant pathway used to form ATP, as summarized in Table 18.

Muscle cells, like neurons, can be excited to produce an action potential that is transmitted along their cell membranes. The electrical events and underlying ionic fluxes in skeletal muscle are similar to neurons. Unlike neurons, however, muscle action potentials initiate a contractile response. The process by which depolarization of the muscle fiber initiates contraction is called *excitation-contraction coupling.*

Muscle contraction is produced by repetitive cycling of the myosin cross-bridges on thick filaments. The cross-bridges attach to actin molecules on the thin filaments and cause the thin filaments to slide over the thick filaments toward the center of the sarcomere. In striated muscle, excitation-contraction coupling is initiated when $Ca^{2+}$ binds to troponin. Troponin causes tropomyosin to move, thereby exposing the actin-binding site to myosin.

In skeletal muscle, $Ca^{2+}$ is released from the sarcoplasmic reticulum (SR) when the muscle fiber depolarizes. In cardiac muscle, $Ca^{2+}$ is released from the SR by the $Ca^{2+}$ that enters the cell during the cardiac action potential. In smooth muscle, excitation-contraction coupling is initiated when $Ca^{2+}$ binds to calmodulin. The $Ca^{2+}$-calmodulin complex activates myosin light chain kinase (MLCK) which, in turn, phosphorylates the 20,000-Da myosin light chains. Cross-bridge cycling begins when the myosin light chains are phosphorylated. When dephosphorylated, the cross-bridges stay attached (or cycle slowly). The attached, slowly cycling cross-bridges are called latch bridges. Latch bridges allow smooth muscle to maintain force while minimizing energy expenditure. A comparison of the properties of skeletal, cardiac, and smooth (single unit and multiunit) muscle is provided in Table 19.

**TABLE 18. SKELETAL MUSCLE FIBER TYPES**

| | Slow-Oxidative Fibers (Type I) | Fast-Oxidative-Glycolytic Fibers (Type IIa) | Fast-Glycolytic Fibers (Type IIb)[a] |
|---|---|---|---|
| Primary source of ATP production | Oxidative phosphorylation | Oxidative phosphorylation | Glycolysis |
| Mitochondria | Many | Many | Few |
| Capillaries | Many | Many | Few |
| Myoglobin content | High (red muscle) | High (red muscle) | Low (white muscle) |
| Glycolytic enzyme activity | Low | Intermediate | High |
| Glycogen content | Low | Intermediate | High |
| Rate of fatigue | Slow | Intermediate | Fast |
| Myosin-ATPase activity | Low | High | High |
| Contraction velocity | Slow | Fast | Fast |
| Fiber diameter | Small | Intermediate | Large |
| Motor unit size | Small | Intermediate | Large |
| Size of motor neuron innervating fiber | Small | Intermediate | Large |

[a]Type IIb fibers are sometimes designated as type IIx in the human muscle physiology literature.
(Reproduced, with permission, from Widmaier EP, Raff H, Strang KT. *Vander's Human Physiology: The Mechanisms of Body Function.* 11th ed. New York, NY: McGraw-Hill; 2008: 276.)

**TABLE 19. COMPARISON OF SKELETAL, SMOOTH, AND CARDIAC MUSCLE**

| Characteristic | Skeletal Muscle | Single Unit Smooth Muscle | Multi Unit Smooth Muscle | Cardiac Muscle |
|---|---|---|---|---|
| Thick and thin filaments | Yes | Yes | Yes | Yes |
| Sarcomeres—banding pattern | Yes | No | No | Yes |
| Transverse tubules | Yes | No | No | Yes |
| Sarcoplasmic reticulum[a] | ++++ | + | + | ++ |
| Gap junctions between cells | No | Yes | Few | Yes |
| Source of activating calcium | SR | SR and extracellular | SR and extracellular | SR and extracellular |
| Site of calcium regulation | Troponin | Myosin | Myosin | Troponin |
| Speed of contraction | Fast-slow | Very slow | Very slow | Slow |
| Spontaneous production of action potentials by pacemakers | No | Yes | No | Yes in certain fibers, but most not spontaneously active |
| Tone (low levels of maintained tension in the absence of external stimuli) | No | Yes | No | No |
| Effect of nerve stimulation | Excitation | Excitation or inhibition | Excitation or inhibition | Excitation or inhibition |
| Physiological effects of hormones on excitability and contraction | No | Yes | Yes | Yes |
| Stretch of cell produces contraction | No | Yes | No | No |

[a]Number of plus signs (+) indicates the relative amount of sarcoplasmic reticulum present in a given muscle type.
(Reproduced, with permission, from Widmaier EP, Raff H, Strang KT. *Vander's Human Physiology: The Mechanisms of Body Function*. 11th ed. New York, NY:McGraw-Hill; 2008: 292.)

# RESPIRATORY PHYSIOLOGY

*(Ganong, pp 647-697. Levitzky, pp 1-264. Widmaier et al, pp 477-523.)*

## Partial Pressures

The primary function of the lungs is $O_2$ and $CO_2$ exchange. When gas exchange at sea level is optimal, the $PO_2$, $PCO_2$, and pH of arterial blood has normal values (range) of 100 mm Hg (80-100 mm Hg), 40 mm Hg (35-45 mm Hg), and 7.40 (7.35-7.45), respectively.

Room air contains 21% $O_2$ and 0.04% $CO_2$; the major constituent of the atmosphere is $N_2$ (~79%). According to Dalton law, the total pressure of a gaseous mixture, such as the atmosphere, is equal to the sum of the partial pressures of the constituent gases. At standard temperature and pressure dry (STPD) (0°C, 760 mm Hg, 0% $H_2O$ vapor), the partial pressure of a gas ($P_{gas}$) is calculated as the product of the total pressure of the gas (ie, atmospheric pressure) and the fractional concentration of the gas ($FI_{gas}$), that is, the percent concentration expressed as a decimal.

$$P_{gas} = (P_{total})(FI_{gas}) = (P_{total})(\%gas/100)$$

Once air is inspired, it becomes warmed and humidified within the respiratory tract. Thus, when determining partial pressures of the gases anywhere in the body (BTPS, 98.6°F [37°C], 760 mm Hg, 100% $H_2O$ vapor), that is, in tracheal (conducting airways), alveolar, and exhaled air and in arterial and venous blood, the $H_2O$ vapor tension ($PH_2O$ at 98.6°F [37°C] is 47 mm Hg) must be subtracted from the total pressure of 760 mm Hg before multiplying by the fractional concentration of a gas, as follows:

$$P_{gas} = (P_{total} - PH_2O)(FI_{gas}) = (P_{total} - 47 \text{ mm Hg})(\%gas/100)$$

A summary of the partial pressures of the respiratory gases at sea level is presented in Table 20. The fractional concentration of the gases in the atmosphere does not change at high altitude, but as one ascends above sea level, the total barometric pressure decreases as the weight of the air above the atmosphere decreases. As a result, the partial pressure of oxygen and the other gases in the atmosphere decrease at high altitude.

The average partial pressure of oxygen in the alveoli is calculated using the alveolar gas equation:

$$P_AO_2 = P_IO_2 - (PaCO_2/R),$$

**TABLE 20.  PARTIAL PRESSURES OF RESPIRATORY GASES AT SEA LEVEL (BP = 760 MM HG)**

| Gases | Dry Inspired Air (Atmospheric) | Humidified Inspired Air (Dead Space) | Alveolar Air | Mixed Expired Air | Arterial Blood | Mixed Venous Blood |
|---|---|---|---|---|---|---|
| $PO_2$ | 159 (20.93) | 149 (20.93) | 104 (14.6) | 120 (16.8) | 100 | 40 |
| $PCO_2$ | 0.3 (0.04) | 0.3 (0.04) | 40 (5.6) | 27 (3.8) | 40 | 46 |
| $PN_2$ | 600 (79) | 563 (79) | 569 (79.8) | 566 (79.4) | 573 | 573 |
| $PH_2O$ | 0.0 (0.0) | 47 | 47 | 47 | 47 | 47 |
| Total | 760 | 760 | 760 | 760 | 760 | 706 |

Note I: The partial pressures are given in mm Hg followed in parenthesis by the percentage concentration.
Note II: $H_2O$ vapor is not expressed as a % of the total because the $PH_2O$ is temperature-dependent, not concentration-dependent. The $PH_2O$ at 98.6°F [37°C] is 47 mm Hg. This value must be subtracted from the total pressure of 760 mm Hg before multiplying by the fractional concentration of a gas when determining partial pressures of the gases anywhere in the body (BTPS), that is, in tracheal (conducting airways), alveolar, and exhaled air and in arterial and venous blood; only inspired atmospheric air is expressed under STPD.
Note III: In arterial and mixed venous blood, the respiratory gases are conventionally expressed in terms of their partial pressure. Therefore, the percentages are not indicated.

where $R$ is the respiratory gas exchange ratio ($\dot{V}CO_2/\dot{V}O_2$). Under normal circumstances its value depends on metabolism and is equal to 0.8.

## Ventilation

The air moving into the lung with each breath is called the *tidal volume* ($V_T$). The amount of air moving into the lung per minute is called the *minute ventilation* ($\dot{V}_E$), which is calculated as the product of the tidal volume and the respiratory rate:

$$\dot{V}_E(mL/min) = V_T(mL) \times \text{respiratory rate (breaths/min)}$$

Functionally, the respiratory tract consists of the conducting airways, which extend from the nose down to the terminal bronchioles, and the gas-exchanging airways, which extend from the respiratory bronchioles to the alveoli. The volume of the conducting airways is referred to as the anatomical dead space ($V_D$), which can be estimated as 1 mL/lb of body weight. The conducting airways do not participate in gas exchange because they are ventilated, but are perfused by systemic blood vessels, not by the pulmonary circulation. Sometimes, there are also alveoli that are ventilated but not perfused, which comprise areas of *alveolar dead space*. The *physiological dead space* is the sum of the anatomical and alveolar dead spaces. The ratio of the physiological dead space volume to the tidal volume ($V_D/V_T$) can be calculated using the Bohr equation, which takes advantage of the fact that any $CO_2$ present in the expired air ($P_ECO_2$) must have come from alveoli that are both ventilated and perfused.

$$V_D/V_T = Paco_2 - P_ECO_2/Paco_2$$

The dead space volume ($V_D$) must be subtracted from the tidal volume to determine the volume of gas that enters the gas-exchanging airways with each breath. The volume of gas going to the gas-exchanging airways each minute is called the *alveolar ventilation* ($\dot{V}_A$), and is calculated as:

$$\text{Alveolar ventilation } (\dot{V}_A) = (V_T - V_D) \times \text{respiratory rate}$$

The average partial pressure of carbon dioxide in the alveoli is proportional to carbon dioxide production and inversely proportional to alveolar ventilation:

$$Paco_2 = \dot{V}CO_2 / \dot{V}_A$$

Thus, at a constant rate of $CO_2$ production,

Normal alveolar ventilation = normal $Paco_2$ (35-45 mm Hg)
Hyperventilation = decreased $Paco_2$ (< 35 mm Hg)
Hypoventilation = increased $Paco_2$ (> 45 mm Hg)

## Mechanics of Breathing

Air is moved in and out of the lungs by the movement of the diaphragm and chest. During inspiration, the diaphragm descends and the rib cage moves up and out. Because the lungs are connected to the chest wall via the pleura, expansion of the chest wall expands the lungs. In accordance with Boyle law, expansion of the lungs creates a subatmospheric intraalveolar pressure, which draws air into the alveoli as air moves down its pressure gradient from an area of higher to lower pressure. Expiration is usually passive due to the elastic recoil of the lungs and chest wall when the inspiratory muscles cease contracting. Gas flow during expiration can be increased by actively contracting the expiratory muscles, but the maximum expiratory flow is limited by airway compression.

The gas moving in and out of the lungs is measured with spirometry. As shown in Figure 10:

- *Tidal volume* is the gas moving in and out of the lungs with each breath.
- The maximum amount of gas that can be expelled from the lungs after breathing in as far as possible is called the *vital capacity.*
- The maximum amount of gas that can be expelled from the lungs after a normal breath is called the *expiratory reserve volume.*
- The maximum amount of gas that can be inspired over and above the tidal volume is the *inspiratory reserve volume.*
- The maximum volume of gas that can be inspired from the resting expiratory level is the *inspiratory capacity.*
- The *total lung capacity* is the volume of gas present in the lungs after a maximum inspiration, and is equal to the sum of the four primary lung volumes.
- The gas remaining in the lung at the end of a quiet (tidal) expiration is the *functional residual capacity (FRC).*
- The amount of gas remaining in the lung at the end of a maximum expiration is the *residual volume.*

The residual volume cannot be measured by spirometry, and neither can the capacities that contain the residual volume, that is, the functional residual capacity and the total lung capacity.

## Lung Volumes and Capacities

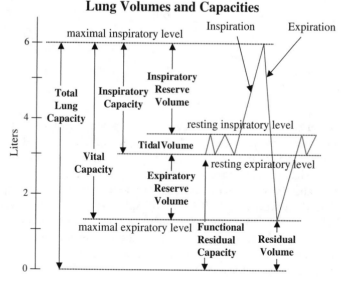

Figure 10

The lungs and chest wall are elastic structures. The lungs tend to recoil inward from the chest wall at all lung volumes, creating a subatmospheric intrapleural pressure, which becomes more negative with increases in lung volume. Intrapleural pressure is normally about −5 cm $H_2O$ at FRC, and decreases to about −30 cm $H_2O$ at TLC. The factors contributing to the lung's elastic recoil properties are elastic fibers and surfactant. The inverse of elastic recoil is compliance, which is defined as $\Delta V/\Delta P$, and represents the slope of a pressure-volume curve of the lung. Lung compliance is increased (elastic recoil is decreased) with alveolar septal departitioning and loss of elastic fibers that occur in emphysema and as part of the normal aging process. Lung compliance is decreased (increased elastic recoil, "stiff" lungs, restrictive lung disease) when normal elastic fibers are replaced by scar tissue (pulmonary interstitial fibrosis), in infiltrative diseases, when the lungs are filled with exudate or fluid, and when there is a deficiency of surfactant.

In addition to the elastic work of breathing, work is required to overcome the resistance to airflow offered by the airways. Airway resistance ($R_{aw}$) is defined as the driving pressure for airflow divided by the flow rate:

$$R_{aw} = \frac{\Delta P}{\dot{V}} = \frac{P_{atm} - P_{alv,} \, cmH_2O}{FlowRate, \, L/sec}$$

$R_{aw}$ can also be defined by Poiseuille law:

$$\frac{\Delta P}{\dot{V}} = \frac{8l\eta}{\pi r^4}$$

where
  $l$ is length.
  $\eta$ is viscosity.
  $r$ is radius.

Measurement of airway resistance requires a body plethysmograph to measure intrathoracic pressures. More frequently, airway resistance is assessed by changes in expiratory flow rates. An increase in airway resistance is the hallmark of obstructive lung disease. The effect of increased airway resistance (airway obstruction) is (1) to ↓ expiratory flow rates (peak flow, forced vital capacity [FVC], forced expiratory volume in 1 second [$FEV_{1.0}$], and $FEV_{1.0}$/FVC) and (2) to increase residual volume, functional residual capacity, and total lung capacity. These effects also cause characteristic changes in the configuration of the maximal expiratory flow-volume curves of the lung as shown in Figure 11.

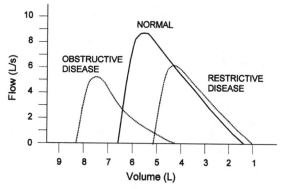

Figure 11

Maximal expiratory flow-volume curves representative of obstructive and restrictive pulmonary diseases. *(Reproduced, with permission, from Levitzky, MG. Pulmonary Physiology. 7th ed. New York, NY: McGraw-Hill;2007: 46.)*

## Hypoxia and Hypoxemia

The causes of tissue hypoxia can be classified into four groups, hypoxic hypoxia (hypoxemia), anemic hypoxia, hypoperfusion or stagnant hypoxia, and histotoxic hypoxia, as summarized in Table 21. There are also four different categories of hypoxemia.

**TABLE 21. TYPES OF HYPOXIA**

| Classification | $PAO_2$ | $PaO_2$ | $CaO_2$ | $PvO_2$ | $CvO_2$ | Corrected with Increased $F_iO_2$? |
|---|---|---|---|---|---|---|
| Hypoxic hypoxia | | | | | | |
| Low alveolar $PO_2$ | Low | Low | Low | Low | Low | Yes |
| Diffusion impairment | N | Low | Low | Low | Low | Yes |
| Right-to-left shunts | N | Low | Low | Low | Low | No |
| V/Q mismatch | N | Low | Low | Low | Low | Yes |
| Anemic hypoxia | N | N | Low | Low | Low | No |
| CO poisoning | N | N | Low | Low | Low | Possibly |
| Hypoperfusion hypoxia | N | N | N | Low | Low | No |
| Histotoxic hypoxia | N | N | N | High | High | No |

N = normal.
(Reproduced, with permission, from Levitzky MG. *Pulmonary Physiology.* 7th ed. New York, NY: McGraw-Hill; 2007.)

# CARDIOVASCULAR PHYSIOLOGY

*(Ganong, pp 80, 547-644. Stead et al, pp 5-9. Widmaier et al, pp 359-425.)*

## Electrical Activity of the Heart

### Action Potential

The contractile response of cardiac muscle begins just after the start of depolarization and lasts about 1.5 times as long as the action potential.

As seen in Figure 12, the initial rapid depolarization and overshoot (phase 0) are produced by the activation of $Na^+$ channels. The initial repolarization (phase 1) is produced by inactivation of $Na^+$ channels. The plateau (phase 2) is caused primarily by the activation of $Ca^{2+}$ channels. During phases 0 to 2 and a portion of phase 3, cardiac muscle cannot be excited again and thus, is in the absolute refractory period. It remains in the relative refractory period until phase 4 (Figure 13).

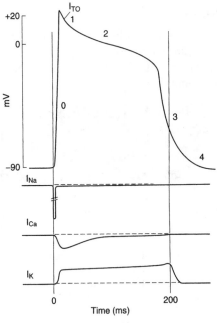

Figure 12

Top: Phases of the action potential of a cardiac muscle fiber. 0, depolarization; 1, initial rapid repolarization; 2, plateau phase; 3, late rapid repolarization; 4, baseline. Bottom: Diagrammatic summary of $Na^+$, $Ca^{2+}$, and cumulative $K^+$ currents during the action potential, Inward current down, outward current up. *(Reproduced, with permission, from Gangong, WF. Review of Medical Physiology, 22nd ed. New York: McGraw-Hill, 2005:80.)*

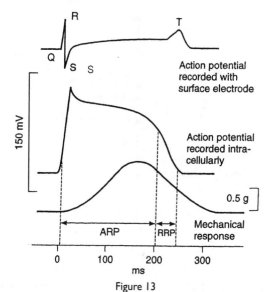

Figure 13

Action potentials and contractile response of mammalian cardiac muscle fiber plotted on the same time axis. ARP, absolute refractory period; RRP, relative refractory period. *(Reproduced, with permission, from Ganong, WF. Review of Medical Physiology, 22nd ed. New York: McGraw-Hill, 2005:80.)*

As such, tetanus does not occur like that seen in skeletal muscle. The downstroke or final repolarization (phase3) to the resting membrane potential (phase 4) is caused by closure (inactivation) of the $Ca^{2+}$ channels and $K^+$ efflux through various types of $K^+$ channels.

### Electrocardiogram

Recording extracellularly, the electrocardiogram (ECG) represents the summed electrical activity of all of the cardiac muscle cells and is represented by the following:

- The P wave is produced by atrial depolarization.
- The QRS complex is produced by ventricular depolarization.
- The ST segment is the time from the end of ventricular depolarization to the start of ventricular repolarization.
- The T wave corresponds to ventricular repolarization.
- The PR interval is the time for atrial depolarization and conduction through the atrioventricular (AV) node.

The mean electrical axis of depolarization (mean QRS vector) can be determined from the standard bipolar and the unipolar limb leads, as seen in Figure 14.

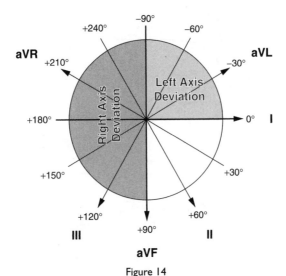

Figure 14
(*Reproduced, with permission, from Stead, LG et al.* First Aid for the Medicine Clerkship, *2nd ed. New York: McGraw-Hill, 2006:7.*)

## Mechanical Events of the Cardiac Cycle

The cardiac action potential triggers a wave of contraction that spreads through the myocardium. The phases of the cardiac cycle are shown in Figure 15 and include:

- Atrial systole
- Ventricular systole, which comprises isovolumetric contraction, rapid ejection, and reduced ejection
- Ventricular relaxation, which includes isovolumetric relaxation, rapid ventricular filling, and reduced ventricular filling

### Arterial Blood Pressure and Cardiac Output

The interaction of the factors controlling arterial blood pressure and cardiac output are summarized in Figure 16.

The heart rate is controlled primarily by the autonomic innervation of the heart, with sympathetic stimulation increasing heart rate by increasing the rate of phase 4 depolarization in the sinoatrial node, and vagal stimulation decreasing heart rate. Blood pressure is maintained by the baroreceptor reflex. Baroreceptors located in the carotid sinus and aortic arch respond to a decrease in blood pressure (eg, due to hemorrhage) by reflexly stimulating sympathetic

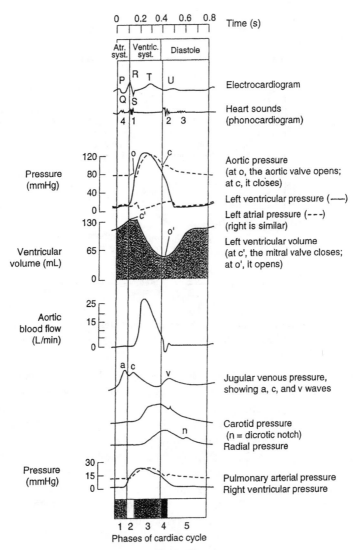

Figure 15

Events of the cardiac cycle at a heart of 75 beats/min. The phases of the cardiac cycle identified by the numbers at the bottom are as follows; 1, atrial systole; 2, isovolumetric ventricular contraction; 3, ventricular ejection; 4, isovolumetric ventricular relaxation; 5, ventricular filling. Note that late in systole, aortic pressure actually exceeds left ventricular pressure. However, the momentum of the blood keeps it flowing out of the ventricle for a short period. The pressure relationships in the right ventricle and pulmonary artery are similar, abbreviations; Atr. syst, atrial systole; Ventric syst., ventricular systole. (Reproduced, with permission, from Ganong WF. Review of Medical Physiology, 22nd ed. New York: McGraw-Hill, 2005:567.)

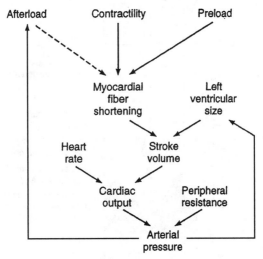

**Figure 16**

Solid arrows indicate increases, and the dashed arrow indicates a decrease. *(Reproduced, with permission, from Ganong WF. Review of Medical Physiology, 22nd ed. NewYork: McGraw-Hill, 2005:572.)*

activity to the heart and blood vessels, which increases heart rate, contractility, total peripheral resistance, and decreases venous compliance (see Figure 17).

Stroke volume (and thus cardiac output) is dependent on preload, afterload, and contractility. The relationship between preload (end-diastolic fiber length) and stroke volume is known as the length-tension relationship, and is represented by a Starling curve. Increases in preload (as measured by such indices as ventricular end-diastolic volume, ventricular end-diastolic pressure, atrial pressure, or central venous pressure) cause increases in the tension developed by cardiac muscle, which increases the stroke volume and cardiac output. The Starling curve is shifted up and to the left by an increase in contractility or a decrease in afterload. The Starling curve is shifted down and to the right by a decrease in contractility or an increase in afterload as shown in Figure 18.

Preload is dependent on blood volume, venous compliance, and total peripheral resistance (TPR). The relationship between these variables is represented by a vascular function curve. Changes in vascular volume or venous compliance cause a parallel shift in the vascular function curves. Changes in TPR cause the slope of the vascular function curve to change as shown in Figure 19.

The change in pressure and volume within the heart during one cardiac cycle can be represented by a pressure-volume loop. The work required to eject the blood is called the stroke work. The stroke work is the

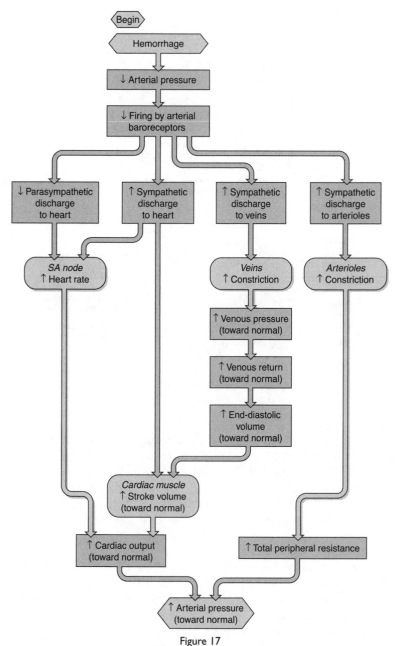

Figure 17
(Reproduced, with permission, from Widmaier E, Hershel R, Strang K. Vander's Human Physiology. 11th ed. New York, NY:McGraw-Hill;2008: 410.)

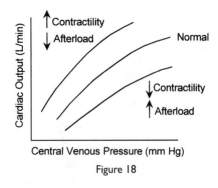

Figure 18

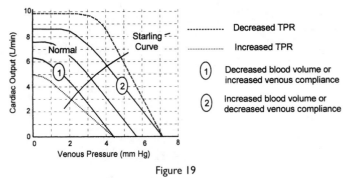

Figure 19

product of mean left ventricular systolic pressure and stroke volume, and is equal to the area within the pressure-volume curve. The energy required to eject the blood is dependent on the stroke work and the wall stress (tension). According to Laplace law, wall stress ($T$) is proportional to the systolic pressure ($P$) and the radius of the ventricle ($r$) and inversely proportional to the thickness of the ventricular wall ($w$):

$$T = P \times r/w$$

Wall stress increases in heart failure because the preload increases to compensate for the decrease in contractility. The increased radius of the enlarged heart causes wall stress to increase, and, therefore, more energy is required to eject blood. If the coronary circulation cannot provide the necessary oxygen, ischemic pain (angina) results (Figure 20).

Blood pressure decreases as blood flows through the circulation. The magnitude of the decrease is proportional to the resistance of each segment of the circulation. The greatest decrease occurs as blood flows through the arterioles. The segments of the circulation are in series with each other. The

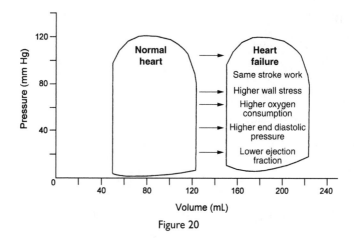

Figure 20

quantity of blood flowing into each organ is inversely proportional to the relative resistance of each organ. For example, at rest approximately 20% of the cardiac output flows through the skeletal muscles. During exercise, when the resistance of the skeletal muscle vessels decreases, over 80% of the cardiac output can flow through the skeletal muscles. The organs in the body are in parallel with each other, with the exception of the lungs, whose blood flow is in series with the systemic circulation.

The velocity ($v$) of blood through a vessel is proportional to the flow of blood through the vessel ($Q$) and inversely proportional to the area of the vessel ($A$):

$$v = Q/A$$

Increasing the velocity of blood can change flow from laminar (streamline) to turbulent (rapid, disorderly), as predicted by a Reynolds number that exceeds 2000. Turbulent flow produces a sound called a murmur if it occurs in the heart or a bruit if it occurs in a blood vessel. Flow through stenotic or incompetent heart valves produces cardiac murmurs. Occlusion of blood vessels by a sclerotic plaque, for example, will produce bruits. Some examples of cardiac murmurs include:

Systolic murmurs

1. Aortic stenosis
2. Pulmonic stenosis
3. Mitral regurgitation
4. Tricuspid regurgitation
5. Ventricular septal defect

Diastolic murmurs

1. Aortic regurgitation
2. Pulmonic regurgitation
3. Mitral stenosis
4. Tricuspid stenosis

## Capillary Fluid Balance

Fluid exchange across capillaries is dependent on the balance between the hydrostatic ($P$) and the osmotic ($\pi$) pressures between the capillaries and interstitial space, and the permeability of the capillary wall ($K_f$), as predicted by Starling law of capillary fluid balance:

$$\text{Filtration} = K_f \left[ (P_{cap} + \pi_i) - (\pi_{cap} + P_i) \right]$$

Excess filtration out of the capillaries causes fluid accumulation in the interstitial space, called edema. Edema can result from:

- An increase in capillary permeability ($K_f$), as during an inflammatory response
- A decrease in plasma proteins, as during malnutrition, which decreases $\pi_{cap}$
- An increase in capillary hydrostatic pressure ($P_{cap}$), as in heart failure
- A decrease in interstitial hydrostatic pressure ($P_i$) as with rapid evacuation of a pneumothorax

Normally, the fluid filtered from the capillaries is returned to the circulation by the lymphatic system, so blockage of the lymphatic circulation can also produce edema.

## GASTROINTESTINAL PHYSIOLOGY

*(Ganong, pp 467-513. Widmaier et al, pp 529-565.)*

The first stage in the digestion and absorption of food is chewing and swallowing. Chewing and swallowing can be initiated voluntarily or involuntarily. Chewing breaks food into small pieces and mixes them with salivary secretions including salivary $\alpha$-amylase. Swallowing is coordinated by a swallowing center in the brain stem. During the oral phase of swallowing, the tongue pushes the food into the pharynx. During the pharyngeal phase, peristaltic contractions and relaxation of the upper esophageal sphincter (UES) allow the food to enter the esophagus. During the esophageal phase, the lower esophageal sphincter (LES) relaxes and the food is propelled into the stomach by primary peristalsis. A secondary peristaltic wave, initiated by the presence of food in the smooth muscle, clears the esophagus of any food not propelled into the stomach by primary peristalsis.

The stomach breaks food into small pieces and mixes the pieces with gastric secretions to produce a paste-like material called chyme. Liquids and chyme are forced through the pylorus by a rise in gastric pressure. Liquids empty from the stomach in one and a half hour. Solids cannot pass through the pyloric sphincter until they are broken into small pieces ($< 1$ mm$^3$), and, therefore, emptying of solids takes from 1 to 3 hours.

Gastric emptying is slowed by the enterogastric reflex and the release of inhibitory hormones. The reflex and the secretion of hormones are evoked by the presence of acid or fats in the duodenum. The secretion of gastric acid by the parietal cells is regulated by paracrine (histamine), neural (vagus nerve), and hormonal (gastrin) influences. The characteristics of major gastrointestinal hormones are summarized in Table 22.

The intestine is responsible for the digestion and absorption of food and nutrients. During the digestive phase, food is slowly moved along the intestine by segmentation. During the interdigestive phase, the intestine is cleared of any nonabsorbed particles by the migrating motor complex.

Carbohydrates, proteins, and fats are digested by several enzymes. Carbohydrate digestion is completed in the small intestine by pancreatic amylase and by oligosaccharides such as maltase, lactase, sucrase, and trehalase which are located in the brush border of the small intestine. Proteins are broken down in the small intestine by enzymes from the pancreas (trypsin, chymotrypsin, elastase, and carboxypeptidase) and from aminopeptidase found in the intestinal brush border. Fat digestion occurs via pancreatic lipase and colipase.

Bile is necessary for the digestion and absorption of fats. However, the amount of bile acids emptied into the proximal small intestine from the gallbladder is insufficient for complete fat digestion and absorption. Receptor-mediated active transport of bile acids in the terminal ileum returns the bile acids via the portal blood to the liver for secretion into the small intestine (this circulation of bile is called the enterohepatic circulation). Approximately 95% of the bile acid pool is recirculated from the intestine and about 5% is lost in the stool.

Water absorption is caused by osmotic forces generated by sodium absorption. The source of water is both exogenous (oral input) and endogenous (GI tract secretion) and averages 8 to 10 L/d. Generally, less than 0.2 L/d is eliminated in the stool. The majority of water absorption occurs in the jejunum and ileum, with less amounts of absorption occurring in the colon.

## TABLE 22. PROPERTIES OF GASTROINTESTINAL HORMONES

| | Gastrin | CCK | Secretin | GIP |
|---|---|---|---|---|
| Chemical class | Peptide | Peptide | Peptide | Peptide |
| Site of production | Antrum of stomach | Small intestine | Small intestine | Small intestine |
| Stimuli for hormone release | Amino acids, peptides in stomach; parasympathetic nerves | Amino acids, fatty acids in small intestine | Acid in small intestine | Glucose, fat in small intestine |
| Factors inhibiting hormone release | Acid in stomach; somatostatin | | | |
| *Target Organ Responses* | | | | |
| *Stomach* | | | | |
| Acid secretion | Stimulates | Inhibits | Inhibits | |
| Motility | Stimulates | Inhibits | Inhibits | |
| Growth | Stimulates | | | |
| *Pancreas* | | | | |
| Bicarbonate secretion | | Potentiates secretin's actions | Stimulates | |
| Enzyme secretion | | Stimulates | Potentiates CCK's actions | |
| Insulin secretion | | | | Stimulates |
| Growth of exocrine pancreas | Stimulates | Stimulates | Stimulates | |
| *Liver (bile ducts)* | | | | |
| Bicarbonate secretion | | Potentiates secretin's actions | Stimulates | |
| *Gallbladder* | | | | |
| Contraction | | Stimulates | | |
| Sphincter of Oddi | | Relaxes | | |
| *Small intestine* | | | | |
| Motility | Stimulates ileum | | | |
| Growth | Stimulates | | | |
| *Large intestine* | Stimulates mass movement | | | |

(Reproduced, with permission, from Widmaier E, Hershel R, Strang K. *Vander's Human Physiology*. 11th ed. New York: McGraw-Hill;2008: 542.)

Some of the key functions of the stomach, small intestine, and colon are summarized below:

Stomach

- Mucus secretion (mucus cells)
- Pepsinogen secretion (chief cells)
- HCL secretion (parietal cells)
- Intrinsic factor secretion (parietal cells)
- Gastrin secretion (G cells in antrum)
- Accommodation (receptive relaxation) and peristalsis

Small intestine

- Iron absorption (duodenum)
- Folate absorption (duodenum)
- Bile acid absorption (ileum)
- Vitamin $B_{12}$ absorption (ileum)
- Water reabsorption
- Carbohydrate, protein, fat absorption
- Segmentation (digestive period) and migrating motor complex-MMC (inter-digestive period)

Colon

- Absorption of sodium and water
- Net secretion of potassium and bicarbonate
- Vitamin synthesis from colonic bacteria
- Segmentation and mass action contraction

## RENAL AND URINARY PHYSIOLOGY

*(Ganong, pp 505-551. Widmaier et al, pp 525-558.)*

The kidney is responsible for maintaining the constancy and volume of the extracellular fluid. The functional unit of the kidney is the glomerulus and its associated nephron. As depicted in Figure 21, the three basic components of renal function are:

- Glomerular filtration
- Tubular reabsorption
- Tubular secretion

Each day, 160 to 180 L of fluid is filtered into the approximately one million nephrons in the human kidney. The glomerular filtration rate (GFR) is dependent on the Starling forces between the glomerular capillaries (cap) and Bowman capsule (BC):

$$GFR = K_f \left[ (P_{cap} + \pi_{BC}) - (\pi_{cap} + P_{BC}) \right]$$

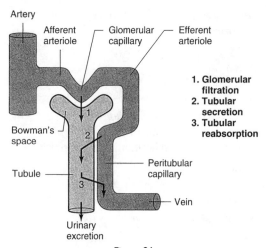

Artery

Afferent arteriole — Glomerular capillary — Efferent arteriole

1. **Glomerular filtration**
2. **Tubular secretion**
3. **Tubular reabsorption**

Bowman's space

Tubule

Peritubular capillary

Vein

Urinary excretion

Figure 21

Basic components of renal function. *(Reproduced with permission, from Widmaier EP et al. Vander's Human Physiology: The Mechanism of Body Function, 10th ed. New York: McGraw-Hill, 2006:531.)*

The amount of material filtered into the proximal tubule is called the filtered load. Approximately 20% of the plasma flowing through the glomerulus (renal plasma flow, RPF) is filtered into the proximal tubule:

**Filtration Fraction GFR/RPF**

The relative quantity of material excreted by the kidney (the renal clearance) is expressed as the volume of plasma that is completely cleared of the material by the kidney:

$$\text{Renal clearance} = (U_{conc} \times V)/P_{conc}$$

where

$U_{conc}$ = Urinary concentration of material
$P_{conc}$ = Plasma concentration of material
$V$ = Urinary flow rate

If a material is filtered but not reabsorbed or secreted, its renal clearance will be equal to the GFR. The clearances of creatinine or insulin are used clinically to measure GFR. If a material is completely cleared from the plasma during its passage through the kidney by a combination of filtration and secretion, its renal clearance will be equal to the renal plasma flow (RPF). The clearance of the organic anion para-aminohippurate (PAH) is used clinically to measure RPF:

$$\text{Renal blood flow (RBF)} = RPF/(1 - \text{hematocrit})$$

| TABLE 23.  PROXIMAL TUBULE REABSORPTION | | |
|---|---|---|
| Material | % Reabsorbed | Mechanism |
| Na⁺ | 60-70 | Na/H exchange Na-nutrient cotransport diffusion |
| K⁺, urea, Cl⁻ | 60-70 | Diffusion and solving drug |
| Glucose, amino acids | 100 | Na-nutrient cotransport |
| Phosphate | 90 | Na-nutrient cotransport |
| Bicarbonate | 85 | Indirectly via Na/H exchange |

### Proximal Tubule, Loop of Henle, Distal Tubule

The proximal tubule is responsible for reabsorbing most of the material filtered from the glomerulus as shown in Table 23.

The loop of Henle is responsible for producing a dilute filtrate. It reabsorbs approximately 25% of the salt and 15% of the water filtered from the glomerulus. The filtrate flowing from the loop of Henle to the distal convoluted tubule has a Na⁺ concentration of approximately 100 mEq/L.

The distal nephron is responsible for regulating salt and water balance. Na⁺ balance is regulated by aldosterone and atrial natriuretic peptide (ANP). Water balance is regulated by antidiuretic hormone (ADH), which is also called arginine vasopressin (AVP). K⁺ balance is regulated by aldosterone.

Aldosterone increases Na⁺ reabsorption and K⁺ secretion by the principal cells of the cortical and medullary collecting ducts. Aldosterone acts on the cell nucleus, increasing Na⁺ conductance of the apical membrane (which, by allowing more Na⁺ to enter the cell, increases Na⁺ reabsorption), the number of Na⁺,K⁺-ATPase pump sites (which, by increasing intracellular K⁺ concentration, increases K⁺ secretion), and the concentration of mitochondrial enzymes.

ANP decreases Na⁺ reabsorption by the renal epithelial cells of the medullary collecting ducts.

ADH increases water reabsorption by the principal cells of the cortical and medullary collecting ducts. ADH upregulates the number of water channels on the apical membrane of the epithelial cells by a cyclic adenosine monophosphate (cAMP)-dependent process.

Changes in renal hydrogen ion excretion are essential to the maintenance of acid-base balance in the body. The mechanisms of renal hydrogen ion excretion include:

- Bicarbonate ion reabsorption
- Titratable acid excretion (tubular secretion of H⁺, which combines with filtered phosphate)
- Ammonium ion excretion (tubular secretion of H⁺, which combines with filtered ammonia)

## ENDOCRINE AND REPRODUCTIVE PHYSIOLOGY

*(Ganong, pp 242-250, 317-453. Widmaier et al, pp 315-358, 567-582, 599-645.)*
Most of the hormones secreted by the endocrine glands are controlled by the hypothalamus and pituitary gland (hypophysis). The posterior pituitary contains the axons of neurons located within the paraventricular and supraoptic nuclei of the hypothalamus. These hypothalamic neurons synthesize:

- Oxytocin (responsible for milk ejection and uterine contraction)
- Antidiuretic hormone (ADH) also known as vasopressin (increases water permeability of renal collecting ducts)

| TABLE 24. ANTERIOR PITUITARY HORMONES | | |
|---|---|---|
| **Pituitary Hormone** | **Hypothalamic Hormone Affecting Pituitary Hormone** | **Major Action of Pituitary Hormone** |
| Thyroid-stimulating hormone (TSH) | Thyroid-releasing hormone (TRH) | Stimulates thyroid hormone synthesis and secretion |
| Adrenocorticotropic hormone (ACTH) | Corticotropin-releasing hormone (CRH) | Stimulates adrenal cortical secretion of glucocorticoids, mineralocorticoids, and sex hormones |
| Growth hormone | Growth hormone-releasing hormone | Stimulates synthesis of somatomedins by liver, which, in turn |
| | Growth hormone inhibitory hormone (somatostatin) | stimulate protein synthesis, organ and bone growth |
| Follicle-stimulating hormone (FSH) | Gonadotropin-releasing hormone (GnRH) | Spermatogenesis (males) Estradiol synthesis (females) |
| Luteinizing hormone (LH) | Gonadotropin-releasing hormone (GnRH) | Testosterone synthesis (males) Ovulation (females) |
| Prolactin | Prolactin-inhibiting factor (dopamine) Thyroid-releasing hormone (TRH) | Breast development and milk production |

The anterior pituitary secretes six major hormones as summarized in Table 24. The synthesis and release of these hormones are controlled by the hypothalamus. The hypothalamic releasing hormones are secreted into the median eminence from which they enter the capillary plexus that coalesces to form the anterior pituitary portal veins. These veins form another capillary plexus within the pituitary from which the releasing factors diffuse to the pituitary endocrine cells.

## Pancreatic Hormones

Insulin and glucagon are two key hormones secreted by the pancreas. Insulin affects carbohydrate, lipid, and protein metabolism in adipose, liver, and muscle tissues. Insulin is secreted by the β-cells of the islets of Langerhans and it increases the entry of glucose, amino acids, and fatty acids into cells. It promotes the storage of these metabolites and inhibits their synthesis and mobilization as shown in Figure 22. Glucagon is secreted by the α-cells of the islets of Langerhans and its effects oppose those of insulin.

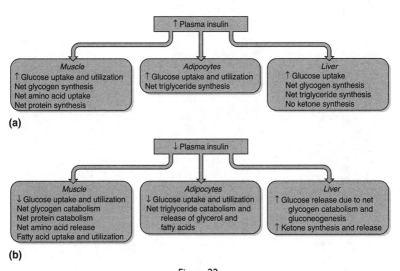

**Figure 22**
Effects of insulin. *(Reproduced, with permission, from Widmaier E, Hershel R, Strang K. Vander's Human Physiology. 11th ed. New York, NY: McGraw-Hill;2008:572).*

The Menstrual Cycle
The key events of the menstrual cycle are summarized in Table 25.

**TABLE 25. SUMMARY OF THE MENSTRUAL CYCLE**

| Day(s) | Major Events |
|---|---|
| 1–5 | Estrogen and progesterone are low because the previous corpus luteum is regressing.<br>*Therefore:* (a) Endometrial lining sloughs<br>(b) Secretion of FSH and LH is released from inhibition, and their plasma concentrations increase.<br>*Therefore:* Several growing follicles are stimulated to mature. |
| 7 | A single follicle (usually) becomes dominant. |
| 7–12 | Plasma estrogen increases because of secretion by the dominant follicle.<br>*Therefore:* Endometrium is stimulated to proliferate. |
| 7–12 | LH and FSH decrease due to estrogen and inhibin negative feedback.<br>*Therefore:* Degeneration (atresia) of nondominant follicles occurs. |
| 12–13 | LH surge is induced by increasing plasma estrogen.<br>*Therefore:* (a) Oocyte is induced to complete its first meiotic division and undergo cytoplasmic maturation.<br>(b) Follicle is stimulated to secrete digestive enzymes and prostaglandins. |
| 14 | Ovulation is mediated by follicular enzymes and prostaglandins. |
| 15–25 | Corpus luteum forms and, under the influence of low but adequate levels of LH, secretes estrogen and progesterone, increasing plasma concentrations of these hormones.<br>*Therefore:* (a) Secretory endometrium develops.<br>(b) Secretion of FSH and LH is inhibited, lowering their plasma concentrations.<br>*Therefore:* No new follicles develop. |
| 25–28 | Corpus luteum degenerates (if implantation of the conceptus does not occur).<br>*Therefore:* Plasma estrogen and progesterone concentrations decrease.<br>*Therefore:* Endometrium begins to slough at conclusion of day 28, and a new cycle begins. |

(Reproduced, with permission, from Widmaier E, Hershel R, Strang K. *Vander's Human Physiology.* 11th ed. New York, NY: McGraw-Hill;2008: 625.)

# General Principles: Cellular Physiology

## Questions

**1.** A 61-year-old man with erectile dysfunction asks his physician to prescribe Viagra® (sildenafil citrate). Sildenafil produces its physiological effects by blocking the enzyme that hydrolyzes the second messenger by which nitric oxide produces its physiological effects. Which of the following is the second messenger?

a. G protein
b. Cyclic GMP
c. Guanylate cyclase
d. cGMP phosphodiesterase
e. Diacylglycerol

**2.** A 42-year-old woman consults a dermatologist to evaluate and treat the frown lines on her forehead just above the nose. After the treatment options are explained to her, the patient asks the dermatologist to administer botulinum type A (Botox). Botox smooths out glabellar lines by which of the following mechanisms?

a. Blocking the release of synaptic transmitter from $\alpha$-motoneurons
b. Preventing the opening of sodium channels on muscle membranes
c. Decreasing the amount of calcium released from the sarcoplasmic reticulum
d. Increasing the flow of blood into the facial muscle
e. Enhancing the enzymatic hydrolysis of acetylcholine at the neuromuscular junction

**3.** In promyelocytic leukemia, fusion of retinoic acid receptor alpha (RAR-α) to other nuclear proteins causes aberrant gene silencing and prevents normal cellular differentiation. Treatment with the hormone retinoic acid reverses this repression and allows cellular differentiation and apoptosis to occur. Which of the following characteristics of a hydrophobic hormone that binds to nuclear receptors is most important in governing its diffusibility through a cell membrane?

a. Molecular weight
b. Electrical charge
c. Lipid solubility
d. Diameter
e. Three-dimensional shape

**4.** An 83-year-old woman with sepsis develops multiorgan failure. Based on her blood urea nitrogen of >100 mg/dL, she is placed on continuous venovenous hemodialysis. Which of the following factors will increase the diffusive clearance of solutes across the semipermeable dialysis membrane?

a. Area of the membrane increases
b. Concentration gradient for the solutes decreases
c. Lipid solubility of the solutes decreases
d. Size of the solute molecules increases
e. Thickness of the membrane increases

**5.** A 48-year-old woman with advanced breast cancer presents with severe nausea, vomiting, and dehydration. She is not undergoing chemotherapy at that time. Laboratory findings reveal elevated serum-ionized calcium. Parathyroid hormone (PTH) levels are undetectable but there is an increase in parathyroid-hormone-related peptide (PTHrP). The increased flow of calcium into the cell is an important component of the upstroke phase of the action potential in which of the following?

a. Cardiac ventricular muscle
b. Intestinal smooth muscle
c. Skeletal muscle
d. Nerve cells
e. Presynaptic nerve terminals

**6.** A 10-year-old boy sprains his ankle while running. History reveals that he has difficulty running, jumping, and keeping up with other children in races. His mother reports that she is also clumsy. Physical examination demonstrates footdrop, weakness, sensory loss, and reduced reflexes. The boy is found to have a decrease in nerve conduction velocity and an X-linked mutation of connexin 32, consistent with Charcot-Marie-Tooth disease. The neuropathy and gait disorder result because connexin is an important component of which of the following?

a. Gap junction
b. Sarcoplasmic reticulum
c. Microtubule
d. Synaptic vesicle
e. Sodium channel

**7.** A 2-day-old infant starts having brief tonic-clonic seizures throughout the day. His neurological function in between seizures is normal, and he has no other medical or neurological problems. The history reveals no readily apparent causes for the seizures though the mother recalled that her first baby also developed seizures shortly after birth that only lasted for 2 weeks, with no subsequent episodes or developmental problems. Genetic analysis revealed a mutation of voltage-gated $K^+$ channels consistent with a diagnosis of benign familial neonatal seizures. Which of the following would cause an immediate reduction in the amount of potassium leaking out of a cell?

a. Increasing the permeability of the membrane to potassium
b. Hyperpolarizing the membrane potential
c. Decreasing the extracellular potassium concentration
d. Reducing the activity of the sodium-potassium pump
e. Decreasing the extracellular sodium concentration

**8.** A 48-year-old executive was referred for a life insurance physical examination for his new corporation. His body mass index was 34, indicating clinical obesity, and his blood pressure was 145/92 mm Hg. Blood tests showed hyperlipidemia and hyperglycemia with normal insulin levels, consistent with type 2 diabetes mellitus (T2DM). T2DM adversely affects many cellular processes. Which of the following transport processes is a passive downhill process?

a. Sodium out of brain cells
b. Calcium into the sarcoplasmic reticulum (SR)
c. Hydrogen into the lumen of canaliculi of the parietal cells of the stomach
d. Glucose into skeletal muscle and fat cells
e. Phosphate into epithelial cells lining the proximal tubule of the kidney

**9.** A 54-year-old woman undergoes a colonoscopy to screen for colon cancer. Biopsy of a polyp removed during the procedure reveals epithelial cell metaplasia, with some cells progressing toward malignant transformation. A high-fiber diet is prescribed to generate more short-chain fatty acids. The figure below illustrates the concentration of protonated short-chain fatty acids on either side of a colonic epithelial cell membrane. If the concentration of fatty acids on the outside surface of the cell doubles, the rate of diffusion of the short-term fatty acids will change from 10 mg/h to which of the following rates?

20 mg/L        10 mg/L

CHAMBER A      CHAMBER B

a. 5 mg/h
b. 10 mg/h
c. 15 mg/h
d. 20 mg/h
e. 30 mg/h

**10.** A 43-year-old pregnant woman develops preeclampsia at 32 weeks' gestation. Magnesium sulfate, which blocks NMDA receptors in the central nervous system, is ordered for the prevention of eclamptic seizures until the fetus can be delivered. Which of the following activates the NMDA receptor?

a. Acetylcholine
b. GABA
c. Glycine
d. Glutamate
e. Kainate

**11.** A 56-year-old woman presents with fatigue and malaise. Hepatomegaly and mild jaundice are evident upon physical examination. Blood tests reveal an increase in aspartate aminotransferase (AST) and the presence of anti-smooth muscle antibodies (SMA), suggestive of autoimmune hepatitis. Which of the steps in the chemical reactions that occur during cross-bridge cycling in smooth muscle shown below is responsible for relaxation of contracted smooth muscle and the formation of latch bridges?

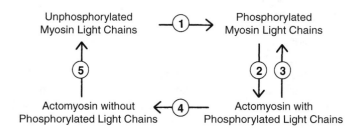

a. Step 1
b. Step 2
c. Step 3
d. Step 4
e. Step 5

**12.** A 23-year-old man is brought to the emergency department after collapsing during basketball practice. On admission he is lethargic and appears confused. His coach reports that it was hot in the gym and he was drinking a lot of water during practice. An increase in which of the following is the most likely cause of his symptoms?

a. Intracellular tonicity
b. Extracellular tonicity
c. Intracellular volume
d. Extracellular volume
e. Plasma volume

**13.** A 14-year-old adolescent girl reports blood in her urine 2 weeks after she had a sore throat. She has uremia and a blood pressure of 160/90 mm Hg with peripheral edema, suggestive of volume expansion secondary to salt and water retention. Which of the following is the approximate extracellular fluid volume of a normal individual?

a. 5% of body mass
b. 10% of body mass
c. 20% of body mass
d. 40% of body mass
e. 60% of body mass

**14.** A previously well 18-year-old woman is admitted to the ICU because of altered mental status. She does not respond to instructions and her arms are postured in a flexor position. Laboratory data reveal a serum sodium concentration of 125 mmol/L. Her friends indicate that the patient had taken ecstasy at a party the night before, and because she was extremely thirsty the next morning, she had consumed a lot of water in a short period of time. Assuming that the reduction in osmolarity is entirely due to water consumption, that her initial weight was 60 kg, and that her initial osmolarity was 300 mOsm/L, which of the following is approximately the quantity of water she would have drank to produce the observed hyponatremia?

a. 2.5 L
b. 3.5 L
c. 5 L
d. 6 L
e. 7 L

**15.** A 49-year-old man in end-stage renal failure is able to perform peritoneal dialysis at home. The osmolality of the solution chosen for peritoneal dialysis will determine the rate of ultrafiltration. Which of the following statements best characterizes a molecule whose osmolality is zero?

a. It will not permeate the membrane.
b. It can only cross the membrane through the lipid bilayer.
c. It causes water to flow across the membrane.
d. It is as diffusible through the membrane as water.
e. It is transported across the membrane by a carrier.

**16.** A 76-year-old woman with a history of uncontrolled hypertension presents in the emergency department with hypotension and shock-like symptoms. Her daughter reports systolic blood pressure near 200 mm Hg earlier in the day and suspects a dissecting aneurysm, which is confirmed with a CT of the chest. Biopsy of the repaired aorta shows giant cell arteritis, and the woman is placed on a regimen of high-dose prednisone. The anti-inflammatory effect of exogenous glucocorticoids is thought to be due to which of the following?

a. Increased capillary membrane permeability
b. Increased formation of leukotrienes
c. Increased release of interleukin-1 (pyrogen) from granulocytes
d. Activation of phospholipase $A_2$
e. Inhibition of the activation of NF-κB

# General Principles: Cellular Physiology

## *Answers*

**1. The answer is b.** (*Ganong, pp 37-38, 43-44, 165, 427-428.*) Erection is initiated by dilation of the arterioles of the penis, which increases blood flow into the erectile tissue of the organ. The increased turgor of the penis also results from compression of the veins, blocking the outflow of blood from the organ. Nitric oxide (NO) is a potent vasodilator that acts by activating guanylyl cyclase, resulting in increased production of the second messenger, cGMP. Sildenafil citrate (Viagra®) is an effective and selective inhibitor of cGMP phosphodiesterase (PDE). By blocking the breakdown of cGMP, sildenafil prolongs the action of NO and erections. Sildenafil is most active against PDE5, the type of PDE found in the corpora cavernosa. Other cGMP PDE5 inhibitors used in the treatment of erectile dysfunction include tadalafil (Cialis®) and vardenafil (Levitra®). Erections are produced by the release of NO, which inhibits the smooth muscle of the corpora cavernosa, allowing blood to fill the penis. Sildenafil is also a potent inhibitor of PDE6 found in the retina, which accounts for the transient blue-green color weakness, one of the side effects of sildenafil. G proteins are coupling molecules that link various receptors to nearby effector molecules, which, in turn, generate second messengers that mediate the hormone's actions. Inositol triphosphate (IP₃) is associated with the membrane phospholipid system for hormonal signal transduction. G-protein activation of the membrane-bound enzyme phospholipase C breaks down membrane phospholipids into diacylglycerol (DAG) and inositol triphosphate. DAG is a potent activator of protein kinase C.

**2. The answer is a.** (*Fauci, pp 842-844. Ganong, pp 87-88.*) Botulinum toxin inhibits the release of acetylcholine from α-motoneurons by blocking one of the proteins responsible for the fusion of the synaptic channel with the presynaptic membrane. Botulinum toxin also inhibits the release of acetylcholine from the neurons of the autonomic nervous system. Botulinum toxins are being employed for a variety of cosmetic and therapeutic purposes. Generalized botulism-like weakness (iatrogenic botulism) is a rare complication of these procedures. Botulinum and tetanus toxin are released from the same class of bacteria (*Clostridium*). Illness begins with cranial nerve involvement and proceeds caudally to involve the extremities. Cases may be classified as food borne, wound botulism, and intestinal botulism. Because of its extraordinary potency, botulinum toxin has also been used as an agent of bioterrorism or biological warfare that could be acquired by inhalation or ingestion. Features of outbreaks suggesting deliberate release of botulinum toxin include infection with an unusual toxin type, outbreak of a large number of cases of acute flaccid paralysis with prominent bulbar palsies with a common geographic factor but without a common dietary exposure, or multiple simultaneous outbreaks without a common source. Tetanus toxin produces an increase in skeletal muscle contraction by blocking the release of inhibitory neurotransmitter from spinal interneurons.

**3. The answer is c.** (*Fauci, pp 2387-2391. Ganong, pp 4, 31. Widmaier, pp 124-125.*) Materials that are not soluble in water can only diffuse across the membrane through the lipid bilayer. The most important factor determining how well a substance can diffuse across the lipid bilayer is the substance's lipid solubility. If two materials have the same lipid solubility, then the permeability of the smaller particle will be greater. Signal transduction pathways differ between water-soluble and lipid-soluble messengers (hormones). Lipid-soluble messengers, including steroid hormones, thyroid hormones, and vitamin derivatives such as retinoids (vitamin A) and vitamin D, interact with intracellular nuclear receptors, in contrast to water-soluble amino acid derivatives and peptide hormones, which interact with cell-surface membrane receptors.

**4. The answer is a.** (*Fauci, pp 1760-1761, 1772-1775. Ganong, pp 4-5. Widmaier, pp 96-100.*) The rate of diffusion is described by the Fick equation, as follows:

$$\text{Net flux} = A \times ([S1] - [S2]) \times D/d.$$

where

| | |
|---|---|
| $A$ | = area available for diffusion |
| $[S1] - [S2]$ | = concentration gradient of the substance across the membrane |
| $d$ | = distance for diffusion, and |
| $D$ | = Diffusion coefficient of the substance = solubility coefficient/square root of gram molecular weight of the substance |

In other words, the flux of a molecule across a membrane is directly proportional to the area of a membrane, the concentration difference of the particles on either side of the membrane, and the lipid solubility of the particle. Net flux is inversely proportional to the thickness of the membrane and the size (specifically, the square root of the gram molecular weight) of the molecule. During acute renal failure, dialysis is often used to support renal function until renal recovery occurs. Hemodialysis relies on the effectiveness of solute diffusion across a semipermeable membrane. There are various modalities of hemodialysis, including intermittent, slow, low-efficiency dialysis, and continuous hemodialysis.

**5. The answer is b.** (*Ganong, pp 58-59, 68, 78, 80, 481. McPhee and Ganong, pp 498-499, 715.*) In intestinal smooth muscle, the upstroke of the action potential is caused by the flow of calcium into the cell. In cells of the cardiac ventricular muscle, the plateau phase of the action potential, but not the upstroke, is accompanied by the flow of calcium into the cells. Skeletal muscle fibers resemble nerve fibers. In both of these cells, the upstroke of the action potential is caused by the flow of sodium into the cell. Hypercalcemia occurs in approximately 10% of all malignancies and is most commonly seen in solid tumors, particularly breast carcinoma, renal carcinoma, and squamous cell carcinomas (eg, esophagus and lung). Solid tumors usually produce hypercalcemia by secreting PTHrP. The resulting humoral hypercalcemia mimics primary hyperthyroidism, but with no elevation in PTH.

**6. The answer is a.** (*Fauci, pp 2662-2664. Ganong, p 17.*) Connexin is a membrane-spanning protein that is used to create gap junction channels. The gap junction channel creates a cytoplasmic passage between two cells. Each cell membrane contains half of the channel. The channel, called a connexon, is constructed from six connexin molecules that form a cylinder with a pore at its center. CMT disease comprises a heterogeneous group of inherited peripheral neuropathies. Approximately 1 in 2500 persons has some form of CMT, making it one of the most frequently occurring inherited neuromuscular disorders. Demyelinating forms of CMT are classified as CMT1 and axonal forms as CMT2. Transmission is most frequently autosomal dominant but it may also be autosomal recessive or X-linked, like the mutation affecting the connexin 32 (Cx32), located in the folds of the Schwann cell cytoplasm around the nodes of Ranvier. This localization suggests a role for gap junctions composed of Cx32 in ion and nutrient transfer around and across the myelin sheath of peripheral nerves.

**7. The answer is b.** (*Ganong, pp 7-8. McPhee and Ganong, pp 144-147, 176-179, 702.*) The amount of potassium moving out of the cell depends on its membrane potential, its concentration gradient, and its membrane conductance. According to the Nernst equation, the electrical gradient for $K^+$ is inward and the concentration gradient is outward. Hyperpolarizing the membrane makes the inside of the cell more negative and therefore makes it more difficult for potassium to flow out of the cell. Answer (c) is incorrect because decreasing the extracellular potassium concentration would increase the flow of potassium out of the cell, as would increasing the permeability of the membrane to potassium (a). Decreasing the activity of the sodium-potassium pump has no immediate effect on potassium efflux, but ultimately results in depolarization of the membrane, resulting in an increased flow of potassium out of the cell. Altering the extracellular sodium concentration has no immediate effect on the flow of potassium across the membrane. Seizures are paroxysmal disturbances in cerebral function caused by an abnormal synchronous discharge of cortical neurons. The epilepsies are a group of disorders characterized by recurrent seizures. Benign familial neonatal seizures constitute a rare type of idiopathic epilepsy linked to autosomal dominant mutations of voltage-gated $K^+$ channels. The seizures are paroxysmal, generally appearing within the first week to month of life, and generally resolve spontaneously within days to weeks after onset. The seizures are brief tonic-clonic seizures with little or no postictal state. There are generally no resultant developmental problems, though there may be a predisposition to developing epilepsy later in life.

**8. The answer is d.** (*Ganong, pp 31-35. Widmaier, pp 104-108, 578-583, 588-589.*) Glucose is transported into skeletal muscle and fat cells by facilitated diffusion and thus does not require the direct or indirect use of energy. Several distinct transporters mediate the facilitated diffusion of glucose. Insulin increases the number of the glucose transporters expressed in skeletal muscle and adipose tissue, and thereby increases the rate of diffusion of glucose, though insulin is not necessary for the diffusion. In diabetes mellitus (DM), when insulin is not available (type 1 DM) or when the cells are unresponsive to insulin (type 2 DM), muscle and adipose tissue cannot efficiently transport glucose across their membranes, leading to the characteristic hyperglycemia that is the hallmark of DM. All of the answer choices describe transport systems that require energy. Sodium is transported out of cells by $Na^+$- $K^+$-ATPase; calcium is transported into the SR by a $Ca^{2+}$-ATPase; and hydrogen is transported from the parietal cells of the stomach by a $H^+$- $K^+$-ATPase. All of these transporters use ATP directly in the transport process. The active transport of $Na^+$ is often coupled to the transport of other substances, a process called secondary active transport. In the proximal tubule, phospate is transported into the luminal cells of the proximal tubule by a $Na^+$- $HPO_4^{2-}$ secondary active transport system. Secondary active transport usually involves the transepithelial movement of ions and other molecules in the gastrointestinal tract, pulmonary airways, renal tubules, and other structures.

**9. The answer is e.** (*Ganong, pp 4-5. McPhee and Ganong, p 364.*) Short-chain fatty acids are released by the action of the colonic microflora on dietary fiber. These short-chain fatty acids promote survival of healthy colonic epithelium while inducing apoptosis in epithelial cells progressing toward malignant transformation. Absorption of protonated short-chain fatty acids into enterocytes occurs by simple diffusion. Fick law states that the net rate of diffusional flux ($J$) of a substance is proportional to its concentration difference ($\Delta c$). Doubling the concentration of protonated short-chain fatty acids outside of the enterocytes from 20 to 40 mg/L causes the concentration difference to increase by threefold from 10 to 30 mg/L. Therefore, the net rate of diffusion would increase from 10 to 30 mg/h.

**10. The answer is c.** (*Fauci, pp 44-45. Ganong, pp 98, 108-110.*) Glutamate is the major neurotransmitter that mediates synaptic excitation in the central nervous system, and glutamate receptors are also known as excitatory amino acid receptors. The NMDA (N-methyl-D-aspartate) receptor channel is one of five different classes of excitatory amino acid receptors. The NMDA receptor is a large channel permeable to $Ca^{2+}$, $K^+$, and $Na^+$. It is activated by glutamate, but unlike other glutamate receptor channels, the NMDA channel is blocked by $Mg^{2+}$ in its resting state. Depolarization of the cell membrane to approximately −40 mV removes the $Mg^{2+}$ blockade. Therefore, the NMDA channel is only opened when the cell is depolarized by other excitatory neurotransmitters. Preeclampsia is the development of high blood pressure during pregnancy. Other signs of preeclampsia include protein in the urine and severe edema (or swelling). The only treatment for preeclampsia is delivery of the baby, which may mean a premature birth. Magnesium sulfate is the treatment of choice for preventing and treating eclamptic seizures. Acetylcholine binding to nicotinic acetylcholine receptors opens ion channels conductive to $Na^+$ and $K^+$. Glycine and GABA are both inhibitory neurotransmitters that act on glycine and $GABA_A$ receptors, respectively, which are ligand-gated $Cl^-$ channels. Binding of GABA to the metabotropic $GABA_B$ receptor activates a G- protein, which leads to activation of $K^+$ channels and inhibition of $Ca^{2+}$ channels. Kainate is another type of glutamate receptor.

**11. The answer is d.** *(Binder, pp 621-628. Ganong, pp 89-90. Widmaier, pp 284-286.)* Smooth muscle relaxes when $Ca^{2+}$ is removed from the myoplasm and latch bridges detach from actin. Latch bridges are unphosphorylated myosin cross-bridges that are bound to actin. These cross-bridges cycle very slowly or not at all and are responsible for the ability of smooth muscle to maintain its tone for a long time without expending energy for cross-bridge cycling. The enzyme myosin light chain phosphatase is responsible for dephosphorylating cross-bridges (step 4). Cross-bridge cycling in smooth muscle cannot begin until the myosin light chains are phosphorylated (step 1). Phosphorylation is enzymatically stimulated by myosin light chain kinase (MLCK).

Smooth muscle autoantibodies (SMA) are found in the sera of patients with autoimmune liver diseases, viral infections, certain cancers, heroin addicts, and female infertility. SMAs are classified according to their reactivity to microfilaments, microtubules, or intermediate filaments. Autoantibodies to actin-like microfilaments appear specific for autoimmune hepatitis, autoantibodies to microtubules occur in infectious mononucleosis, an autoantibodies to intermediate filaments occur in infectious hepatitis, chickenpox, measles, and mumps. Autoimmune hepatitis is positive for both SMA and antinuclear antibodies (ANA), whereas systemic lupus erythematosus (SLE) is positive for ANA but not SMA. A possible pathogenic role for SMAs seems unlikely because the autoantibodies are in the serum and the cytoskeletal antigens are in the cytoplasm. However, observations that serum autoimmune complexes may activate complement raise the possibility of antibody-mediated tissue damage by complement lysis.

**12. The answer is c.** (*Fauci, pp 277-279. Ganong, pp 6-7, 241-242, 729. Stead, p 226.*) Drinking water after losing a significant volume of water as sweat decreases the osmolality of the extracellular fluid because the salt lost from the extracellular fluid in sweat is not replaced by the ingested water. When the extracellular osmolality is decreased, water flows from the extracellular to the intracellular body compartment, causing intracellular volume to increase. The patient's symptoms are caused by swelling of the brain.

**13. The answer is c.** (*Fauci, pp 1784-1787. Ganong, pp 1-3, 6-7. Stead, p 226.*) Sixty percent of the body mass is water. Of this water, one-third (20% of body mass) is extracellular and two-thirds (40% of body mass) is intracellular. The extracellular water is further divided into interstitial water (80% of extracellular fluid, or 15% of body mass) and plasma water (20% of extracellular fluid, or 5% of body mass). The percentage of water in the body is a function of body fat. The greater the percentage of body fat, the lower the percentage of body water. About three-fourths of the lean body mass (mass excluding fat) is water. The distribution of extracellular and intracellular water is a function of the extracellular osmolality. If the osmolality of the extracellular fluid is above normal, the proportion of water in the extracellular fluid, in comparison to that in the intracellular water, increases; hypotonicity of the extracellular water decreases the proportion of water in the extracellular fluid. Poststreptococcal glomerulonephritis is an acute nephritic syndrome that typically affects children between the age of 2 and 14 years, although 10% of cases are patients older than 40. Throat infections with certain M-type streptococci antedate the glomerular disease by 1 to 3 weeks. Findings include hematuria, proteinuria and pyuria, red blood cell casts, edema, hypertension, and oliguric renal failure. Antibiotic treatment for streptococcus should be given to the patient and all cohabitants, as incidence in cohabitants is as high as 40%.

**14. The answer is e.** (*Ganong, pp 1, 5-6, 729. Widmaier, pp 108-112.*) When water is ingested from the intestine, it enters the plasma and rapidly achieves osmotic equilibrium with the interstitial and intracellular compartments. Assuming that she had a normal osmolarity of 300 mOsmol/L initially, at her initial body weight of 60 kg, with 60% of body weight being water, her initial volume was 36 L. A sodium concentration of 125 mM is equivalent to an osmolarity of 250 mOsmol/L. Assuming that her normal osmolarity of 300 mOsm was reduced to 250 mOsm by the ingestion of water, she drank approximately 7 L.

$$\text{Osmolarity} = \text{mOsmol/volume}$$
$$300 \text{ mOsm/L} = 60 \text{ kg} \times 60\% \times 300/\text{initial volume}$$
$$\text{Initial volume} = 10{,}800 \text{ mOsmol}/300 \text{ mOsm/L} = 36 \text{ L}$$
$$250 \text{ mOsm/L} = 60 \text{ kg} \times 60\% \times 300/\text{new volume}$$
$$\text{New volume} = 10{,}800 \text{ mOsmol}/250 \text{ mOsmol/L} \cong 43 \text{ L}$$
$$\text{Volume consumed} = \text{new volume} - \text{initial volume}$$
$$= 43 \text{ L} - 36 \text{ L} = 7 \text{ L}$$

The amount of water ingested by the patient was not likely this high because she probably lost significant amount of salt as sweat while under the influence of ecstasy. Her signs and symptoms are due to the brain swelling caused by hypotonicity.

**15. The answer is d.** *(Fauci, pp 1761, 1772-1775. Ganong, pp 56.)* The osmolality of a substance is the number of osmoles per kg of solvent. One osmole (Osm) equals the gram molecular weight of a substance divided by the number of free-moving particles that each molecule liberates in solution. Osmotically active substances in the body are dissolved in water, and the density of water is 1. Thus, osmolar concentrations can be expressed as osmoles (or milliosmoles) per liter of water. If the osmolality is zero, there are no free-moving particles and thus, the molecule is as diffusible as water through the membrane. Dialysis is often used for the treatment of either acute or chronic kidney disease. Commonly accepted criteria for initiating patients on maintenance dialysis include marked uremia and reductions in glomerular filtration rate, hyperkalemia and/or acidosis that are unresponsive to medication, and persistent extravascular fluid expansion despite diuretic therapy. Hemodialysis is used in >90% of patients with end-stage renal disease (ESRD) in the United States, but no large-scale clinical trials have been completed to compare outcomes among patients randomized to either hemodialysis or peritoneal dialysis.

**16. The answer is e.** *(Ganong, pp 371-372, 636.)* Evidence is accumulating that the transcription factor, nuclear factor-κB (NF-κB), plays a key role in the inflammatory response. NF-κB is a heterodimer that normally exists in the cytoplasm of cells bound to IκBα, which renders it inactive. Stimuli such as viruses, cytokines, and oxidants separate NF-$\kappa$B from I$\kappa$B$\alpha$, and NF-$\kappa$B moves to the nucleus where it binds to DNA of the genes for numerous inflammatory mediators, resulting in their increased production and secretion. Glucocorticoids inhibit the activation of NF-$\kappa$B by increasing the production of I$\kappa$B$\alpha$, and this is probably the main basis of their anti-inflammatory action. The anti-inflammatory effects of exogenous glucocorticoids are due to their ability to decrease capillary membrane permeability and probably also to their ability to stabilize lysosomal membranes and decrease the formation of bradykinin. Glucocorticoids inhibit the enzyme phospholipase $A_2$; this decreases the release of arachidonic acid and the variety of substances produced from it, such as leukotrienes, prostaglandins, thromboxanes, and prostacyclin. Cortisol owes its fever-reducing action to the hormone's ability to decrease the release of pyrogen (interleukin 1) from granulocytes. However, only in massive doses will the hormone achieve the effects described. Endogenous cortisol does not exert a significant anti-inflammatory action.

# General Principles: Multisystem Processes

## Questions

**17.** A 62-year-old man presents to the emergency room with an acute onset of aphasia and hemiparesis. A computed tomography (CT) scan reveals an increase in intracranial fluid. Which of the following solutions will be most effective in reducing intracranial pressure following a large hemispheric stroke?

a. 150 mmol sodium chloride
b. 250 mmol glycerol
c. 250 mmol glucose
d. 350 mmol urea
e. 350 mmol mannitol

**18.** An 82-year-old woman is brought to the emergency department complaining of nausea, vomiting, muscle cramps, and generalized weakness. Laboratory analysis reveals significant hyperkalemia. Elevations of extracellular potassium ion concentration will have which of the following effects on nerve membranes?

a. The membrane will become more excitable.
b. The membrane potential will become more negative.
c. The activity of the $Na^+$- $K^+$ pump will decrease.
d. Potassium conductance will increase.
e. Sodium conductance will increase.

**19.** A 65-year-old man being treated with a beta blocker and an angiotensin-converting enzyme (ACE) inhibitor for his heart failure presents to his cardiologist's office complaining of fatigue, weakness, shortness of breath, and an irregular heart beat. An ECG reveals atrial fibrillation, so his cardiologist adds digoxin to his treatment regimen, but tells the patient that he will need to get his blood drawn to check for low $K^+$ on a regular basis. Hypokalemia will increase the risk and severity of digitalis toxicity because of which of the following?

a. Hypopolarization of cardiac muscle membranes
b. Increased inhibition of the $Na^+$- $K^+$ pump
c. Increased excitability of cardiac muscle cells
d. Increased amplitude of cardiac muscle action potentials
e. Increased removal of cardiac cytosolic $Ca^{2+}$ via the $Na^+$- $Ca^{2+}$ exchanger

**20.** A 19-year-old man is found comatose in his garage by his father who calls 911. Blood work drawn in the emergency department shows: $PaO_2$ = 105 mm Hg, $PaCO_2$ = 24 mm Hg, pH = 7.31, $SaO_2$ = 98%, $Na^+$ = 135 mEq/L, $K^+$ = 5 mEq/L, $Cl^-$ = 100 mEq/L, $HCO_3^-$ = 5 mEq/L, BUN = 15 mg/dL, Cr = 1.2 mg/dL, glucose = 95 mg/dL. Which of the following is the most likely diagnosis?

a. Carbon monoxide poisoning
b. Diabetes mellitus
c. Ethylene glycol ingestion
d. Renal tubular acidosis
e. Respiratory arrest

**21.** A 55-year-old obese man with type 2 diabetes mellitus presents for his annual checkup. Serum lipoprotein analysis done after a 12-hour fast shows elevated low- and very-low-density lipoproteins (LDL and VLDL), elevated triglycerides, and decreased high-density lipoprotein (HDL) cholesterol. What contributes to the lipid abnormalities in type 2 diabetes mellitus?

a. Hyperglycemia increases triglyceride uptake into adipose tissue.
b. Insulin resistance increases triglyceride uptake into adipose tissue.
c. Insufficient insulin action increases LDL receptor activity.
d. Insufficient insulin action in adipose tissue decreases lipoprotein lipase activity.
e. Insulin resistance and hyperglycemia decrease fatty acid flux to the liver and lipolysis.

**22.** The friends of a 26-year-old man, who is scheduled to be married in a month, plan a bachelor's party for him in Las Vegas. After a round of golf in 100°F weather, the group heads to the pool. They order several rounds of drinks over the next 4 hours and also order lunch poolside. Most of the group orders hamburgers and french fries, but the groom-to-be is watching his weight and opts for a club sandwich and a side of coleslaw. Later that night, they go for dinner and to the casinos, where they imbibe some more. Early next morning, the groom-to-be becomes ill. He thinks it is just a hangover, but presents to the emergency department 36 hours later with persistent vomiting and orthostatic hypotension. Which of the following metabolic abnormalities are most likely present in this patient?

a. Hypokalemia, hypochloremia, and metabolic alkalosis
b. Hypokalemia, hypochloremia, and metabolic acidosis
c. Hyperkalemia, hyperchloremia, and metabolic alkalosis
d. Hyperkalemia, hyperchloremia, and metabolic acidosis
e. Normal serum electrolytes and acid-base balance

**23.** A 58-year-old man is transported to the emergency department due to impaired breathing and shortness of breath. Arterial blood gases show a pH = 7.35, $Pa_{CO_2}$ = 60 mm Hg, and [$HCO_3^-$] = 31 mEq/L. Which of the following is the most likely diagnosis of this patient?

a. Anxiety-induced hyperventilation
b. Chronic obstructive pulmonary disease (COPD)
c. Alcoholic ketoacidosis
d. Narcotic overdose
e. Salicylate overdose

**24.** A 22-year-old woman professional golfer faints and slips into a coma while waiting to tee off on the 16th hole of the LPGA Jamie Farr Classic Tournament in Toledo, OH. The EMTs and tournament physicians arrive on the scene in a mobile clinic. The patient has a respiratory rate of 22 breaths/min, a heart rate of 110 beats/min, a temperature of 99°F, and reactive pupils. They interview her caddy about the golfer's medical history. He reports that he was assigned as a replacement caddy that morning when the regular caddy became ill. He states that the golfer had been very focused on her round and had not had anything to eat or drink for the past 4 hours, even though the temperature was in the upper 80's and the humidity was 85%. He said she was complaining of being light-headed and was making frequent trips to the bathroom during and in between holes. As they were walking up a hill to the 16th tee, she asked him why he was carrying her clubs and where was her caddy. A stat blood sample showed a pH of 7.2, a high anion gap, and a serum osmolality of 340 mOsm/L. Which of the following is a likely diagnosis?

a. Heat exhaustion
b. Heat stroke
c. Vomiting
d. Diarrhea
e. Diabetes mellitus

**25.** A 10-month-old well-nourished, lethargic infant is brought to the emergency department with a history of vomiting and profuse watery diarrhea for 5 days. His mother reports that he has also had a marked decrease in urine output. Serum sodium is 190 mmol/L (normal range = 135-142 mmol/L), urine sodium is 18 mmol/L (normal range = 20-40 mmol/L), and urine osmolality is 75 mOsm/kg (normal = 100 mOsm/kg). The infant is treated for gastroenteritis and a saline drip is started. After 3 days, he appears well and alert and his diarrhea and vomiting have subsided. However, he still has hypernatremia, polyuria, and low urine sodium. His persistent clinical signs are most likely due to which of the following?

a. Hyperaldosteronism
b. Diabetes insipidus
c. Diabetes mellitus
d. Renal failure
e. Hypothyroidism

**26.** A 28-year-old student goes to Cancun for his spring break. After running the beach the morning he was to return, he feels so thirsty he takes a drink of water from a garden hose at the hotel. After his return, the man presents in the Student Medical Center reporting foul-smelling diarrhea and flatulence over the past 5 days. Stool cultures confirm an infection with the protozoan *Giardia lamblia*. Which of the following arterial blood gases would be expected in this patient?

| | Pa$CO_2$ | [$HCO_3^-$] | Anion Gap |
|---|---|---|---|
| pH | mm Hg | mEq/L | mEq/L |
| a. 7.22 | 30 | 15 | 12 |
| b. 7.22 | 30 | 15 | 25 |
| c. 7.38 | 37 | 25 | 16 |
| d. 7.51 | 49 | 38 | 12 |
| e. 7.51 | 25 | 22 | 25 |

**27.** A 48-year-old woman suffering from a severe tension headache is brought to the emergency department after her husband discovered her unresponsive and barely breathing when he stopped at home from work during his lunch hour. A bottle of narcotic analgesic (Vicodin) was found next to the bathroom sink. Which of the following arterial blood gases are most consistent with her clinical presentation?

a. pH = 7.02, Pa$CO_2$ = 60 mm Hg, [$HCO_3^-$] = 15 mEq/L, anion gap = 12 mEq/L
b. pH = 7.10, Pa$CO_2$ = 20 mm Hg, [$HCO_3^-$] = 6 mEq/L, anion gap = 30 mEq/L
c. pH = 7.27, Pa$CO_2$ = 60 mm Hg, [$HCO_3^-$] = 26 mEq/L, anion gap = 12 mEq/L
d. pH = 7.40, Pa$CO_2$ = 20 mm Hg, [$HCO_3^-$] = 10 mEq/L, anion gap = 30 mEq/L
e. pH = 7.51, Pa$CO_2$ = 49 mm Hg, [$HCO_3^-$] = 38 mEq/L, anion gap = 12 mEq/L

**28.** A 22-year-old man is planning to run a marathon when he goes to visit his brother in Denver. Because of the high altitude, he decides to leave for Denver early to train for the event. While in Denver, he visits an urgent care center after experiencing extensive spasms and cramping in his calf muscles while running, symptoms that he seldom experienced at sea level. Laboratory analysis reveals hypocalcemia. Which of the following is the reason high altitude predisposes to tetany?

a. Low oxygen tension causes a decrease in skeletal muscle blood flow.
b. Low oxygen tension causes an increase in skeletal muscle lactate.
c. Plasma protein concentration is reduced by hypoxia.
d. Stimulation of $Na^+$- $K^+$-ATPase reduces the plasma concentration of free ionized $Ca^{2+}$.
e. Plasma proteins are more ionized under alkalotic conditions, which provide more protein anion to bind with $Ca^{2+}$.

**29.** A 29-year-old man presents with recurring episodes of edema accompanied by chills and fever. A history reveals prolonged travel in the Far East and a diagnosis of parasites that block the lymph vessels. Which of the following characteristics of vessels is most different when comparing the vascular and lymphatic systems?

a. Spontaneous vasomotor activity
b. Absorption of proteins from the interstitial fluid
c. Absorption of nutrients from the gastrointestinal (GI) tract
d. Backflow of fluid is prevented by valves
e. Endothelial cells form the vessel walls

**30.** A 35-year-old man presents in the emergency department with altered mental status. Blood glucose concentration is 600 mEq/L. Hyperglycemia is accompanied by an abnormal increase in which of the following physiological variables?

a. Arterial pH
b. Alveolar $P_{CO_2}$
c. Intracellular volume
d. Plasma sodium concentration
e. Urine volume

**31.** A 72-year-old woman with a history of hypertension presents to the emergency department with generalized weakness. Her medications include potassium-sparing diuretics and an ACE inhibitor. Serum creatinine and BUN are elevated, and an ECG reveals peaked T waves. Which of the following electrolyte disturbances should be corrected to return the ECG to normal?

a. Hyperkalemia
b. Hypokalemia
c. Hypercalcemia
d. Hypocalcemia
e. Hypermagnesemia

**32.** A 49-year-old man is brought to the emergency department with severe gastric pain after ingesting a large quantity of unknown fluid. His blood pressure is 90/60 mm Hg and his pulse rate is 106 beats/min. Laboratory results show the following:

$$pH = 7.03$$
$$\text{Bicarbonate} = 12 \text{ mEq/L}$$
$$\text{Potassium} = 6.3 \text{ mEq/L}$$
$$\text{Anion gap} = 32 \text{ mEq/L}$$
$$\text{Ionized calcium} = 1 \text{ mM}$$

The high anion gap is most likely caused by an elevated plasma concentration of which of the following?

a. Hydrogen ion
b. Potassium
c. Chloride
d. Lactate
e. Citrate

**33.** A 54-year-old man goes out to shovel the snow so that he can drive his wife to her doctor's appointment. After getting some chest pain and feeling short of breath, he thinks he better go in and rest a while before finishing the task. When his wife comes downstairs, she finds him sitting with his head down on the morning paper at the kitchen table. When the ambulance arrives, he is still responsive, but has a cardiac and respiratory arrest en route to the hospital. Which of the following arterial blood gases would be expected given these findings?

a. pH = 7.22, $PaCO_2$ = 60 mm Hg, $[HCO_3^-]$ = 26 mEq/L, anion gap = 12 mEq/L
b. pH = 7.05, $PaCO_2$ = 60 mm Hg, $[HCO_3^-]$ = 15 mEq/L, anion gap = 25 mEq/L
c. pH = 7.10, $PaCO_2$ = 20 mm Hg, $[HCO_3^-]$ = 6 mEq/L, anion gap = 30 mEq/L
d. pH = 7.51, $PaCO_2$ = 49 mm Hg, $[HCO_3^-]$ = 38 mEq/L, anion gap = 14 mEq/L
e. pH = 7.40, $PaCO_2$ = 20 mm Hg, $[HCO_3^-]$ = 10 mEq/L, anion gap = 26 mEq/L

**34.** A 21-year-old woman is admitted to the emergency department after ingesting a large dose of aspirin to try to get rid of her headache. The patient is diaphoretic and has the following blood gases: pH of 7.45, $PaCO_2$ of 17 mm Hg, and $[HCO_3^-]$ of 13 mmol/L. Which of the following treatment options would be most deleterious to this patient?

a. Gastric lavage
b. Intravenous glucose
c. Decreasing alveolar ventilation
d. Increasing fluid volume
e. Administering activated charcoal

**35.** A child makes a blue slush drink using a container of windshield wiper fluid in the garage. The arterial blood gases shown below indicate that the child has which of the following?

$$pH = 7.32$$
$$PaCO_2 = 28 \text{ mm Hg}$$
$$[HCO_3^-] = 16 \text{ mEq/L}$$
$$\text{Anion gap} = 28 \text{ mEq/L}$$

a. Respiratory alkalosis
b. Respiratory acidosis
c. Metabolic alkalosis
d. Metabolic acidosis
e. Respiratory and metabolic acidosis

**36.** A patient with Guillain-Barré syndrome develops paralysis of the respiratory muscles that increases $Pa_{CO_2}$ from 40 to 60 mm Hg and increases the concentration of hydrogen ion in arterial blood from 40 mEq/L (pH 7.4) to 50 mEq/L (pH 7.3). As a result, which of the following would happen?

a. The plasma $[HCO_3^-]$ would decrease.
b. The pH of the urine would increase.
c. The amount of ammonium excreted in the urine would decrease.
d. The central chemoreceptors would be stimulated.
e. The peripheral chemoreceptors would be inhibited.

**37.** A 65-year-old man is admitted to the hospital because of profound muscle weakness. His blood glucose is 485 mg/dL and his serum potassium is 8.2 mmol/L. He is diagnosed with diabetic ketoacidosis and hyperkalemia. In addition to the serum glucose and potassium, which of the following laboratory values would most likely be above normal?

a. Serum $[HCO_3^-]$
b. Anion gap
c. Arterial $P_{CO_2}$
d. Plasma pH
e. Blood volume

**38.** An 84-year-old woman presents with muscle weakness, cramping, irritability, and neuromuscular excitability. Electrolytes reveal hypokalemia and a higher than normal plasma bicarbonate concentration. Which of the following conditions causes metabolic alkalosis?

a. Diarrhea
b. Hypoaldosteronism
c. Hypoxemia
d. Renal failure
e. Treatment with a loop diuretic

**39.** A 23-year-old woman is admitted to the hospital with a 3-month history of malaise and generalized muscle cramps. Laboratory results reveal serum sodium of 144 mmol/L, serum potassium of 2.0 mmol/L, serum bicarbonate of 40 mmol/L, and arterial pH of 7.5. Which of the following is the most likely cause of this patient's hypokalemic alkalemia?

a. Hyperaldosteronism
b. Hyperventilation
c. Persistent diarrhea
d. Renal failure
e. Diabetes

**40.** A 20-year-old woman goes to the emergency department due to symptoms of palpitations, dizziness, sweating, and paresthesia that have not resolved over the past several days. Her history suggests an anxiety disorder, and blood gases and electrolytes are ordered. Her doctor prescribes a benzodiazepine after a positron emission tomography (PET) scan shows increased perfusion in the anterior end of each temporal lobe. Which of the following blood gases would be expected at the time of admission of this patient?

a. pH = 7.28, $Pa_{CO_2}$ = 20 mm Hg, $[HCO_3^-]$ = 16 mEq/L, anion gap = 25 mEq/L
b. pH = 7.28, $Pa_{CO_2}$ = 60 mm Hg, $[HCO_3^-]$ = 26 mEq/L, anion gap = 12 mEq/L
c. pH = 7.44, $Pa_{CO_2}$ = 25 mm Hg, $[HCO_3^-]$ = 16 mEq/L, anion gap = 12 mEq/L
d. pH = 7.51, $Pa_{CO_2}$ = 20 mm Hg, $[HCO_3^-]$ = 24 mEq/L, anion gap = 12 mEq/L
e. pH = 7.51, $Pa_{CO_2}$ = 49 mm Hg, $[HCO_3^-]$ = 38 mEq/L, anion gap = 12 mEq/L

**41.** A 25-year-old man training for a 10-km race runs at a moderate level of approximately 25% of his maximal oxygen consumption. During the increase in aerobic metabolism in the exercising skeletal muscles, most of the volatile acid entering the blood is buffered by which of the following?

a. Bicarbonate
b. Plasma proteins
c. Hemoglobin
d. Phosphates
e. Lactate

**42.** A 64-year-old man with a long history of type 2 diabetes mellitus presents at his internist's office with a chief complaint of weakness and fatigue. Serum chemistries are: Na$^+$: 130 mEq/L; K$^+$: 6.3 mEq/L; HCO$_3$$^-$: 18 mEq/L; BUN: 43 mg/dL; creatinine: 2.9 mg/dL; glucose: 198 mg/dL. The only medication the patient is currently taking is 5 mg glyburide twice daily. These electrolyte and acid-base disturbances are most likely the result of which of the following?

a. Hypoventilation
b. Hyperreninemia
c. Hypovolemia
d. Hypocalcemia
e. Hypoaldosteronism

**43.** An 18-year-old man presents with symptoms of vitamin B$_{12}$ deficiency. Further diagnostic tests reveal that he has pernicious anemia. The underlying problem in pernicious anemia is which of the following?

a. Iron deficiency
b. Inadequate dietary intake of cyanocobalamin
c. Pancreatic insufficiency
d. Crohn disease
e. Autoimmune destruction of parietal cells in the gastric mucosa

**44.** A 65-year-old man with type I diabetes presents to the emergency department with impaired mental status and generalized muscle weakness. Laboratory tests reveal a blood glucose concentration of 500 mg/dL, an anion gap of 22 mmol/L, and a bicarbonate ion concentration of 14 mmol/L. Other expected blood values in this patient include an increase in which of the following?

a. Insulin
b. K$^+$
c. Na$^+$
d. Pa$_{CO_2}$
e. pH

**45.** A 49-year-old man is brought to the emergency department with weakness, confusion, and shortness of breath. The ECG reveals QRS widening and flattened P waves typical of serum potassium concentrations exceeding 7.5 mEq/L. Which of the following conditions results in hyperkalemia?

a. Adrenal medullary stimulation
b. Diuretic therapy
c. Insulin administration
d. Metabolic alkalosis
e. Volume depletion

**46.** A patient comes into the emergency department exhibiting signs of hyperkalemia. The extracellular potassium of a hyperkalemic patient can be decreased by administering which of the following drugs?

a. Atropine
b. Epinephrine
c. Glucagon
d. Lactic acid
e. Isotonic saline

**47.** A 22-year-old woman presents to the emergency department with nausea, abdominal pain, and vomiting, which has gotten progressively worse over the past 24 hours. On physical examination, her abdomen is soft and tender, but there is no guarding or rebound tenderness. Her temperature = 99.1°F, heart rate = 110 beats/min, respiratory rate = 16 breaths/min, and blood pressure = 135/85 mm Hg when lying down and 112/70 mm Hg while standing. Laboratory findings are: WBC = 7.5, Hb = 12 g/dL, $Na^+$ = 140 mEq/L, $K^+$ = 3.2 mEq/L, $Cl^-$ = 95 mEq/L, and $HCO_3^-$ = 37 mEq/L. Which of the following $Paco_2$ and pH values are consistent with these findings?

| $Paco_2$ (mm Hg) | pH |
|---|---|
| a. 25 | 7.70 |
| b. 47 | 7.52 |
| c. 40 | 7.40 |
| d. 28 | 7.32 |
| e. 60 | 7.20 |

**48.** A 25-year-old man, who is a medical student living in Rochester, MN, decides to go backcountry skiing in Colorado over spring break. Which of the following points on the graph below best represents the blood gas values obtained from the student 72 hours after his arrival in Aspen (base altitude = 7945 ft)?

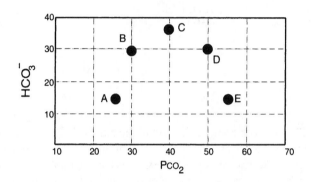

a. A
b. B
c. C
d. D
e. E

**49.** A 69-year-old man is brought to the emergency department by his son because of headache, nausea, and fatigue. The patient has smoked two packs of cigarettes a day for past 50 years before stopping 1 year ago, when he was diagnosed with small cell carcinoma of the lung. Laboratory tests reveal: WBC = 8.3, glucose = 106 mg/dL, $Na^+$ = 122 mEq/L, $K^+$ = 4.1 mEq/L. His hyponatremia may be a result of excess secretion of which of the following?

a. Aldosterone
b. Arginine vasopressin
c. Atrial natriuretic hormone
d. Insulin
e. Norepinephrine

**50.** A 39-year-old man presents to the emergency room complaining of tingling in his hands and muscle twitching. On admission, the patient is alert and stable, with an initial examination remarkable only for carpopedal spasm. Which of the following blood gas values will most likely be observed in this patient?

| | Pa$CO_2$<br>(mm Hg) | [$HCO_3^-$]<br>(mM) |
|---|---|---|
| a. | 50 | 40 |
| b. | 60 | 20 |
| c. | 40 | 30 |
| d. | 30 | 15 |
| e. | 20 | 20 |

**51.** A 27-year-old patient with insulin-dependent diabetes mellitus tells his roommate that he cannot afford to refill his insulin prescription until he gets a paycheck. The roommate offers to get it for him, but the patient assures him that he can wait until after the weekend. When the roommate returns from a weekend trip on Sunday evening, he finds the man unresponsive on the couch. He calls 911. Which of the following arterial blood gases taken in the emergency department would be expected in this diabetic coma patient?

a. pH = 7.10, Pa$CO_2$ = 25 mm Hg, [$HCO_3^-$] = 15 mEq/L, anion gap = 12 mEq/L
b. pH = 7.10, Pa$CO_2$ = 25 mm Hg, [$HCO_3^-$] = 15 mEq/L, anion gap = 30 mEq/L
c. pH = 7.10, Pa$CO_2$ = 80 mm Hg, [$HCO_3^-$] = 25 mEq/L, anion gap = 12 mEq/L
d. pH = 7.45, Pa$CO_2$ = 25 mm Hg, [$HCO_3^-$] = 15 mEq/L, anion gap = 12 mEq/L
e. pH = 7.45, Pa$CO_2$ = 50 mm Hg, [$HCO_3^-$] = 40 mEq/L, anion gap = 30 mEq/L

**52.** A 27-year-old man presents to the emergency department with asthmatic bronchitis that started 3 days ago. He is given an aerosolized bronchodilator treatment, which relieves his symptoms. Arterial blood gases following bronchodilator therapy demonstrate metabolic acidosis with a normal anion gap. These findings can be attributed to which of the following?

a. A laboratory error
b. A decrease in plasma chloride concentration resulting from the chloride shift after the treatment restored alveolar ventilation
c. A decrease in plasma bicarbonate due to renal compensation for the respiratory alkalosis that existed prior to treatment
d. An increase in lactic acid secondary to the hypoxemia that existed prior to treatment
e. An increase in citrate from the vehicle used in the bronchodilator preparation

**53.** A group of medical students in the Wilderness Medicine Club leave right after their organ systems midterm exam to go on a spring break trip hiking in the Rocky Mountains. They arrive at their lodge in Denver by 2 PM mountain time, and then drive to the base camp (10,000 ft), where they camp for the night. The next day, several of the students experience mental and muscle fatigue, and complain of headaches, nausea, and dyspnea, so the guide decides to acclimate at 10,000 ft for another day. Three of the students grow impatient and announce that they are going to climb to Mt. Elbert, the highest mountain in Colorado (14,400 ft altitude, barometric pressure = 447 mm Hg). About 3 hours later, one of the students returns in a panic to get medical help because his friends are disoriented, ataxic, short of breath, and vomiting. The guide calls for the search and rescue helicopter, which locates the hikers and takes them to the nearest emergency department. A diagnostic workup will likely show a decrease in which of the following values?

a. pH
b. $Pa_{CO_2}$
c. Pulmonary vascular resistance
d. 2,3-Bisphosphoglycerate
e. Erythropoietin

**54.** A 19-year-old man presents at the emergency department complaining of shortness of breath. His oxyhemoglobin dissociation curve was shifted from that for normal hemoglobin A depicted in curve A in the figure below to curve B. This finding is consistent with which of the following conditions?

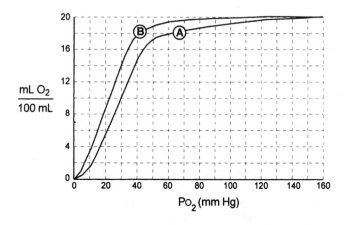

a. Increased body temperature
b. Hypoventilation
c. Carbon monoxide poisoning
d. Exercise
e. Recent transfusion with banked blood

**55.** A 28-year-old pregnant woman develops placental insufficiency at 27-weeks' gestation. It is determined that a preterm caesarian section will be required. To determine how soon the delivery can be done, a sample of amniotic fluid is aspirated. Measurement of the lecithin-sphingomyelin (L-S) ratio in amniotic fluid assesses which of the following?

a. Fetal adrenal function
b. Fetal brain development
c. Fetal kidney development
d. Fetal lung maturity
e. Placenta gas exchange

**56.** A 25-year-old man, who is a fourth-year medical student at Louisiana State University School of Medicine in New Orleans, LA, enrolls in a month-long clinical elective at the University of Colorado School of Medicine in Denver, CO. Which of the following values will return toward normal after the student has acclimatized to the change in altitude?

a. Arterial oxygen tension
b. Plasma bicarbonate concentration
c. Hemoglobin concentration
d. Alveolar ventilation
e. Cardiac output

**57.** A 27-year-old woman presents with nausea, vomiting, and tachypnea. Arterial blood gases reveal a $Pa_{O_2}$ of 105 mm Hg, a $Pa_{CO_2}$ of 30 mm Hg, and a pH of 7.47. These findings are consistent with which of the following conditions?

a. Anemia
b. Compensated metabolic alkalosis
c. Exercise hyperpnea
d. Pregnancy
e. Too rapid of ascent to high altitude

**58.** An 86-year-old man waiting to see his doctor is sitting in an examination room in which the air temperature is 21°C (70°F). He is wearing only a thin gown that is open in the back. The majority of his body heat will be lost by which of the following mechanisms?

a. Radiation and conduction
b. Vaporization of sweat
c. Breathing
d. Horripilation
e. Cutaneous vasoconstriction

**59.** A 69-year-old man is brought to the emergency department by his wife after he blacks out and falls, hitting his head on the kitchen floor. She indicates that he has been drinking beer all afternoon while watching the baseball game on television. Measurement of serum $Na^+$, glucose, BUN, and osmolality indicates an osmolar gap between calculated and measured osmolarity. Which of the following changes in arterial blood gas values are consistent with a presentation of ethanol-induced coma?

|  | pH | $Paco_2$ | Anion Gap |
|---|---|---|---|
| A. | ↑ | ↑ | ↑ |
| B. | ↓ | ↑ | ↑ |
| C. | ↑ | ↑ | ↓ |
| D. | ↓ | ↓ | ↑ |
| E. | ↑ | ↓ | ↓ |

a. A
b. B
c. C
d. D
e. E

**60.** A 23-year-old woman, who is a medical student, presents at Student Health Services with headache, muscle aches, fatigue, and alternating sweating and chills. Her temperature is 101.5°F. The physician proceeds to rule out meningitis but the patient does not report any neck stiffness or photophobia. Upon further questioning, she indicates that she has recently returned from a medical mission trip to Zambia in sub-Saharan Africa, and that she has completed all of the recommended travel precautions, including malaria prophylaxis. She has lost 8 lb in the last week because she has not felt like eating due to her general malaise and abdominal discomfort. At concentrations present in the diet, which of the following vitamins is absorbed primarily by diffusion?

a. Folate
b. Niacin
c. Vitamin $B_{12}$
d. Vitamin C
e. Vitamin D

**61.** A 64-year-old patient with COPD develops jugular venous distention, ascites, and peripheral edema. A chest X-ray reveals cardiomegaly with marked enlargement of the right ventricle. A decrease in which of the following variables is the major cause of cor pulmonale in COPD?

a. Alveolar $P_{CO_2}$
b. Alveolar $P_{O_2}$
c. Arterial [$H^+$]
d. Pulmonary artery pressure
e. Pulmonary vascular resistance

# General Principles: Multisystem Processes

## Answers

**17. The answer is e.** *(Fauci, pp 274-275, 1720-1723, 1734. Ganong, pp 6, 718-719.)* Swelling or edema of the brain with a resultant elevation of intracranial pressure (ICP) occurs with many types of brain injury. Interventions to lower ICP are ideally based on the underlying mechanism responsible for the elevated ICP. In head trauma, stroke, or brain metastases, use of osmotic diuretics to treat cytotoxic edema becomes an appropriate early step. Rapid removal of fluid from the brain can be produced by the administration of a fluid that increases the osmotic pressure difference between the brain and the cerebral vessels. The appropriate solution must have a higher-than-normal osmolarity (ie, >300 mOsm) and be composed of a solute that is impermeable to the blood-brain barrier. Of the solutions listed, only urea and mannitol are hyperosmotic and of these, only mannitol is impermeable to the blood-brain barrier.

**18. The answer is d.** *(Fauci, pp 283-285, 1375. Ganong, p 81. Stead, pp 231-232.)* Because the resting membrane potential is related to the ratio of ICF to ECF K$^+$ concentration, an increase in extracellular K$^+$ partially depolarizes the cell membrane, that is, makes the membrane potential more positive. Depolarizing the membrane opens K$^+$ channels, causing an increase in membrane conductance to potassium. Prolonged depolarization, whether caused by an increase in extracellular K$^+$ or by an action potential, inactivates Na$^+$ channels and decreases the excitability of the nerve membrane, which is manifest as weakness, and which may progress to flaccid paralysis. The activity of the Na$^+$- K$^+$ pump is reduced in hypokalemia, not hyperkalemia.

**19. The answer is b.** *(Fauci, pp 1448-1453. Ganong, pp 81, 574. Stead, p 230.)* Digoxin is used to treat atrial fibrillation in patients with heart failure because it increases vagal tone and cardiac contractility. Digoxin produces its physiological effects by inhibiting Na$^+$- K$^+$-ATPase by blocking the K$^+$ binding site on the enzyme. As a result, intracellular Na$^+$ concentration increases, which reverses the direction of the $Na^+$, $Ca^{2+}$ exchanger, such that less $Ca^{2+}$ is removed from the cell and the cytosolic $Ca^{2+}$ concentration is increased, which increases the developed force in cardiac muscle. When the extracellular $K^+$ concentration is low, digoxin produces a greater inhibition of the $Na^+$- $K^+$ pump. Hypokalemia results in hyperpolarization of the cardiac membrane.

**20. The answer is c.** *(Fauci, pp 288-295. Ganong, pp 338, 563-564. Levitzky, pp 171-185. Stead, pp 221-225.)* This patient has a high anion gap metabolic acidosis. The anion gap is equal to the difference between the plasma concentration of sodium, the major cation in the plasma, and the sum of the concentrations of plasma chloride and bicarbonate, the major measured anions in the plasma.

$$\text{Anion gap} = [Na^+] - ([Cl^-] + [HCO_3^-])$$
$$= 135 \text{ mEq/L} - (100 \text{ mEq/L} + 5 \text{ mEq/L})$$
$$= 30 \text{ mEq/L}$$

The normal anion gap is from 8 to 16 mEq/L. The anion gap is elevated when the concentration of unmeasured anions in the plasma increases. With antifreeze ingestion, the high anion gap metabolic acidosis is caused by the accumulation of the metabolic byproducts of ethylene glycol, namely, oxalic and glycolic acid. Diabetic ketoacidosis also causes a high anion gap metabolic acidosis, but the characteristic hyperglycemia is not present. Renal tubular acidosis results in a normal anion gap metabolic acidosis. Renal failure with uremia is another cause of high anion gap metabolic acidosis, but renal function is normal in this patient. Carbon monoxide poisoning and consequent lactic acidosis causes a high anion gap metabolic acidosis, but the requisite decline in oxygen saturation is not present. Respiratory arrest can be ruled out on the basis of the reduced $Paco_2$ and thus the absence of respiratory acidosis.

**21. The answer is d.** *(Ganong, pp 303-305, 342. McPhee and Ganong, pp 534-536.)* Increased serum lipid levels may result from increased production, decreased clearance, or both. The principal lipid abnormality in diabetes is hypertriglyceridemia, which is due to increased VLDLs. VLDL levels are increased because of insufficient insulin action in adipose tissue, which results in decreased VLDL clearance as a result of decreased lipoprotein lipase activity. Triglyceride uptake into adipose tissue from plasma lipoproteins requires hydrolysis of triglyceride to fatty acids and glycerol by lipoprotein lipase, which is bound to the vascular endothelial surface. The activity of lipoprotein lipase varies in reciprocal fashion with that of cytoplasmic hormone-sensitive lipase, and thus is enhanced by insulin and decreased by catecholamines. Lipoprotein lipase is present in nearly every tissue and acts at the capillary surface as it does in adipose tissue.

**22. The answer is a.** (*Ganong, pp 491-492, 723-724, 729-730, 734-736. Stead, pp 221, 224-225, 230.*) Analysis of serum electrolytes reveals low potassium (hypokalemia), low chloride (hypochloremia), and metabolic alkalosis. These abnormalities arise from two sources. First, gastric juice contains hydrogen, potassium, and chloride in concentrations higher than found in the plasma. Loss of gastric juice through vomiting or drainage leads to depletion of these electrolytes from the plasma. Second, the metabolic abnormalities are exacerbated by the individual's dehydration. Contraction of the vascular volume leads to orthostatic hypotension and the activation of renal mechanisms important for conserving volume. As a result, water, sodium, and bicarbonate are reabsorbed at the expense of increased potassium and hydrogen excretion.

**23. The answer is b.** (*Ganong, pp 734-738. Levitzky, pp 171-181. Stead, pp 221, 223-225, 262-263.*) The interpretation of the arterial blood gas is compensated respiratory acidosis. The primary disturbance is an elevation in arterial $P_{CO_2}$ due to alveolar hypoventilation from the impaired mechanics of breathing in COPD. The hypercapnia lowers the ratio of $HCO_3^-$ to dissolved $CO_2$ in the plasma, and thus lowers the pH according to the Henderson-Hasselbalch equation. To compensate for the acidosis, the kidneys increase the net excretion of $H^+$, which increases the plasma $HCO_3^-$ concentration, returning the pH back into the normal range. Narcotic overdose would be associated with an acute, uncompensated respiratory acidosis. Anxiety-induced hyperventilation would lower arterial $P_{CO_2}$ and increase arterial pH, characteristic of respiratory alkalosis. Ketoacidosis secondary to excessive alcohol ingestion, starvation, or diabetes would cause a metabolic acidosis with a compensatory decrease in arterial $P_{CO_2}$. Salicylate toxicity results in a combined respiratory alkalosis (due to direct stimulation of the medullary respiratory center) and metabolic acidosis (due to accumulation of organic acid).

**24. The answer is e.** *(Fauci, pp 288-292, 1714-1719. Ganong, pp 735-736. Levitzky, pp 174-176, 180-181. Stead, pp 222, 375.)* The anion gap is useful in differentiating the causes of the metabolic acidosis. The anion gap is equal to the difference between the plasma concentration of sodium, the major cation in the plasma, and the sum of the concentrations of plasma chloride and bicarbonate, the major measured anions in the plasma.

$$\text{Anion gap} = [Na^+] - ([Cl^-] + [HCO_3^-])$$

The normal plasma concentrations of $Na^+$, $Cl^-$, and $HCO_3^-$ are 142, 105, and 24 mEq/L, respectively. The normal anion gap is about 12 mEq/L, and is comprised minor ions, such as lactate, phosphate, and sulfate. High anion gap metabolic acidosis results from an increase in unmeasured organic anions, such as occurs with the accumulation of ketoacids in diabetes and its resultant coma. Other causes of high anion gap metabolic acidosis include lactic acidosis accompanying tissue hypoxia or an increase in organic anions or their metabolic byproducts produced from such ingested toxins as ethylene glycol, methanol, and salicylates. In normal anion gap metabolic acidosis, the decline in plasma bicarbonate ion is replaced by an increase in plasma chloride concentration with the concentration of unmeasured minor anions remaining normal, such as occurs with renal or gastrointestinal (GI) bicarbonate losses (eg, diarrhea). Vomiting causes metabolic alkalosis due to the loss of acid. Neither heat exhaustion nor heatstroke is associated with an increased anion gap. Heatstroke results from a failure of thermoregulation and an increase in core body temperature. Core temperature is normal in heat exhaustion.

**25. The answer is b.** *(Ganong, pp 247, 713. Stead, pp 76-77.)* Diabetes insipidus (DI) is a disease caused by decreased release of ADH from the posterior pituitary or the inability of the kidney to respond to ADH. It is characterized by high serum $Na^+$, polyuria, and low urine osmolarity. The low urine osmolarity in the presence of the volume depletion points to DI. The diagnosis is confirmed by the persistent polyuria and low urine sodium after the baby's volume is returned to normal. DI is either central (idiopathic, traumatic, systemic) or nephrogenic in etiology. Nephrogenic DI can either be acquired (renal disease, drugs, hypokalemia, hypercalcemia) or familial.

**26. The answer is a.** (*Stead, pp 139-141, 221-222.*) Diarrhea causes a loss of bicarbonate, which increases plasma hydrogen ion concentration leading to metabolic acidosis, as evidenced by a reduction in plasma bicarbonate and a reduction in pH. Respiratory compensation as a result of peripheral chemoreceptor stimulation by the increased arterial [H$^+$] causes the arterial Pa$CO_2$ to be decreased. Diarrhea is a normal anion gap type of metabolic acidosis because the loss of bicarbonate is replaced by an increase in serum chloride concentration, with no increase in the concentration of unmeasured anions, which makes choice (**a**) the correct answer rather than the high anion gap type of metabolic acidosis represented by choice (**b**), such that you might see in type 1 diabetes mellitus or lactic acidosis. Choice (**d**) is a metabolic alkalosis with respiratory compensation and the interpretation of choice (**e**) is respiratory alkalosis combined with high anion gap metabolic acidosis. Choice (**c**) is normal acid-base status.

**27. The answer is c.** (*Ganong, pp 734-738. Stead, pp 221, 223-225, 262-263, 321.*) Narcotics used for the treatment of severe headache may depress the medullary respiratory center causing alveolar hypoventilation, as evidenced by an elevation in arterial P$CO_2$. The hypercapnia lowers the ratio of $HCO_3^-$ to dissolved $CO_2$ in the plasma, and thus lowers the pH according to the Henderson-Hasselbalch equation. Renal compensation for respiratory acidosis takes hours to start and days to be complete, and thus there has not been sufficient time for the body's compensatory mechanisms to take effect and for plasma [$HCO_3^-$] to rise. Thus, the scenario is most consistent with an acute, uncompensated respiratory acidosis. The slight rise in plasma bicarbonate concentration can be attributed to extracellular buffering of the excess H$^+$.

**28. The answer is e.** (*Ganong, pp 35, 59, 382, 692, 736. Levitzky, pp 172-173. Stead, pp 232-233.*) A decrease in extracellular Ca$^{2+}$ exerts a net excitatory effect on nerve and muscle cells, leading to hypocalcemic tetany, which is characterized by extensive spasms of skeletal muscle. Symptoms of tetany appear at much higher total calcium levels when pH is high, which occurs at high altitude due to hyperventilation. Plasma proteins are more ionized in an alkalotic environment, providing more protein anion to bind with Ca$^{2+}$. The extent of Ca$^{2+}$ binding by plasma proteins is proportionate to the plasma protein level, so a decreased level of plasma proteins would decrease binding and increase the extracellular Ca$^{2+}$. Low oxygen tension leads to peripheral vasodilation and increased blood flow to skeletal muscle. An increase in lactate would lower pH. In heart but not skeletal muscle, $Na^+$- $K^+$ ATPase indirectly affects $Ca^{2+}$ transport via an antiport in the cardiac muscle membranes, which normally exchanges intracellular $Ca^{2+}$ for extracellular $Na^+$.

**29. The answer is b.** *(Fauci, pp 232-233. Ganong, pp 593-594.)* The primary function of the lymphatic vessels is to absorb the proteins that enter the interstitial fluid from the systemic capillaries. Vascular and lymphatic vessels share many characteristics: terminal arterials and lymphatics display vasomotor activity, both are involved in absorbing nutrients from the GI tract, both have valves, and the capillary vessels in both systems are composed of endothelial cells.

**30. The answer is e.** *(Ganong, pp 340-343.)* The increase in blood glucose concentration will result in a filtered load of glucose in excess of what the proximal tubule is able to absorb. As a result, glucose will remain in the filtrate, where it will act as an osmotic diuretic increasing urinary flow. The excess blood glucose will cause water to shift from the intracellular compartment to the extracellular compartment, causing a decrease in intracellular volume and, by dilution, a decrease in plasma sodium concentration. The accompanying increase in ketoacid production will result in a metabolic acidosis (low pH) and a compensatory increase in alveolar ventilation, lowering alveolar $P_{CO_2}$.

**31. The answer is a.** *(Ganong, pp 563-564. Stead, pp 231-232.)* Several different types of drugs, most notably potassium-sparing diuretics and ACE inhibitors, can cause hyperkalemia, which can produce significant changes in the ECG. In elderly persons, a decline in renal function may also lead to hyperkalemia. Hyperkalemia can be a life-threatening emergency. Normal plasma $[K^+]$ is 3.5 to 5 mEq/L. Mild hyperkalemia is 5 to 5.5 mEq/L. Severe hyperkalemia $[K^+]$ is $\geq 7$ mEq/L. As the plasma $K^+$ level rises, the first change on the ECG is the appearance of tall, peaked T waves. The peaked T waves are produced by an accelerated repolarization of ventricular muscle. Potentially fatal hyperkalemia can be treated by administering insulin (along with glucose), which helps $K^+$ transport into cells and therefore lowers extracellular $K^+$, but the effect is temporary. Calcium administration produces cardiac membrane stabilization within minutes, but is contraindicated in patients on digoxin. Removal of potassium from the body can be accomplished with dialysis or with a cation exchange resin, such as sodium polystyrene sulfonate (Kayexalate), but takes hours to work. Hypokalemia is associated with U waves. Hypocalcemia may present with prolonged QT intervals and prolonged ST intervals. Hypercalcemia is associated with a shortened QT interval and widened T waves. Hypermagnesemia presents with prolonged QT and ST intervals, and increased QRS duration.

**32. The answer is e.** (*Fauci, pp 289-266. Ganong, pp 735-736. Levitzky, pp 179-180. Stead, p 222.*) The anion gap is the difference between the concentration of $Na^+$ and the concentration of the major plasma anions, $Cl^-$ and $HCO_3^-$. The minor ions, lactate, phosphate, and sulfate, comprise the normal anion gap. Increases in lactate or citrate could have produced the increased anion gap. The low calcium favors citrate as the cause of the anion gap because citrate complexes with calcium. The low calcium inhibits contraction of vascular smooth muscle, accounting for the low blood pressure. The high serum potassium concentration results from the acidosis, which causes a shift of $K^+$ from the intracellular to the extracellular space.

**33. The answer is b.** (*Fauci, pp 288-295. Ganong, pp 637, 692, 731, 734. Levitzky, pp 171-175, 180-183. Stead, pp 222-223.*) A cardiac and respiratory arrest generates a mixed acid-base disorder, with the coexistence of two primary acid-base disorders, namely respiratory and metabolic acidosis. The respiratory acidosis is due to the alveolar hypoventilation, which increases arterial $P_{CO_2}$ and decreases pH. Cardiac arrest decreases cardiac output and thus oxygen delivery to the tissues, resulting in stagnant (hypoperfusion) hypoxia. The resultant increase in anaerobic glycolysis produces large amounts of lactic acid, which lowers plasma $[HCO_3^-]$ and decreases pH. The normal anion gap of about 12 mEq/L, calculated as the difference between the concentration of $Na^+$ and the concentration of the major plasma anions, $Cl^- + HCO_3^-$, increases due to the increase in the unmeasured organic anion, lactate. Because both independently existing disorders cause acidosis, mixed respiratory and metabolic acidosis may cause dangerously low pH levels and a poor outcome.

**34. The answer is c.** (*Fauci, pp 288-291. Ganong, pp 253, 614-615.*) Although reducing alveolar ventilation would increase $P_{CO_2}$ toward its normal value, it is an inappropriate therapy in this circumstance. Aspirin has a p$Ka$ of 3.5 and will rapidly cross the blood-brain barrier when it is in an unionized state. The alkaline pH resulting from the hyperventilation is keeping most of the aspirin in an ionized form so it cannot easily cross the blood-brain barrier. If the patient is placed on a ventilator to prevent muscle fatigue, it is important to maintain hypocapnic alkalosis or the aspirin will cross the blood-brain barrier and the situation may become far worse. Gastric lavage with isotonic saline followed by administration of activated charcoal is indicated. Excessive insensible water loss from vaporization of sweat may cause severe volume depletion, requiring fluid replacement. Glucose should be administered to prevent hypoglycemia.

**35. The answer is d.** *(Fauci, pp 288-295. Ganong, pp 735-736. Stead, p 222.)* The interpretation of the arterial blood gas is partially compensated metabolic acidosis. The primary disturbance is a decrease in the plasma [$HCO_3^-$], which lowers the ratio of $HCO_3^-$ to dissolved $CO_2$ in the plasma, and thus lowers the pH according to the Henderson-Hasselbalch equation. To compensate for the metabolic acidosis, the lungs increase the rate of alveolar ventilation, which decreases Pa$CO_2$ and also dissolved $CO_2$ and returns the pH toward the normal range. The differential diagnosis of metabolic acidosis is divided into high anion gap and normal anion gap (hyperchloremic) acidosis. The increased anion gap of 28 mEq/L compared to a normal value of approximately 12 mEq/L is consistent with an increase in glycolic acid, a metabolite of ethylene glycol, which is a constituent of antifreeze.

**36. The answer is d.** *(Fauci, pp 288-295. Ganong, pp 672-677, 734-735. Levitzky, pp 171-180, 202-209.)* Increasing arterial Pa$CO_2$ stimulates both the central and peripheral chemoreceptors. In respiratory acidosis, the increase in $CO_2$ drives the $CO_2$ hydrolysis equation to the right, with dissociation of carbonic acid into $H^+$ and $HCO_3^-$. The ratio of $HCO_3^-$ to dissolved $CO_2$ decreases, causing a fall in pH, but the absolute concentration of plasma $HCO_3^-$ increases slightly (1 mmol/L per 10 mm Hg increase in Pa$CO_2$) because some of the hydrogen ions are buffered by nonbicarbonate buffers. In renal compensation for the respiratory acidosis, the increased arterial hydrogen ion concentration increases $H^+$ secretion by the distal tubule, lowering the pH of the urine and increasing $NH_4^+$ excretion. The excretion of $H^+$ is accompanied by the generation of new bicarbonate, causing the plasma bicarbonate ion concentration to increase to a greater extent

(4 mmol/L per 10 mm Hg increase in $Pa_{CO_2}$), which helps to return the pH toward normal.

**37. The answer is b.** (*Stead, pp 63-68, 221-222.*) In diabetic ketoacidosis, there is an increased production of acetoacetic and $\beta$-hydroxybutyric acids, which leads to an increase in plasma concentration of hydrogen ion. These fixed acids are buffered by all body buffers but mainly by bicarbonate. The concentration of plasma $HCO_3^-$ is therefore below normal. The consumption of bicarbonate and the addition of the anions of the fixed acids to the plasma cause an elevation of the anion gap. The anion gap is equal to plasma $[Na^+]$ − (plasma $[HCO_3^-]$ + plasma $[Cl^-]$) and is normally about 12 mEq/L. The acidosis would stimulate the carotid body chemoreceptors to cause an increase in ventilation, which decreases arterial $P_{CO_2}$. Although blood volume is not affected by metabolic acidosis, the osmotic diuresis that accompanies untreated diabetes may lead to a loss of blood volume.

**38. The answer is e.** (*Fauci, pp 288-294. Levitzky, pp 174-175.*) Loop diuretics, such as furosemide (Lasix), act by inhibiting the Na-K-2Cl symporter in the thick ascending limb of the loop of Henle. By inhibiting the transporter, loop diuretics reduce the reabsorption of NaCl and thus water, and also promote $K^+$ excretion. As a result, treatment with a loop diuretic causes hypokalemia and can cause metabolic alkalosis by inducing volume depletion. Volume depletion activates the renin-angiotensin-aldosterone system. Angiotensin II increases bicarbonate reabsorption in the proximal tubule by increasing Na/H exchange, and aldosterone increases distal bicarbonate reabsorption by promoting $H^+$ secretion. Hypoaldosteronism would have the opposite effect. Loop diuretic therapy also tends to generate alkalosis and hypokalemia by increasing distal tubule salt delivery, which stimulates both $K^+$ and $H^+$ secretion. Renal failure, hypoxemia, and diarrhea all produce metabolic acidosis accompanied by a decreased plasma bicarbonate concentration.

**39. The answer is a.** (*Fauci, pp 280-284, 288-294. Ganong, pp 380-381. Stead, pp 93-94, 221-225, 230.*) Aldosterone promotes the loss of both $H^+$ and $K^+$, producing metabolic alkalosis and hypokalemia. Persistent diarrhea will cause the loss of bicarbonate from the body, resulting in metabolic acidosis. Renal failure is often accompanied by metabolic acidosis because of the inability to excrete $H^+$. Diabetes also causes metabolic acidosis because of the accumulation of ketoacids. Hyperventilation results in a respiratory alkalosis, which is compensated for by a decreased bicarbonate concentration.

**40. The answer is c.** *(Fauci, pp 288-289, 295. Ganong, p 259. Levitzky, pp 172-181. Stead, pp 223-224.)* Anxiety causes hyperventilation, which lowers $Pa_{CO_2}$ and increases arterial pH, that is, respiratory alkalosis. Because the condition has persisted for several days, there has been adequate time for renal compensation to occur. In order to compensate for the increased pH, the kidneys decrease the secretion of hydrogen ions and decrease bicarbonate reabsorption. The resultant decrease in plasma bicarbonate concentration in compensated respiratory alkalosis helps to bring the pH back toward normal, making (**c**) the correct answer over (**d**), which is acute, uncompensated respiratory alkalosis. The anion gap is normal in acute and compensted respiratory alkalosis. Choice (**e**) is metabolic alkalosis. Choice (**a**) is metabolic acidosis with respiratory compensation present. Choice (**b**) is an acute, uncompensated respiratory acidosis.

**41. The answer is c.** *(Fauci, pp 287-288. Ganong, pp 730-734. Levitzky, pp 165-167.)* Aerobic metabolism produces 13,000 to 24,000 mmol of volatile acid $(CO_2)$ per day. This yields close to that amount of $H^+$ ions produced per day via the reaction $CO_2 + H_2O \leftrightarrow H_2CO_3 \leftrightarrow H^+ + HCO_3^-$. The lungs excrete almost all of the $CO_2$ as it is formed. At the tissues, $CO_2$ diffuses into the red blood cells, where the enzyme carbonic anhydrase accelerates the above reaction. Nonbicarbonate buffers, primarily hemoglobin, buffer any $CO_2$ that accumulates in the blood. Phosphate, lactate, and plasma proteins are also nonbicarbonate buffers, but they buffer only a small portion of the volatile acid dissolving in the blood. Bicarbonate is not an effective buffer of volatile acid (from $CO_2$).

**42. The answer is e.** *(McPhee and Ganong, pp 598, 608-615, 621-622, 723. Stead, pp 89-91, 230-233.)* This patient probably has hyporeninemic hypoaldosteronism (type IV renal tubular acidosis), a disorder characterized by hyperkalemia and metabolic acidosis in association with mild chronic renal insufficiency, as evidenced by the elevate BUN and serum creatinine. The syndrome is thought to be due to impairment of renin secretion by the juxtaglomerular apparatus, associated with underlying renal disease, a common sequel to diabetes. As a result of the decreased renin

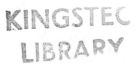

concentration, mineralocorticoid deficiency occurs. The principal function of aldosterone is to increase sodium reabsorption in the distal tubule and collecting ducts, which causes secretion of potassium and hydrogen ions. Hypoaldosteronism therefore results in a decrease in $H^+$ secretion, which leads to the production of metabolic acidosis (and hyperkalemia and hyponatremia). Hypoventilation would produce respiratory, not metabolic, acidosis. Hypovolemia causes an increase in aldosterone secretion, which can lead to an increase in $H^+$ secretion and metabolic alkalosis. Hypocalcemia does not directly affect acid-base balance.

**43. The answer is e.** (*Ganong, pp 31, 315, 496. Stead, pp 150-151.*) Patients with pancreatic insufficiency, as well as patients with Crohn disease, bacterial overgrowth, or who have undergone partial gastrectomy or ileal resection, may exhibit vitamin $B_{12}$ deficiency, but the cause of the vitamin $B_{12}$ deficiency in pernicious anemia is impaired uptake of vitamin $B_{12}$ due to the lack of intrinsic factor (IF) in the gastric mucosa as a result of autoimmune destruction of the gastric parietal cells. Cobalamin, also known as vitamin $B_{12}$, is an essential vitamin found in such foods as liver, fish, and dairy products. Absorption of cobalamin occurs exclusively from the ileum, where specific receptors on ileal enterocytes bind a complex of cobalamin and intrinsic factor. Although intrinsic factor is secreted by gastric parietal cells, binding of the vitamin to intrinsic factor occurs primarily in the proximal small intestine. The acidic environment of the gastric lumen favors the binding of cobalamin to R protein-type binding proteins that originate from salivary and gastric secretions. Pancreatic proteases in the small intestine degrade the R proteins, and the rise in pH favors rapid and complete transfer of the vitamin to intrinsic factor.

**44. The answer is b.** (*Ganong, pp 340-343. Stead, pp 63-65.*) Hyperkalemia is frequently observed in patients with uncontrolled diabetic ketoacidosis. The hyperosmotic extracellular fluid draws water out of cells and $K^+$ follows the water by solvent drag. Additionally, the lack of insulin decreases the ability of $K^+$ to enter cells. The normal compensation for metabolic acidosis is hyperventilation and decreased $P_{CO_2}$.

**45. The answer is e.** (*Fauci, pp 283-285. Ganong, pp 723-724. Stead, pp 231-232.*) Hyperkalemia can result from an increased $K^+$ load, decreased $K^+$ excretion, or shift of $K^+$ from the intra- to the extracellular fluid. Volume depletion decreases distal tubular flow and NaCl delivery to the distal tubule, which decreases K⁺ excretion, leading to hyperkalemia. Metabolic acidosis, insulin administration, and elevated epinephrine levels from stimulation of the adrenal medulla all promote the movement of K⁺ into cells, and thus hypokalemia. Diuretic therapy may be associated with hypokalemia as a result of increased K⁺ excretion, though K⁺-sparing agents may maintain normokalemia. The most common cause of elevated potassium in laboratory results is a laboratory error called pseudohyperkalemia, a falsely elevated measurement due to hemolysis of the blood specimen with leakage of potassium from the lysed cells. The test should be repeated if you suspect pseudohyperkalemia.

**46. The answer is b.** *(Fauci, pp 283-285. Stead, pp 231-232.)* The movement of K⁺ into cells is facilitated by the presence of insulin and epinephrine. During exercise, epinephrine hastens the movement of K⁺ into muscle cells, preventing the accumulation of K⁺ in the extracellular space around active muscle cells. In cases of life-threatening hyperkalemia, insulin is often injected (along with glucose) to reduce the plasma K⁺ concentration.

**47. The answer is b.** *(Fauci, pp 292-294. Ganong, pp 734-736. Levitzky, pp 175-180. Stead, pp 221-225.)* The patient likely has a viral gastroenteritis with metabolic alkalosis (high bicarbonate, high pH) due to a loss of HCl from vomiting. There is also a higher than normal arterial $P_{CO_2}$ (>45 mm Hg) produced by respiratory compensation for the alkalemia. The orthostatic blood pressure changes are indicative of volume depletion, which is a hallmark of saline-sensitive metabolic alkalosis.

**48. The answer is a.** *(Ganong, pp 684-686. Levitzky, pp 234-240.)* As barometric pressure decreases with ascent to high altitude, the partial pressure of inspired oxygen decreases below normal (21% of lower barometric pressure). The resultant decrease in alveolar $P_{O_2}$ leads to a decrease in arterial $P_{O_2}$, a condition classified as hypoxic hypoxia or hypoxemia. Hypoxemia stimulates the peripheral chemoreceptors to increase ventilation, causing arterial $P_{CO_2}$ to decrease and arterial pH to rise (respiratory alkalosis). After 72 hours, renal compensation for the respiratory alkalosis causes a decrease in renal H⁺ excretion, which lowers plasma bicarbonate concentration.

**49. The answer is b.** (*Ganong, pp 244-247, 716. Stead, pp 77-78.*) Arginine vasopressin (AVP), also known as antidiuretic hormone (ADH), increases water reabsorption from the cortical and medullary collecting ducts in the kidney. ADH is normally released in response to a rise in plasma $Na^+$ concentration, and therefore the increased water reabsorption appropriately restores extracellular osmolarity toward normal. When excess ADH is excreted, the water reabsorption dilutes the extracellular fluid, producing a hypotonic hyponatremia accompanied by an increase in urinary sodium and urine osmolality. This condition is called the syndrome of inappropriate ADH secretion (SIADH) and can be life threatening. The etiology of SIADH includes idiopathic overproduction associated with CNS disorders (head trauma, stroke, encephalitis) and pulmonary disease (tuberculosis, pneumonia), ectopic ADH production by malignant tumors, and drug-induced stimulation of the hypothalamic-pituitary axis (vincristine, carbamezine, chlorpropamide). Patients with SIADH usually improve with fluid restriction.

**50. The answer is e.** (*Ganong, pp 382, 392. Stead, pp 223-224.*) The patient's condition is caused by a decrease in the serum concentration of ionized calcium ($Ca^{2+}$), which increases nerve and muscle excitability, leading to spontaneous axonal discharges and muscle contractions, called hypocalcemic tetany. Decreased serum-ionized calcium and thus the symptoms of tetany can appear at higher total calcium levels when respiratory alkalosis is present because the $H^+$ that dissociates from plasma proteins in the presence of a high pH is replaced by $Ca^{2+}$. Although both a $Paco_2$ of 30 mm Hg and a $Paco_2$ of 15 mm Hg are consistent with respiratory alkalosis, only the combination of a $Paco_2$ of 20 mm Hg and an $HCO_3^-$ of 20 mM produces an alkaline pH (7.6). The combination of a $Paco_2$ of 30 mm Hg and an $HCO_3^-$ of 15 mM is metabolic acidosis.

**51. The answer is b.** (*Fauci, pp 287-290. Ganong, pp 735-736. Stead, p 222.*) In untreated type 1 diabetes mellitus, the generation of ketoacids produces metabolic acidosis. The primary disturbance is a decrease in the plasma $[HCO_3^-]$, which lowers the ratio of $HCO_3^-$ to dissolved $CO_2$ in the plasma, and thus lowers the pH according to the Henderson-Hasselbalch equation. To compensate for the metabolic acidosis, the lungs increase the rate of alveolar ventilation, which decreases $Paco_2$ and also dissolved $CO_2$ and returns the pH toward the normal range. The body does not overcompensate for an acid-base disturbance, and thus compensatory hyperventilation for metabolic acidosis would not increase pH above 7.4. The differential diagnosis of metabolic acidosis is divided into high anion gap and normal anion gap (hyperchloremic) acidosis. The increased anion gap of 30 mEq/L compared to a normal value of approximately 12 mEq/L is consistent with an increase in ketoacids, that is, acetoacetic acid and β-hydroxybutyric acid, in the diabetic patient.

**52. The answer is c.** *(Levitzky, p 172-181. Stead, p 265.)* During the early stages of an asthmatic attack, patients often hyperventilate, producing a decrease in arterial $CO_2$ concentration (hypocapnia) and an increase in pH (respiratory alkalosis). Over 3 days, the kidneys compensate for the respiratory alkalosis by lowering bicarbonate. When the respiratory problem is resolved, the patient will be left with the decreased bicarbonate and a normal anion gap metabolic acidosis. Although hypoxemia may produce lactic acidosis, that would be accompanied by an increased anion gap.

**53. The answer is b.** *(Ganong, pp 684-686. Levitzky, pp 234-239.)* Hypoxemia at high altitude stimulates the peripheral chemoreceptors to increase ventilation, causing arterial $P_{CO_2}$ to decrease and arterial pH to rise (respiratory alkalosis). Tissue hypoxia also stimulates erythropoietin production, which increases the number of red blood cells and the hemoglobin concentration, which increases arterial oxygen content, and thus tissue oxygen delivery. Hypoxia also increases the concentration of 2,3-bisphosphoglycerate, which decreases hemoglobin's affinity for oxygen, thereby increasing oxygen release to the tissues. Alveolar hypoxia constricts the pulmonary vessels at high altitude, causing an increase in pulmonary vascular resistance and pulmonary artery pressure (pulmonary hypertension).

**54. The answer is e.** *(Ganong, pp 666-669. Levitzky, pp 145-155.)* Bank blood is low in 2,3-bisphosphoglycerate (2,3-BPG), which results in a higher affinity of hemoglobin for oxygen and a shift in the oxyhemoglobin dissociation curve to the left. An increase in body temperature or an increase in $P_{aCO_2}$ resulting from hypoventilation shift the oxyhemoglobin dissociation to the right. During exercise, there is an increase in muscle temperature, carbon dioxide, and $H^+$, all of which shift the oxyhemoglobin curve to the right and enhance oxygen release to the tissues. Although carbon monoxide shifts the curve to the left, it does so at a reduced oxygen content (mL $O_2$/100 mL blood) because of a lower than normal % $O_2$ saturation.

**55. The answer is d.** (*Ganong, pp 655-657. Levitzky, pp 26-28.*) The surface active component of the lung extract that is essential for stability of the lung during extrauterine respiration, is surfactant. Surfactant is a complex consisting of 10% to 15% proteins and 85% to 90% lipids, 85% of which is phospholipid (lecithin), and approximately 75% of which is dipalmitoyl phosphatidylcholine. The synthesis of lecithin increases as the fetus matures and thus the measurement of lecithin concentration in the amniotic fluid provides an index of fetal lung maturity. Sphingomyelin is another choline phospholipid found in a variety of tissues in the fetus. The lecithin-sphingomyelin (L/S) ratio has been reported to provide a more accurate assessment of fetal lung maturity than lecithin concentration alone. An L/S ratio ≥2 is indicative of biochemical maturation of the lung. Infants born with L/S ratios <2 have an increased incidence of respiratory distress syndrome (RDS) of the newborn, also known as hyaline membrane disease.

**56. The answer is e.** (*Levitzky, pp 237-239.*) Cardiac output, heart rate, and blood pressure initially increase upon ascent to high altitude, but return to normal after a few days. The arterial $P_{O_2}$ remains low at high altitude due to the low inspired and alveolar $P_{O_2}$ levels. The hypoxemia stimulates alveolar ventilation, which remains elevated at high altitude. To compensate for the respiratory alkalosis, plasma bicarbonate concentration decreases after several days at high altitude, and remains low. Hemoglobin concentration increases secondary to hypoxia-induced erythropoietin production.

**57. The answer is d.** (*Ganong, p 444. Levitzky, pp 172-177.*) The alveolar and arterial $P_{CO_2}$ are determined by the rate of $CO_2$ production ($V_{CO_2}$) divided by the rate of alveolar ventilation. Thus, at any given metabolic rate, hyperventilation is by definition a decrease in $Pa_{CO_2}$. Pregnancy produces hyperventilation because progesterone stimulates the brain stem respiratory centers to increase alveolar ventilation. The compensatory response to metabolic alkalosis is a decrease in alveolar ventilation (increased $Pa_{CO_2}$). During most levels of exercise, alveolar ventilation increases in proportion to carbon dioxide production such that the arterial

$P_{CO_2}$ remains normal; thus the increased rate of alveolar ventilation in exercise is not hyperventilation, but it has been given a special term, called exercise hyperpnea. At high altitude, $PaO_2$ would be lower than normal.

**58. The answer is a.** *(Ganong, pp 251-255, 760.)* Radiation and conduction account for 70% of heat lost when the environmental temperature is below body temperature. Insensible water loss from the vaporization of sweat accounts for another 27% of heat loss under these conditions. The remaining heat is normally lost by respiration (2%) and urination and defecation (1%). Cutaneous vasoconstriction would decrease heat loss.

**59. The answer is d.** *(Ganong, pp 734-736. Levitzky, p 178. Stead, pp 221-222.)* Alcoholic ketoacidosis is associated with a high anion gap metabolic acidosis with a compensatory rise in alveolar ventilation, which lowers the arterial $P_{CO_2}$.

**60. The answer is e.** *(Fauci, pp 1280-1294. Ganong, p 477.)* Absorption of vitamin D increases linearly as the intraluminal concentration increases, suggesting absorption by a nonsaturable passive-diffusion mechanism. The term vitamin D refers to a family of essentially water-insoluble compounds involved primarily in the regulation of calcium homeostasis. Water-soluble vitamins, including vitamin C, folate, niacin, and vitamin $B_{12}$, are a diverse group of organic compounds that are essential for normal growth and development. At the low concentrations present in the diet (1 to 100 nM), transport of the water-soluble vitamins across the brush border occurs by specialized mechanisms, such as membrane carriers, active transport systems, and membrane-binding proteins and receptors specific for a particular vitamin. Malaria is a protozoan disease transmitted by the bite of infected *Anopheles* mosquitoes. It is the most important of the parasitic diseases of humans, and occurs throughout most of the tropical regions of the world. The first symptoms of malaria are nonspecific, similar to the symptoms of a minor viral illness. Malaria does not have the neck stiffness, photophobia, or rash like those seen in meningitis.

**61. The answer is b.** *(Fauci, pp 362, 1453-1455.)* Cor pulmonale is defined as dilation and hypertrophy of the right ventricle in response to diseases of the pulmonary vasculature and/or lung parenchyma that are sufficient to cause pulmonary hypertension. Pulmonary hypertension is an increase in pulmonary artery pressure due to a rise in pulmonary vascular resistance. The major cause of pulmonary hypertension in COPD is increased pulmonary vasoconstriction due to alveolar hypoxia. Alveolar hypercapnia and acidosis in COPD also contribute to the development of pulmonary hypertension and cor pulmonale. COPD accounts for approximately half of the cases of cor pulmonale in North America.

# Physiology of the Hematopoeitic and Lymphoreticular Systems

## Questions

**62.** A 52-year-old man is brought to the emergency department with severe chest pain. Angiography demonstrates a severe coronary occlusion. A thrombolytic agent is administered to reestablish perfusion. Which of the following does the thrombolytic agent activate?

a. Heparin
b. Plasminogen
c. Thrombin
d. Kininogen
e. Prothrombin

**63.** A 42-year-old patient is scheduled for surgery that will likely require a transfusion. Because the patient has a rare blood type, an autologous blood transfusion is planned. Prior to surgery, 1500 mL of blood is collected. The collection tubes contain calcium citrate to prevent coagulation. Which of the following is the mechanism for citrate's anticoagulative action?

a. Blocking thrombin
b. Binding factor XII
c. Binding vitamin K
d. Chelating calcium
e. Activating plasminogen

**64.** Prior to having his first colonoscopy, a 50-year-old man undergoes a bleeding time test to rule out any clotting disorders. Bleeding time is determined by nicking the skin superficially with a scalpel blade and measuring the time required for hemostasis. It will be markedly abnormal (prolonged) in a person who has which of the following?

a. Anemia
b. Vitamin K deficiency
c. Thrombocytopenia
d. Leukopenia
e. Hemophilia

**65.** A 67-year-old woman with a history of venous thromboembolism is placed on warfarin (Coumadin) prophylactically. The blood concentration of Coumadin becomes too high and bleeding occurs. The bleeding can best be treated by the administration of which of the following?

a. Fibrinogen
b. Thrombin
c. Platelets
d. Protein C
e. Vitamin K

**66.** A 27-year-old HIV+ man presents with fever, waxing and waning mental status, and hematuria. Blood analysis shows thrombocytopenia and hemolytic anemia, but a normal prothrombin time and partial thromboplastin time. Which of the following is the most likely basis for the pathogenesis of these findings?

a. Decreased activity of plasma metalloproteinase
b. Abnormal sequestration of platelets in the spleen
c. Immune-mediated platelet destruction
d. Drug-induced antibody binding of platelets
e. A lack of von Willebrand factor protein

**67.** A 44-year-old woman with a history of excessive menstrual bleeding and menstrual cycles that generally last over 7 days complains of increasing fatigue and cold extremities. Laboratory results reveal a hemoglobin (Hb) concentration of 6 g/dL. In this patient with anemia, which of the following would be reduced?

a. Arterial $P_{O_2}$
b. Total arterial oxygen content
c. Dissolved oxygen content
d. Percent $O_2$ saturation in the arterial blood
e. Oxygen extraction

**68.** A 48-year-old man presents to the emergency department with chest pain and shortness of breath. His ECG shows ST segment elevation and cardiac enzymes are elevated. After cardiac catheterization revealed 90% occlusion of his left anterior descending coronary artery, the patient is scheduled for coronary artery bypass graft (CABG) surgery. During surgery, his oxygen saturation curve shifts from a to b, as shown in the figure below. Which of the following can best account for this shift?

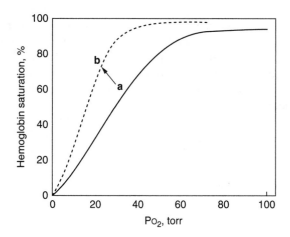

a. A change in pH from 7.4 to 7.3
b. A change in $P_{CO_2}$ from 40 to 46 mm Hg
c. A decrease in core body temperature from 37°C to 32°C
d. An increase in erythrocyte 2,3-bisphosphoglycerate (BPG)
e. Transfusion of blood with a higher $P_{50}$ than normal

**69.** A 24-year-old woman presents to her family physician with intractable hiccups. The patient is instructed to breathe into and out of a bag in order to rebreathe exhaled $CO_2$. In the blood, the majority of $CO_2$ is transported as which of the following?

a. Dissolved $CO_2$
b. Carbonic acid
c. Carbaminohemoglobin
d. Carboxyhemoglobin
e. Bicarbonate

**70.** A 37-year-old man presents with low exercise tolerance. Blood work shows a normal hematocrit and hemoglobin concentration but a decreased $P_{50}$. Which would be true of his oxyhemoglobin transport and dissociation?

a. Hemoglobin's affinity for oxygen is increased.
b. There is less loading of $O_2$ at the alveolar-capillary level than normal.
c. Oxygen unloading is increased at the tissue level.
d. Hemoglobin's saturation with oxygen is lower than normal at any $Pa_{O_2}$.
e. The differential diagnosis includes a point mutation resulting in increased binding of 2,3-bisphosphoglycerate to his hemoglobin chains.

**71.** A 45-year-old woman presents to her family physician's office with fatigue of at least 3 months' duration. Her only explanation is that keeping up with her twin 4-year-olds really tires her out, and she does not even have enough energy to make nutritious meals for her and her husband. Vital signs and ECG are normal, but a third heart sound is heard with auscultation and she is pale. Blood results show Hb: 8 g/dL, Hct: 30%, MCV = 115 fL, WBC = 8000/µL, platelets: 200,000/µL. A deficiency of which of the following substances can most likely account for these findings?

a. Iron
b. Folate
c. Glucose-6-phosphatase
d. Niacin
e. Zinc

**72.** A 65-year-old slightly cyanotic man presents to his physician complaining of pruritus and nose bleeds. A blood test reveals a Hct of 62%, leading to the diagnosis of polycythemia vera. Treatment includes aspirin to prevent thrombosis and periodic phlebotomy to reduce the hematocrit. The reduction in hematocrit is beneficial because it does which of the following?

a. Reduces blood viscosity
b. Increases arterial oxygen saturation
c. Reduces blood velocity
d. Decreases cardiac output
e. Increases arterial oxygen content

**73.** A 65-year-old man with chronic bronchitis is admitted to the emergency department with cyanosis and shortness of breath. Arterial and venous blood samples show the following:

| | |
|---|---|
| $Pa_{O_2}$ | 50 mm Hg |
| $Pa_{CO_2}$ | 67 mm Hg |
| $Pv_{O_2}$ | 30 mm Hg |
| $Sa_{O_2}$ | 80% |
| $Sv_{O_2}$ | 50% |
| Hb | 20 g/dL |

What do these data reveal about the patient's gas exchange and transport?

a. Arteriovenous oxygen content difference is lower than normal.
b. Dissolved oxygen content in the venous blood is higher than normal.
c. Dissolved $CO_2$ content in the arterial blood is lower than normal.
d. Oxygen extraction is higher than normal.
e. Oxyhemoglobin content in the arterial blood is lower than normal.

**74.** A 23-year-old man with a ruddy complexion presents with chief complaints of headache, dizziness, and lethargy. Blood analysis shows erythrocytosis and a $P_{50}$ of 20 mm Hg. He denies any history of tobacco smoking and is unaware of any other exposure to carbon monoxide or nitrites. Which of the following is a probable cause for these findings?

a. High-$O_2$ affinity hemoglobinopathy
b. Low-$O_2$ affinity hemoglobinopathy
c. Sickle cell trait
d. $\alpha$-Thalassemia-2
e. $\beta$-Thalassemia major

**75.** A 42-year-old woman presents to her doctor's office with heavy menstrual bleeding for up to 2 weeks' duration for each of the past five cycles. She also reports that she has a tendency to bruise easily, and has had several episodes of epistaxis over the past couple of months. Blood analysis shows: Hb = 8 g/dL, Hct = 24%, MCV = 70, platelet count = 230,000/$\mu$L. Which of the following is a likely cause of her bleeding disorder?

a. Aplastic anemia
b. Hemophilia
c. Nonsteroidal anti-inflammatory drugs
d. Vitamin $B_{12}$ deficiency
e. von Willebrand disease

**76.** A 61-year-old man presents to his family physician with the chief complaint of frequent diarrhea accompanied by weight loss. He reports a tendency to bruise easily and laboratory data reveal a prothrombin time of 19 seconds (normal = 11 to 14 seconds). The bruising and prolonged prothrombin time can be explained by a decrease in which of the following vitamins?

a. Vitamin A
b. Vitamin C
c. Vitamin D
d. Vitamin E
e. Vitamin K

**77.** A 26-year-old woman presents at the obstetrician's office for her second trimester evaluation. Which of the following values would normally be less in the fetus than in the mother?

a. Hemoglobin concentration
b. Affinity of hemoglobin for oxygen
c. Erythrocyte binding of 2,3-biphosphoglycerate
d. Cardiac output/kg body weight
e. Cardiac glycogen content

**78.** A 21-year-old woman presents to her doctor's office indicating that she has felt very tired for the past 2 weeks and has recently developed a sore throat, enlarged tonsils, fever, and a rash on her chest and abdomen. Urine output has been normal. Her temperature is 100.7°F (38.1°C) and blood pressure is 100/70 mm Hg. Lung fields are clear on auscultation but there are exudates on the pharynx, the posterior cervical nodes are enlarged and tender, and she has splenomegaly. The white blood cell count is 20,000/μL with lymphocytosis and greater than 10% atypical lymphocytes. Rapid antigen testing for Gram-negative bacteria is negative and serologic testing shows a positive reaction for heterophile antibody. Based on these findings, the most likely diagnosis is which of the following?

a. β-Hemolytic *Streptococcus* infection
b. Hepatitis B
c. Infectious mononucleosis
d. Measles
e. Toxic shock syndrome

**79.** A 32-year-old woman presents to the emergency department with a chief complaint of acute shortness of breath and right-sided chest pain, which increases during inspiration. She does not have a cough or fever, and does not have a history of asthma or other respiratory disease. She has not been ill or immobile, but reports having taken oral contraceptives for 8 years until shortly before conceiving her first child about 2 years ago. The family history is notable for her mother who died of a pulmonary embolism. Her respiratory rate is 25 breaths/min and her heart rate is 110 beats/min. Chest x-ray is normal, but a ventilation/perfusion scan reveals a possible pulmonary embolism. Which of the following blood disorders is associated with a hypercoagulable state?

a. Activated protein C resistance
b. Antithrombin III excess
c. Disseminated intravascular coagulation
d. Hypoprothrombinemia
e. Idiopathic thrombocytopenic purpura

**80.** A 9-year-old African American boy is brought to the emergency department by his mother who states that he was complaining of muscle aches and pain while playing basketball, which became worse whenever he was running up and down the court. She reports that he was sick with a fever last week, but she thought he was feeling better so she let him go to his summer basketball camp. Blood tests show anemia, increased reticulocyte count, and sickle-shaped cells. Hemoglobin electrophoresis confirms the presence of HbS. The primary mechanism for the change in RBC shape during a sickle cell crisis is which of the following?

a. The presence of antibodies against the red blood cell membrane
b. Low levels of erythropoietin
c. A decrease in erythrocyte volume during dehydration
d. A rightward shift in the oxyhemoglobin dissociation curve of HbS compared to normal
e. Polymerization of HbS when cellular oxygen consumption is high

**81.** A 67-year-old man with chronic bronchitis is brought to the emergency department exhibiting labored breathing and cyanosis. The clinical sign of cyanosis is caused by which of the following?

a. An increase in the affinity of hemoglobin for oxygen
b. A decrease in the percent of red blood cells (hematocrit)
c. An increase in the concentration of carbon monoxide in the venous blood
d. A decrease in the concentration of iron in the red blood cells
e. An increase in the concentration of deoxygenated hemoglobin

**82.** A 26-year-old pregnant woman is diagnosed with placenta previa, which requires premature delivery of her fetus of 28-weeks' gestation. A blood sample is taken from both the mother and the newborn infant for determination of the oxyhemoglobin saturation curve. If curve N in the figure below is the oxyhemoglobin saturation curve of the mother who has normal HbA, which of the curves is most likely obtained from the premature infant?

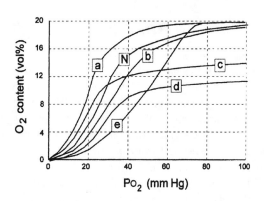

a.  a
b.  b
c.  c
d.  d
e.  e

# Physiology of the Hematopoeitic and Lymphoreticular Systems

## *Answers*

**62. The answer is b.** *(Ganong, pp 540-545.)* Plasminogen is the inactive precursor of plasmin, the proteolytic enzyme involved in clot dissolution. An infusion of tissue plasminogen activator (tPA) soon after a heart attack (and possibly a thrombolytic stroke) can lessen the chances of permanent damage. Thrombin, the enzyme ultimately responsible for the formation of fibrin monomers, is generated from prothrombin by activated factor X. Activation of factor X occurs via both extrinsic and intrinsic pathways. Kininogens are enzymes responsible for the production of peptides (kinins) associated with inflammation. Heparin is an anticlotting agent found on endothelial cell surfaces.

**63. The answer is d.** *(Ganong, pp 542-544. Stead, p 160.)* The citrate ion has three anionic carboxylate groups that avidly chelate calcium and reduce the concentration of free calcium in blood. Because free calcium ($Ca^{2+}$) is required for multiple steps in both coagulation pathways, citrate is a useful anticoagulant in vitro. The citrate ion is rapidly metabolized; thus, blood anticoagulated with citrate can be infused into the body without untoward effects. Oxalate, another calcium-chelating anticoagulant, is toxic to cells.

**64. The answer is c.** *(Stead, pp 161-163.)* An abnormally small number of platelets in the blood is called thrombocytopenia. Bleeding time is used to distinguish hemostatic abnormalities caused by a reduced number of platelets from those caused by coagulation defects. Hemostasis following blood vessel injury depends on (1) vascular spasm, (2) formation of a platelet plug, and (3) clot formation. The time for a small cut to stop bleeding depends on the concentration of platelets. A deficiency of vitamin K would result in increased prothrombin time (PT) and increased partial thromboplastin time (PTT) and normal bleeding time. Hemophilia results in increased PTT, but a normal bleeding time.

**65. The answer is e.** *(Fauci, pp 743-745. Ganong, p 544. Stead, pp 159-161.)* Warfarin is often prescribed for patients at risk for thromboembolic episodes. Vitamin K is necessary for the conversion of prothrombin to thrombin. Thrombin is an important intermediate in the coagulation cascade. It converts fibrinogen to fibrin and is a powerful activator of platelets. Warfarin interferes with the activity of vitamin K, and therefore reduces the likelihood of clot formation. Administering vitamin K can restore coagulation if warfarin therapy leads to excessive bleeding.

**66. The answer is a.** *(Fauci, pp 718-725. Stead, pp 161-165.)* The findings describe the presentation of thrombotic thrombocytopenic purpura (TTP). The pathogenesis of TTP is related to a deficiency of, or antibodies to, a plasma metalloproteinase, called ADAMTS13, which cleaves the ultrahigh molecular weight multimers of von Willebrand factor (vWF) produced by endothelial cells into smaller multimers. The ultrahigh molecular weight multimers of vWF initiate platelet aggregation and thrombosis. TTP is more common in HIV infection and pregnant women. Plasmapheresis is the treatment of choice and transfusion with platelets is contraindicated.

**67. The answer is b.** *(Fauci, pp 329-335, 2203. Ganong, pp 666-667, 683, 690. Levitzky, pp 153-154.)* A reduction in the concentration of hemoglobin reduces the oxyhemoglobin content, and thus the total arterial oxygen content. Oxygen extraction by the tissues increases to compensate for the reduced tissue oxygen delivery. Arterial $P_{O_2}$, dissolved oxygen, and the percent saturation of hemoglobin with oxygen are all normal in anemia.

**68. The answer is c.** *(Ganong, pp 666-669. Levitzky, pp 146-152.)* Hypothermia increases hemoglobin's affinity for oxygen, causing the oxyhemoglobin dissociation curve to shift to the left. With a leftward shift, the saturation of hemoglobin with oxygen is greater than normal at any $P_{O_2}$, as denoted by a lower $P_{50}$ value than normal. Acidosis, hypercapnia (increased $P_{CO_2}$), and an increase in erythrocyte [2,3-BPG] all cause rightward shifts of the oxyhemoglobin dissociation curve. Although bank blood has decreased 2,3-BPG, if the transfused blood has a higher $P_{50}$ than normal, then one would expect no shift or a rightward shift.

**69. The answer is e.** *(Ganong, pp 669-670.)* $CO_2$ is transported in arterial blood in three forms: as physically dissolved $CO_2$ (about 5%), in combination with the amino groups of hemoglobin as carbaminohemoglobin (about 10%), and as bicarbonate ion, ie, $HCO_3^-$ (about 85%). The amount of $CO_2$ actually carried as carbonic acid, $H_2CO_3$, is negligible. Carboxyhemoglobin refers to the combination of carbon monoxide (CO) and hemoglobin.

**70. The answer is a.** *(Fauci, pp 635-636. Ganong, pp 666-669.)* A decreased $P_{50}$ denotes a leftward shift of the oxyhemoglobin dissociation curve and an increase in hemoglobin's affinity for oxygen. A leftward shift indicates that more oxygen is loaded at the alveolar-capillary level, and that there is less oxygen unloading at the tissue level because hemoglobin binds the oxygen more tightly than normal. With a decreased $P_{50}$, oxygen saturation is higher than normal at any $PO_2$. Increased 2,3-BPG shifts the oxyhemoglobin dissociation curve to the right.

**71. The answer is b.** *(Fauci, pp 356-362, 441-450. McPhee and Ganong, pp 118, 123-129, 336, 380. Stead, pp 149-153.)* This patient has a macrocytic anemia found with folate or vitamin $B_{12}$ deficiency. Iron-deficiency anemia, the most common type of anemia, and glucose-6-phosphate deficiency, the most common metabolic disorder of red blood cells, are both associated with microcytosis (low MCV). Niacin (vitamin $B_3$) and zinc deficiencies are causes of malabsorption. Niacin deficiency also presents with pellagra.

**72. The answer is a.** *(Fauci, pp 672-674. Stead, pp 158-159.)* Polycythemia vera is a primary bone marrow disease in which an abnormally large number of red blood cells are produced. Patients with polycythemia vera often have high blood pressure (because of increased blood volume) and cyanosis (because of increased oxygen extraction from blood flowing slowly through capillaries). Reduction of the red cell mass by phlebotomy is the first principle of therapy in polycythemia vera because it reduces blood viscosity, which removes a major source of complications and may also alleviate systemic hypertension, pruritus, and splenomegaly.

**73. The answer is d.** *(Ganong, pp 666-667. Levitzky, pp 146-147, 180-183.)* The lower-than-normal levels of venous oxygen tension and saturation indicate that the tissues have extracted more oxygen than normal. $O_2$ extraction is the arteriovenous oxygen content difference, and could be calculated from the data given, though that would not be necessary to answer this question. Total oxygen content is the sum of the dissolved oxygen ($PO_2$ in mm Hg × 0.003 mL $O_2$/100 mL blood/mm Hg $PO_2$) and the oxyhemoglobin content ([Hb] × 1.34 mL $O_2$/g% Hb × % $O_2$ saturation). Arterial oxygen content in this patient is therefore 21.6 mL $O_2$/100 mL blood and venous oxygen content is 13.5 mL $O_2$/100 mL blood, with the a-v $O_2$ = 8.1 mL $O_2$/100 mL blood, compared to a normal value of approximately 5 mL $O_2$/100 mL blood.

**74. The answer is a.** *(Fauci, pp 636-643. Ganong, p 667. Levitzky, p 142-156.)* The $P_{50}$ of the oxyhemoglobin curve is the oxygen tension at which half of the hemoglobin is saturated with oxygen. The normal $P_{50}$ of hemoglobin A is 27 mm Hg. A decreased $P_{50}$ of 22 mm Hg indicates a higher-than-normal affinity for $O_2$, such as may occur with a number of inherited variants of hemoglobin. The thalassemia syndromes are inherited disorders of hemoglobin's globin chains. Severity is highly variable, but findings generally include hypochromia and microcytosis with varying degrees of anemia. Persons with sickle cell trait inherit the gene for normal Hb A from one parent and the abnormal gene for HbS from the other parent. People with sickle cell trait generally have no manifestations of the disease, but can pass it on to their children.

**75. The answer is e.** *(McPhee and Ganong, pp 115-143. Stead, pp 148-152.)* Because platelet count is normal, causes of thrombocytopenia, including aplastic anemia, vitamin $B_{12}$ deficiency, and NSAIDs can be ruled out, whereas a defect in platelet function is a likely cause of the bleeding disorder. von Willebrand disease is the most common inherited bleeding disorder. Hemophilia A is an X-linked recessive trait leading to a decrease in factor VIII. Females with the trait generally have 50% of the normal amount of the factor with no bleeding problems.

**76. The answer is e.** *(Ganong, pp 313, 509, 544-545. Stead, p 374.)* Vitamin K denotes a group of lipophilic, hydrophobic vitamins that are essential for maintaining normal clotting of blood. Vitamin K is required for hepatic synthesis of seven proteins involved in blood coagulation, (prothrombin [factor II], factors VII, IX, X, proteins C, S, and Z). Vitamin K is involved in the carboxylation of certain glutamate residues in these proteins to form gamma carboxyglutamate (Gla) residues that are involved in calcium binding. Vitamin $K_1$ (phylloquinone) and vitamin $K_2$ (menaquinone) are normally produced by bacteria in the large intestine. Common causes of vitamin K deficiency include cholestasis and factors that limit fat absorption. Dietary deficiency is rare unless there is decreased production by normal flora, as may be seen in broad-spectrum antibiotic use.

**77. The answer is c.** (*Ganong, p 669. Levitzky, pp 154-155.*) Fetal hemoglobin (hemoglobin F) is chemically different from adult hemoglobin (hemoglobin A) in that it has two $\alpha$ and two $\gamma$ chains instead of two $\alpha$ and two $\beta$ chains. The $\gamma$ chains of HbF do not bind 2,3-BPG, resulting in an increased affinity for oxygen, and a leftward shift of the oxygen dissociation curve of HbF. The greater affinity of hemoglobin for oxygen is advantageous in the placental exchange of $O_2$ from maternal blood ($Pa_{O_2}$ = 100 mm Hg) to fetal blood ($Pa_{O_2}$ = 25 mm Hg). Despite the low arterial $Po_2$, the fetus is not hypoxic. Oxygen delivery in the fetus is enhanced by a higher hemoglobin concentration than in the adult and a cardiac output that is two to four times higher than in the adult on a milliliter per kilogram basis. The fetal heart is protected by an increased cardiac glycogen content.

**78. The answer is c.** (*Fauci, pp 210-211, 761-766, 1106-1109. McPhee and Ganong, pp 59-88. Stead, p 346-347.*) Millions visit primary care providers each year complaining of sore throat. The overwhelming majority of patients with a new sore throat have acute pharyngitis of viral or bacterial etiology. The signs and symptoms accompanying acute pharyngitis are not reliable predictors of the etiologic agent, but the clinical presentation may be helpful in narrowing the possibilities. The primary goal of diagnostic testing is to separate streptococcal pharyngitis from other etiologies so that antibiotics can be prescribed more efficiently and judiciously. The diagnosis of infectious mononucleosis caused by the Epstein-Barr virus (EBV) depends primarily on the detection of antibodies to the virus with a heterophile agglutination assay (monospot slide test). Lymphocytosis with atypical lymphocytes are also common laboratory findings in infectious mononucleosis.

**79. The answer is a.** (*McPhee and Ganong, pp 115-143, 700-701. Stead, pp 159-163.*) Activated protein C resistance is the most common inherited hypercoagulable state. Up to 25% of patients who have venous thrombosis without an inciting event are found to have activated protein C resistance. Most of the cases are due to a single DNA base pair mutation in the gene for factor V in the coagulation cascade, known as factor V Leiden. Antithrombin III (AT-III) inhibits the coagulation cascade at a different site than protein C; a deficiency of AT-III results in a hypercoagulable state due to an inability to inactivate factors II, IX, XI, and XII. Hyperprothrombinemia (not hypo) is the second most common cause of hereditary hypercoagulable state and the only one known to cause an overproduction of procoagulant factors, rather than a lack of adequate anticoagulation. Disseminated intravascular coagulation (DIC) is an acquired coagulation defect that results in consumption of coagulation factors I, V, VIII, and XIII, causing bleeding and thrombosis. ITP is another bleeding disorder due to immune-mediated thrombocytopenia of unknown etiology.

**80. The answer is e.** (*McPhee and Ganong, p 123. Stead, p 155.*) Persons with sickle cell anemia have a homozygous substitution of valine for glutamine in the sixth position of the β-hemoglobin chain. During periods of high oxygen consumption, the abnormal HbS polymerizes and distorts the normal shape of red blood cells. The sickled cells cause vaso-occlusion in multiple organs, leading to renal papillary necrosis and hematuria, acute chest syndrome, ischemic retinopathy, and functional asplenism and splenomegaly.

**81. The answer is e.** (*Fauci, pp 230-231. Ganong, p 684. Levitzky, p 156. Stead, pp 262-263.*) Cyanosis is the blue color of the skin produced by desaturated hemoglobin. Cyanosis appears when 5 g of hemoglobin per 100 mL of blood are desaturated. For a person with a normal hemoglobin concentration of 15 g/100 mL, cyanosis appears when one-third of the blood is desaturated. For a person with polycythemia (a higher-than-normal concentration of hemoglobin), cyanosis may appear when only one-fourth of the hemoglobin is desaturated (eg, if hemoglobin concentration is 20 g/100 mL). This individual may not be hypoxic because of the high concentration of saturated hemoglobin. On the other hand, a person with anemia (a lower-than-normal concentration of hemoglobin) may have a significant portion of the hemoglobin desaturated without displaying cyanosis. This individual will not appear cyanotic but may be hypoxic.

**82. The answer is a.** (*Ganong, p 669. Levitzky, pp 154-155.*) The oxyhemoglobin ($HbO_2$) dissociation curve represents the relationship between the partial pressure of oxygen and the amount of oxygen bound to hemoglobin (Hb). Normal Hb is 50% saturated at a $Po_2$ of approximately 27 mm Hg (the $P_{50}$), 75% saturated at a $Po_2$ of 40 mm Hg (the normal $Po_2$ of mixed venous blood), and 97% saturated at a $Po_2$ of 100 mm Hg (the normal arterial $Po_2$). Fetal blood has a higher-than-normal oxygen affinity and therefore is represented by the curve labeled a. Increasing the affinity of Hb for $O_2$ shifts the $HbO_2$ saturation curve to the left and decreases the $P_{50}$. HbA has two $\alpha$ and two $\beta$ globin chains, whereas HbF has two $\alpha$ and two $\gamma$ chains. The $\gamma$ chains in HbF do not bind 2,3-BPG, which results in the higher affinity for oxygen.

# Neurophysiology

## Questions

**83.** A 10-year-old girl with type I diabetes develops a neuropathy limited to sensory neurons with free nerve endings. Quantitative sensory testing will reveal higher-than-normal thresholds for the detection of which of the following?

a. Fine touch
b. Vibration
c. Pressure
d. Temperature
e. Muscle length

**84.** A 16-year-old adolescent boy is brought to the emergency room by ambulance after suffering a concussion during a football game. When he awoke, there was no difficulty with his speech and he was able to understand and follow commands, including repeating language spoken to him, but he had difficulty understanding written language and pictures. His condition is most likely caused by damage to which of the following?

a. The hippocampus
b. Angular gyrus in the categorical hemisphere
c. Broca area in the frontal lobe
d. Wernicke area at the posterior end of the superior temporal gyrus
e. The arcuate fasciculus connecting Broca and Wernicke areas

**85.** A 13-year-old adolescent boy has no movement in his legs after falling out of a tree. Neurological examination shows absence of both the myotatic (stretch) and reverse myotatic reflexes in the lower extremities. Which of the following is the most important role of the $\gamma$-motoneurons?

a. Stimulate skeletal muscle fibers to contract
b. Maintain Ia afferent activity during contraction of muscle
c. Generate activity in Ib afferent fibers
d. Detect the length of resting skeletal muscle
e. Prevent muscles from producing too much force

**86.** A 72-year-old man visits his physician because he finds it difficult to hold his hand steady when painting. Examination reveals a resting tremor and rigidity. The symptoms are relieved by a single dose of levodopa. This patient's neurological signs are most likely related to a lesion within which of the following?

a. The cerebellum
b. The substantia nigra
c. The premotor area
d. The caudate nucleus and putamen
e. The hippocampus

**87.** A 53-year-old man develops loss of pain and temperature sensation in his right leg and loss of proprioception in his left leg (Brown-Séquard syndrome). These symptoms appear 6 weeks following total prostatectomy for prostate cancer. A bone CT scan reveals metastases compressing the patient's left hemicord. His urologist refers him to a neurologist who wishes to confirm normal proprioception in the left leg. In the figure below, which part illustrates the train of action potentials normally seen in a sensory nerve encoding the velocity of limb movement in response to sudden movement?

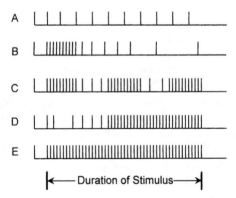

a. A
b. B
c. C
d. D
e. E

**88.** A 72-year-old man develops selective loss of the large pyramidal cells in the precentral gyrus and degeneration of the corticospinal and cortico-bulbar projections. Other neuronal systems are spared. He is told that the progression of the disease is variable, and that the worst prognosis is about a 3-year survival. The precentral gyrus and corticospinal and corticobulbar tracts are essential for which of the following?

a. Vision
b. Olfaction
c. Auditory identification
d. Kinesthesia
e. Voluntary movement

**89.** A 28-year-old woman hits her head on the windshield in an auto-mobile accident. She becomes confused, and develops urinary inconti-nence and a gait disorder. An MRI of the brain reveals enlarged ventricles, suggestive of normal-pressure hydrocephalus. Lumbar puncture confirms normal intracranial pressure, and her symptoms are found to improve after removal of a volume of her cerebrospinal fluid (CSF). Which of the follow-ing best describes the CSF?

a. It is absorbed by the choroid plexus.
b. It circulates in the epidural space.
c. It has a higher protein concentration than plasma.
d. It has a lower glucose concentration than plasma.
e. Its absorption is independent of CSF pressure.

**90.** A 72-year-old man is evaluated by a physiatrist after a stroke. The patient is observed to suffer from dysmetria, ataxia, and an intention tremor. These neurological signs are most likely related to a lesion within which of the following regions of the brain?

a. Basal ganglia
b. Cerebellum
c. Cortical motor strip
d. Eighth cranial nerve
e. Medulla

**91.** A 41-year-old man is seen by his physician complaining of "always feeling tired" and having "vivid dreams when he is sleeping." He is referred to the hospital's sleep center for evaluation. He is diagnosed with narcolepsy based on his clinical history and the presence of rapid eye movements (REM) as soon as he falls asleep. Which of the following signs will be observed when the patient is exhibiting REM sleep?

a. Hyperventilation
b. Periods of loss of skeletal muscle tone
c. Slow but steady heart rate
d. High-amplitude EEG wave
e. Decreased brain metabolism

**92.** A 43-year-old woman has a chief complaint of muscle weakness. The distribution of muscle weakness and the presence of hyperactive tendon reflexes is consistent with pyramidal tract disease. Tapping the patella tendon elicits a reflex contraction of the quadriceps muscle. Which of the following occurs during the contraction of the quadriceps muscle?

a. The Ib afferents from the Golgi tendon organ increase their rate of firing.
b. The Ia afferents from the muscle spindle increase their rate of firing.
c. The $\alpha$-motoneurons innervating the extrafusal muscle fibers decrease their rate of firing.
d. The $\gamma$-motoneurons innervating the intrafusal muscle fibers increase their rate of firing.
e. The $\alpha$-motoneurons to the antagonistic muscles increase their rate of firing.

**93.** A 64-year-old female patient is referred to a neurologist because her sister and brother both suffered recent strokes. She is diagnosed with an antiphospholipid antibody syndrome, and placed on warfarin. Despite the anticoagulation therapy she develops a thrombotic cerebral infarct, which leads to spasticity of her left wrist, elbow, and knee. The lesion most likely affected which of the following?

a. Ia afferent fibers
b. Corticoreticular fibers
c. Corticospinal fibers
d. Reticulospinal fibers
e. Vestibulospinal fibers

**94.** A 27-year-old patient with a chief complaint of mild vertigo of 3-months' duration is seen by a neurologist. Examination reveals a positional (horizontal and vertical) nystagmus that is bidirectional. The patient reports the absence of tinnitus. Which of the following is the most likely etiology of the vertigo?

a. Labyrinthitis
b. Ménière syndrome
c. Lesion of the flocculonodular lobe of the cerebellum
d. Lesion of the spinocerebellum
e. Psychogenic

**95.** A 16-year-old adolescent girl with epilepsy has an electroencephalogram (EEG) recording done during a routine visit to her neurologist. The α-rhythm appearing on an EEG has which of the following characteristics?

a. It produces 20 to 30 waves per second.
b. It disappears when a patient's eyes open.
c. It is replaced by slower, larger waves during REM sleep.
d. It represents activity that is most pronounced in the frontal region of the brain.
e. It is associated with deep sleep.

**96.** A 24-year-old woman goes to her ophthalmologist for an annual examination. The image distance of a normal relaxed eye is indicated in the figure below. If an object is placed 25 cm away from the eye, the image will be focused on the retina if the refractive power of the eye is increased to which of the following?

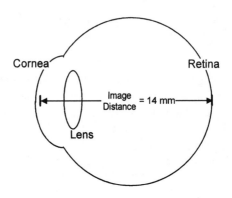

a. 40 diopters
b. 44 diopters
c. 56 diopters
d. 71 diopters
e. 75 diopters

**97.** A 59-year-old woman is admitted to the hospital because of agitation and aggression. Three years prior to admission, her irregular, flinging movements had become so severe that she could not walk or assist in her own care. Huntington chorea is a hereditary disease affecting neurons within which of the following areas of the brain?

a. Anterior cerebellum
b. Subthalamus
c. Substantia nigra
d. Striatum
e. Limbic system

**98.** A 22-year-old woman presents at the student medical center with tachycardia and palpitations. She reports that she has been taking a diet supplement containing ephedrine that she purchased from an Internet site. Activation of the sympathetic nervous system by ephedrine causes smooth muscle contraction in which of the following?

a. Bronchioles
b. Pupils
c. Intestines
d. Arterioles
e. Ciliary bodies

**99.** A 22-year-old musician visits an otolaryngologist complaining of ringing in his ear. An audiometry test reveals a high-frequency hearing loss in which the threshold for hearing high-frequency sounds is raised by 1000 times. If a patient is unable to hear high-frequency sounds, the damage to the basilar membrane is closest to which of the following structures?

a. Oval window
b. Helicotrema
c. Stria vascularis
d. Modiolus
e. Spiral ganglion

**100.** An 86-year-old woman presents to her cardiologist's office complaining of hemiparesis that has worsened over the past 3 days. She is on anticoagulant therapy for her pacemaker. A CT of the brain reveals a subdural hematoma. On physical examination, stroking the plantar surface of her foot produces a reflex extension of the large toe rather than the expected flexion. The Babinski sign elicited by the physician indicates damage to which of the following?

a. Basal ganglia
b. Brain stem
c. Cerebellum
d. Lower motor neurons
e. Upper motor neurons

**101.** A 41-year-old man complains to his physician about jet lag whenever he flies long distances to meetings. Melatonin is prescribed as a way to reset his circadian rhythm. The circadian rhythm is controlled by which of the following nuclei?

a. Arcuate
b. Lateral
c. Paraventricular
d. Suprachiasmatic
e. Ventromedial

**102.** A 48-year-old woman with multiple sclerosis and increasing spasticity is treated with an intrathecal infusion of baclofen, a GABA$_B$ agonist which mediates presynaptic inhibition. Presynaptic inhibition in the central nervous system affects the firing rate of $\alpha$-motoneurons by which of the following mechanisms?

a. Increasing the chloride permeability of the presynaptic nerve ending
b. Decreasing the potassium permeability of the $\alpha$-motoneuron
c. Decreasing the frequency of action potentials by the presynaptic nerve ending
d. Hyperpolarizing the membrane potential of the $\alpha$-motoneuron
e. Increasing the amount of the neurotransmitter released by the presynaptic nerve ending

**103.** A 29-year-old woman presents at the ophthalmologist's office complaining of slowly progressive loss of vision. Based on the visual field defect shown here, the ophthalmologist determines that the patient has a right-sided homonymous hemianopia. She refers the patient to a neurologist who orders a CT scan of the head. The CT scan demonstrates a high-density, space-occupying lesion, which is compressing which area of the brain?

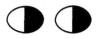

a. The right lateral geniculate nucleus
b. The left optic nerve
c. The right visual cortex
d. The optic chiasm
e. The left optic tract

**104.** A 62-year-old woman is referred to a neurologist by her family physician because of a recent loss of initiative, lethargy, memory problems, and a loss of vision. She is diagnosed with primary hypothyroidism and an enlarged pituitary gland. She is referred to an endocrinologist for treatment of her thyroid problem and to a neuro-ophthalmologist for visual field evaluation. Which of the following visual field defects is most likely to be found?

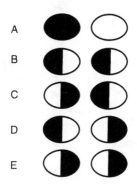

a. A
b. B
c. C
d. D
e. E

**105.** A 34-year-old woman, who has been immobilized with a sprained ankle for the past 4 days, develops a throbbing pain that has spread to her entire left leg. History reveals that she has been taking oral contraceptives for 15 years. Compared to localized pain, such as one might experience from a needle stick, which of the following characterizes ischemic pain?

a. Ischemic pain sensory fibers are classified as A delta (Aδ) sensory fibers.
b. Ischemic pain is produced by overstimulating somatic touch receptors.
c. Ischemic pain is transmitted to the brain through the neospinothalamic tract.
d. Ischemic pain receptors quickly adapt to a painful stimulus.
e. Ischemic pain sensory fibers terminate within the substantia gelatinosa of the spinal cord.

**106.** A 17-year-old boy is admitted to the hospital with a traumatic brain injury, sustained when he fell off his motorcycle. He develops a fever of 102.2°F (39°C), which is unrelated to an infection or inflammation. The fever is most likely due to a lesion of which of the following?

a. The lateral hypothalamus
b. The arcuate nucleus
c. The posterior nucleus
d. The paraventricular nucleus
e. The anterior hypothalamus

**107.** A 29-year-old man is brought to the emergency room after a traffic accident causing a traumatic brain injury. Within several hours he begins eating objects such as paper, is unable to maintain attention, and displays increased sexual activity. He is diagnosed with Klüver-Bucy syndrome. A diagnostic MRI is ordered to confirm bilateral lesions of which of the following regions of the brain?

a. Temporal lobe
b. Hypothalamus
c. Olfactory lobe
d. Hippocampus
e. Cingulate gyrus

**108.** A medical student is working in a sensory physiology laboratory during the summer after her first year. She is responsible for conducting electrophysiologic recordings from several types of sensory receptor cells. The intracellular recording shown in the figure below was obtained from a receptor cell in response to a specific stimulus. From which of the following sensory systems was this recording obtained?

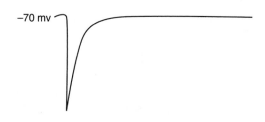

a. Hearing
b. Smell
c. Taste
d. Touch
e. Vision

**109.** A 22-year-old man sees his ophthalmologist because it is becoming increasingly difficult for him to read the newspaper. His vision problem most likely results from an inability to contract which of the following?

a. The iris
b. The ciliary body
c. The suspensory ligaments
d. The extraocular muscles
e. The pupil

**110.** At a first-grade parent-teacher conference, the teacher of a 6-year-old boy indicates that the boy seems to have difficulty hearing. His parents take him to the pediatrician, who refers the boy to an otolaryngologist. The boy is found to have a significant hearing deficit accompanying a middle ear infection that also involves the middle ear bones. Which of the following is the primary function of the middle ear bones?

a. To amplify sounds
b. To filter high-frequency sounds
c. To localize a sound
d. To enhance frequency discrimination
e. To protect the ear from load sounds

**111.** The morning after a rock concert, a 20-year-old college student notices difficulty hearing his professor during lecture. The physician at the student health center suspects possible damage to his hair cells by the loud music. Depolarization of the hair cells in the cochlea is caused primarily by the flow of which of the following?

a. $K^+$ into the hair cell
b. $Na^+$ into the hair cell
c. $Cl^-$ out of the hair cell
d. $Ca^{2+}$ into the hair cell
e. $K^+$ out of the hair cell

**112.** A 62-year-old man with a history of hypertension and hyperlipidemia is admitted to the hospital for evaluation after demonstrating signs and symptoms of a stroke. Subsequent CT scans, perceptual tests, and a neurological examination provide evidence for impairment of the otolith pathways. The otolith organs (utricle and saccule) are responsible for which of the following?

a. Producing the vestibular-ocular reflex
b. Detecting the position of the head in space
c. Producing rotary nystagmus
d. Detecting angular acceleration
e. Producing the stretch reflex

**113.** A 68-year-old man presents with a chief complaint of night blindness (nyctalopia). He is found to have avitaminosis A, which underlies the impairment of rod function. Which of the reactions in the retinal rods is caused directly by the absorption of light energy?

a. Dissociation of scotopsin and metarhodopsin
b. Decomposition of scotopsin
c. Transformation of 11-*cis* retinal to all-*trans* retinal
d. Transformation of metarhodopsin to lumirhodopsin
e. Transformation of vitamin A to retinene

**114.** A 20-year-old boxer presents at a neurologist's office complaining of dizziness and a problem with his balance. He indicates that in a recent match, he suffered several blows to the ears. Which of the following normally happens when a person slowly rotates toward the right?

a. The stereocilia on the hair cells in the right horizontal semicircular canal bend away from the kinocilium.
b. Both the left and right eyes deviate toward the left.
c. The hair cells in the left horizontal semicircular canal become depolarized.
d. The visual image on the retina becomes unfocused.
e. The endolymph in the left and right horizontal semicircular canals moves in opposite directions.

**115.** A 58-year-old woman goes to her physician because she is having difficulty threading needles. An eye examination leads to the diagnosis of presbyopia (old eyes). Her condition is most likely caused by which of the following?

a. Clouding of the vitreous
b. Retinal detachment
c. Ciliary muscle paralysis
d. Stiffening of the lens
e. Degeneration of the macula

**116.** An 8-year-old boy is hit in the head by a baseline drive during a little league game. His father, a doctor, rushes out on the field to do a neurological assessment, including use of his penlight to check reactivity of the pupils. When light strikes the eye, which of the following normally increases?

a. The activity of transducin
b. The amount of transmitter released from the photoreceptors
c. The concentration of all-*trans* retinal within the photoreceptors
d. The concentration of calcium within the photoreceptors
e. The activity of guanylyl cyclase

**117.** A 59-year-old woman with bilateral glaucoma is treated with drops of the parasympathetic agent pilocarpine. Cholinergic stimulation of the pupil causes which of the following?

a. Pupillary dilation (mydriasis)
b. Pupillary constriction (miosis)
c. Inequality of pupil size
d. Tonic pupil (slow redilation after exposure to light)
e. Absence of the pupillary response to light

**118.** A 20-year-old woman complains of altered taste following extraction of her wisdom teeth. Which of the following is the most likely cause of the dysgeusia?

a. A disturbed salivary milieu
b. Injury to the taste receptor cells
c. Impaired transport of the tastant to the receptor cells in the taste bud
d. Damage to the gustatory afferent nerves
e. Damage to the central gustatory pathways

**119.** A 52-year-old male smoker complains of the inability to smell. Which of the following is the most likely cause of his anosmia?

a. Interference with transport of odorants to the receptor cells
b. Carbon monoxide-induced damage to the olfactory afferent nerves
c. Metaplasia of the olfactory neuroepithelium
d. Nicotine-induced damage to the central olfactory pathways
e. A neoplasm of the inferior frontal region

**120.** A Jewish couple presents at the wife's obstetrician's office with questions about screening for the neurodegenerative disorder Tay-Sachs disease. What percentage of the human genome is involved in the formation and function of the nervous system?

a. 20
b. 40
c. 60
d. 80
e. >90

**121.** A 24-year-old male medical student develops apprehension, restlessness, tachycardia, and tachypnea as he enters the testing center for his initial licensure examination. Activation of which of the following receptors would be expected to decrease his anxiety?

a. Neuropeptide Y
b. Glutamate
c. $GABA_A$
d. Histamine
e. Neurokinin 1 (NK-1, substance P)

**122.** An 85-year-old man is brought to his doctor by his daughter. She reports that he has memory loss, is often confused, and has been having increasing difficulty with routine activities that he used to do on his own, such as paying bills and going grocery shopping. She wonders if this is just old age or a more serious problem. Which of the following would provide the definitive diagnosis of Alzheimer disease?

a. Nonspecific slowing of the EEG
b. Presence of an apolipoprotein ε4 (Apo ε4) allele on chromosome 19
c. Improved symptoms with cholinesterase inhibitors
d. Cerebral cortical atrophy on CT or MRI
e. Neuritic plaques containing A-beta (Aβ) amyloid bodies

**123.** A 26-year-old African American female medical student goes to the emergency department when she sees flashes of light, moving spots, and has reduced visual acuity. An ophthalmology consult reveals that she is myopic, does not have eye pain, and has a scotoma in the peripheral vision field of her right eye. There is no cherry red spot on the fovea. Which of the following is the most likely cause for her acute vision loss?

a. Central retinal artery embolism
b. Retinal detachment
c. Optic neuritis
d. Glaucoma
e. Macular degeneration

**124.** After sitting with one leg crossed under the other for several hours while working on a document at her computer terminal, a 52-year-old woman tries to stand up, but is unable to walk on the crossed leg, and feels tingling and pain in it. Which of the following explains the loss of motor function without the loss of pain sensation in the peripheral nerves?

a. $A\beta$ fibers are more sensitive to pressure than C fibers.
b. C fibers are more sensitive to pressure than $A\beta$ fibers.
c. C fibers are more susceptible to hypoxia than B fibers.
d. A fibers are more susceptible to local anesthetics than C fibers.
e. C fibers have higher conduction velocities than A fibers.

**125.** Three weeks following a GI infection with *Campylobacter jejuni*, a 60-year-old man develops weakness and tingling in his legs. Over the next few days, his legs and face become paralyzed, and he is hospitalized for Guillain-Barré syndrome. Which of the following is the most likely underlying cause of his motor paralysis?

a. Antibodies against nerve growth factor
b. Antibodies against oligodendrogliocytes
c. Demyelination of $A\beta$ fibers
d. Demyelination of B fibers
e. Demyelination of C fibers

**126.** A 32-year-old woman from the IT department presents to the employee health clinic late in the afternoon complaining of fatigue, muscular weakness, and double vision. She indicates that the symptoms have been getting worse over the past 2 months and that she gets worse the longer she works at the computer screen. Cranial nerve examination discloses impaired movement of the right eye and bilateral ptosis, which worsen with repetitive eye movements. An MRI of the chest shows enlargement of the thymus gland. The neuropathy of this clinical presentation is most likely caused by antibodies against which of the following?

a. Acetylcholine
b. Acetylcholinesterase
c. Postsynaptic muscarinic acetylcholine receptors
d. Presynaptic nicotinic acetylcholine receptors in autonomic ganglia
e. Postsynaptic nicotinic acetylcholine receptors on the motor end plate

**127.** A 26-year-old woman presents with unilateral facial weakness. She states that whenever she tries to close her eyes, the upper eyelid on the affected side rolls upward. Electromyography on the affected side shows evidence of axonal degeneration. Which of the following characteristics of an axon is most dependent on its diameter?

a. The magnitude of its resting potential
b. The duration of its refractory period
c. The conduction velocity of its action potential
d. The overshoot of its action potential
e. The activity of its sodium-potassium pump

**128.** An 80-year-old farmer presented with complaints of weakness and fatigue, aching, orthostatic hypotension, constipation, and sleep disturbances. His family physician told him that he was just getting old, and would have to get used to it. His bradykinesia worsened and he couldn't pick up his feet when he walked. When he was no longer able to plow his own fields, he got depressed, and his wife said he would just sit at the table and rub his thumb along his fingers. She called her son-in-law, a neurologist, and asked him if he'd come out to the country to evaluate "Pops." The pathophysiology of Parkinson disease can be attributed to a paucity of which of the following neurotransmitters?

a. Acetylcholine
b. Dopamine
c. Glutamate
d. Neuropeptide Y
e. Serotonin

**129.** A 62-year-old man with COPD presents to the emergency room in respiratory distress. The attending physician uses succinylcholine to produce skeletal muscle relaxation prior to tracheal intubation. Soon after infusion of the succinylcholine, the patient develops a severe bradycardia. Which of the following drugs would counteract the bradycardia without affecting muscle relaxation?

a. Curare
b. Atropine
c. Epinephrine
d. Acetylcholine
e. Dopamine

**130.** A fireman suffers extensive burns, resulting in a fluid and electrolyte imbalance. Which of the following conditions will produce a decrease in the magnitude of a nerve membrane action potential?

a. Hyperkalemia
b. Hypokalemia
c. Hypernatremia
d. Hyponatremia
e. Hypocalcemia

**131.** An 18-year-old man, who became ill after eating mushrooms, is brought to the emergency department, where he is treated for muscarinic poisoning. Which of the following signs is consistent with muscarinic poisoning?

a. Skeletal muscle contractures
b. Bradycardia
c. Dilation of the pupils
d. Hypertension
e. Diuresis

**132.** A 19-year-old woman with a history of diplopia and paresthesia is diagnosed with multiple sclerosis (MS). Immersion of an affected limb in a cold bath restores nerve conduction in many MS patients. The explanation often cited for this effect is that cold increases the duration of the action potential. Which of the following best explains why increasing the duration of the action potential can restore nerve conduction in patients with MS?

a. The capacitance of the nerve fiber membrane is increased.
b. The duration of the refractory period is increased.
c. The potassium conductance of the membrane is increased.
d. The amount of sodium entering the nerve with each action potential increases.
e. The membrane potential becomes more positive.

**133.** A 37-year-old woman presents with severe migraine headaches that are accompanied by hemiparalysis. Genetic analysis confirms the suspicion of an inherited channelopathy. The membrane potential will depolarize by the greatest amount if the membrane permeability increases for which of the following ions?

a. Chloride
b. Potassium
c. Sodium
d. Chloride and potassium
e. Sodium and potassium

**134.** A 65-year-old postgastrectomy patient presents to his gastroenterologist's office with fatigue, weakness in his legs, and frequent falls over the past several months. His physical examination demonstrates increased deep tendon reflexes and decreased vibratory sense in his toes. Laboratory analysis reveals megaloblastic anemia and vitamin $B_{12}$ deficiency. Which of the following mechanisms cause the neurological deficits characteristic of vitamin $B_{12}$ deficiency?

a. Decreased folate concentration
b. Decreased myelin synthesis
c. Decreased $Na^+$-$K^+$ pump activity
d. Increased hyperphosphorylated microtubule protein tau
e. Production of anti-nerve antibodies (ANA)

**135.** A 52-year-old man presents at the oral surgeon's office with an abscessed tooth. Prior to surgery to extract the tooth, the patient is given a shot of procaine. Preventing the inactivation of sodium channels by local anesthetics will decrease which of the following?

a. The relative refractory period of nerve cells
b. The upstroke velocity of nerve cell action potentials
c. The downstroke velocity of nerve cell action potentials
d. The magnitude of the overshoot in nerve cell action potentials
e. The duration of nerve cell action potentials

**136.** A 13-year-old boy on the junior high wrestling team experienced attacks of proximal muscle weakness that lasted from 30 minutes to as long as 4 hours following exercise and fasting. The trainer attributed it to the symptoms of fatigue, but his mother recalled having similar symptoms when she was dieting. Genetic testing revealed an inherited channelopathy. Electrically excitable gates are normally involved in which of the following?

a. The depolarization of the end-plate membrane by acetylcholine
b. Hyperpolarization of rods by light
c. Release of calcium from ventricular muscle sarcoplasmic reticulum (SR)
d. Transport of glucose into cells by a sodium-dependent, secondary active transport system
e. Increase in nerve cell potassium conductance caused by membrane depolarization

**137.** A 58-year-old man with a history of hypertension and renal disease presents at his physician's office with a complaint of headaches. His blood pressure is 190/115 mm Hg and laboratory results show an elevated plasma renin activity with hypernatremia. Which of the following best describes the sodium gradient across the nerve cell membrane?

a. It is a result of the Donnan equilibrium.
b. It is significantly changed during an action potential.
c. It is used as a source of energy for the transport of other ions.
d. It is the primary determinant of the resting membrane potential.
e. It is maintained by a $Na^+/Ca^{2+}$ exchanger.

**138.** A 19-year-old sexually active woman presents with lower abdominal pain for 1 week. Physical examination reveals a temperature of 101°F (38.33°C), tenderness on pelvic examination, and a mucopurulent vaginal discharge. Synaptic transmission between pain fibers from the pelvis and spinal cord neurons is mediated by which of the following?

a. Acetylcholine
b. Substance P
c. Endorphins
d. Somatostatin
e. Serotonin

**139.** At which point on the action potential shown in the figure below is the membrane closest to the Na⁺ equilibrium potential?

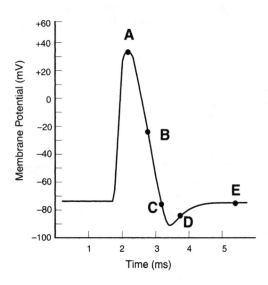

a. Point A
b. Point B
c. Point C
d. Point D
e. Point E

**140.** A 16-year-old, highly allergic girl who is stung by a bee gives herself a shot of epinephrine prescribed by her physician. Because epinephrine activates β-adrenergic receptors, it will relieve the effects of the bee sting by decreasing which of the following?

a. The contraction of airway smooth muscle
b. The strength of ventricular muscle contraction
c. The rate of depolarization in the SA node
d. The transport of calcium into skeletal muscle fibers
e. The rate of glycogenolysis in the liver

**141.** An 86-year-old woman develops unilateral vesicular eruption on the trunk in a $T_8$ dermatomal pattern. Staining of the skin scrapings confirms a diagnosis of herpes zoster. The woman complains of significant pain, as well as increased sensitivity to touch. Which of the following receptors is responsible for measuring the intensity of a steady pressure on the skin surface?

a. Pacinian corpuscle
b. Ruffini ending
c. Merkel disk
d. Meissner corpuscle
e. Krause ending

**142.** A 24-year-old man complains of fatigue, increased daytime somnolence, and periodic sudden loss of muscle tone. Polysomnography confirms the diagnosis of narcolepsy. Narcolepsy is associated with which of the following?

a. Increased discharge of noradrenergic neurons in the locus ceruleus
b. Increased discharge of serotonergic neurons in the midbrain raphé
c. Decreased adenosine levels in the reticular formation
d. The presence of prions
e. Hypothalamic dysfunction with decreased CSF levels of orexins

# Neurophysiology

## Answers

**83. The answer is d.** *(Ganong, pp 141-143.)* Free nerve endings contain receptors for temperature, pain, and crude touch. However, fine touch, pressure, and vibration are detected by nerve endings contained within specialized capsules that transmit the stimulus to the sensory receptors. Muscle length is encoded by the primary nerve endings of Ia fibers, which are located on intrafusal fibers within the muscle spindle.

**84. The answer is b.** *(Fauci, pp 161-167. Ganong, pp 272-275.)* Aphasias are language disorders in which a person is unable to properly express or understand certain aspects of written or spoken language. Aphasias are caused by lesions to the language centers, which are located in the categorical hemisphere of the neocortex. There are a number of different classifications of aphasias, but one divides them into fluent, nonfluent, and anomic aphasias. In this case, the boy developed an anomic aphasia, in which there was no difficulty with his speech and he was able to understand and follow commands, but he had difficulty understanding written language and pictures. Anomic aphasia is the single most common language disturbance seen in head trauma, metabolic encephalopathy, and Alzheimer disease. Anomic aphasia can be caused by lesions anywhere within the language network, but often is caused by damage to the angular gyrus without damage to Broca or Wernicke areas. A lesion in Broca area leads to nonfluent aphasia, such as seen in Pick disease. Fluent aphasias are due to lesions to Wernicke area or to lesions in and around the auditory cortex. Language disorders caused by memory loss, which could be the result of a hippocampal lesion, are not classified as aphasias, nor are language disorders caused by vision or hearing abnormalities or motor paralysis. Damage to the arcuate fasciculus would be incorrect because the patient was able to verbally repeat language spoken to him.

**85. The answer is b.** *(Ganong, pp 130-133.)* The γ-motoneurons innervate the intrafusal fibers of the muscle spindle. When a skeletal muscle contracts, the intrafusal muscle fiber becomes slack and the Ia afferents stop firing. By stimulating the intrafusal muscle fibers during a contraction, the γ-motoneurons prevent the intrafusal muscle fibers from becoming slack and thus maintain Ia firing during the contraction.

**86. The answer is b.** *(Fauci, pp 2549-2565. Ganong, pp 202-222. Stead, pp 325-326. Widmaier, pp 307-308.)* These findings are consistent with the presence of Parkinson disease, which is characterized by resting tremor rigidity and akinesia. It is caused by destruction of the dopamine secreting neurons within the substantia nigra of the basal ganglia. Levo (L)-dopa is a precursor for dopamine. L-dopa, rather than dopamine, is administered because it can cross the blood-brain barrier, but dopamine cannot. In contrast to the resting tremor of Parkinson disease, cerebellar disease is characterized by an intention tremor. In contrast to damage to the nigrostriatal dopaminergic system in Parkinson disease, Huntington disease results in a loss of the intrastriatal GABAergic and cholinergic neurons in the caudate nucleus and putamen of the basal ganglion.

**87. The answer is b.** *(Fauci, pp 147, 154-158, 2588-2590. Ganong, pp 129-132. McPhee and Ganong, pp 148-162. Widmaier, pp 299-305.)* The Ia afferents, which innervate the muscle spindles, have a phasic and tonic component. **B** illustrates the response of Ia afferents to sudden movement of a limb. The high-frequency burst of action potentials encodes the velocity of the initial movement, whereas the steady firing encodes the position of the limb when the movement is completed. **A** and **E** illustrate the behavior of a tonic receptor, which discharges at the same rate for as long as the stimulus is present. The patterns of sensory loss are often indicative of the level of nervous system involvement. In the spinal cord, segregation of fiber tracts and the somatotopic arrangement of fibers give rise to distinct patterns of sensory loss. Lesions that involve one-half of the spinal cord lead to loss of proprioception on the ipsilateral side and loss of pain and temperature sensation on the contralateral side. This presentation is called Brown-Séquard syndrome, which may be accompanied by contralateral hemiparesis with lesions in the high cervical spinal cord.

**88. The answer is e.** *(Fauci, pp 2575. McPhee and Ganong, pp 151-154. Ganong, pp 202-205.)* The precentral gyrus is the motor area of the cortex that contains the cell bodies of the neurons that form the corticospinal tract (also referred to as the pyramidal tract). The corticospinal tract contains axons that cross to the contralateral side of the brain within the pyramids and end within the motor areas of the spinal cord. These structures are essential for the generation of fine voluntary movements. Kinesthesia, the sense of movement and position of the limbs, is handled primarily by the Ia and Ib afferents that innervate the muscle spindles and Golgi tendon organs, respectively, and by the parietal lobe. Primary lateral sclerosis (PLS) is a rare disorder arising sporadically in mid-to-late life. PLS is characterized clinically by progressive spastic weakness of the limbs, preceded or followed by spastic dysarthria and dysphagia, indicating combined involvement of corticospinal and corticobulbar tracts. Sensory changes are absent and neither EMG nor muscle biopsy shows denervation.

**89. The answer is d.** (*Ganong, pp 612-614. Stead, pp 326-327.*) The concentrations of protein and glucose within the cerebrospinal fluid (CSF) are much lower than those of plasma. Changes in the CSF concentrations of these substances are helpful in detecting pathologic processes, such as tumor or infection, in which the blood-brain barrier is disrupted. Cerebrospinal fluid, which is in osmotic equilibrium with the extracellular fluid of the brain and spinal cord, is formed primarily in the choroid plexus by an active secretory process. It circulates through the subarachnoid space between the arachnoid mater and pia mater and is absorbed into the circulation by the arachnoid villi. The epidural space, which lies outside the dura mater, may be used clinically for instillation of anesthetics.

**90. The answer is b.** (*Fauci, pp 151-153, 2560-2561. Ganong, pp 221-222. Widmaier, p 307.*) Ataxia, dysmetria, and an intention tremor all are classic findings in a patient with a lesion involving the cerebellum. Affected persons also exhibit adiadochokinesia, which is a loss of ability to accomplish a swift succession of oscillatory movements, such as moving a finger rapidly up and down. Lesions in the basal ganglia more commonly present with a resting tremor, such as seen in Parkinson disease. Lesions in the medulla may compromise respiration and other autonomic functions. Damage to the eighth (vestibulocochlear) nerve can result in symptoms such as hearing loss, nystagmus, and vertigo.

**91. The answer is b.** (*Fauci, pp 171-179. Ganong, pp 195-201.*) In a normal sleep cycle, a person passes through the four stages of slow-wave sleep before entering REM sleep. In narcolepsy, a person may pass directly from the waking state to REM sleep. REM sleep is characterized by irregular heart beats and respiration and by periods of atonia (loss of muscle tone). Hypoventilation is characteristic of both REM and non-REM sleep because sleep depresses the central chemoreceptors. Brain activity during REM sleep is higher than during wakefulness so there is an increase in brain metabolism. It is also the state of sleep in which dreaming occurs. High-amplitude EEG waves occur in the late stages of slow-wave sleep.

**92. The answer is a.** (*Ganong, pp 129-133.*) The Ib afferents innervating the quadriceps muscles are activated when the quadriceps contracts in response to tapping the patella tendon. Stretching the patella tendon stretches the intrafusal muscle fibers within the quadriceps muscle and causes an increase in Ia afferent activity. The increase in Ia afferent activity causes an increase in α-motoneuron activity, which results in contraction of the quadriceps muscle. When the muscle contracts, the intrafusal muscle fibers are unloaded and the Ia afferent activity is reduced.

**93. The answer is b.** (*Fauci, pp 147, 151.*) Spasticity results from overactivity of the α-motoneurons innervating the skeletal musculature. Under normal circumstances, these α-motoneurons are tonically stimulated by reticulospinal and vestibulospinal fibers originating in the brain stem. These brain stem fibers are normally inhibited by fibers originating in the cortex. Cutting the corticoreticular fibers releases the brain stem fibers from inhibition and results in spasticity. Cutting the fibers from the reticular formation, vestibular nuclei, or the Ia afferents will reduce the spasticity.

**94. The answer is c.** (*Fauci, pp 130-133, 176. Ganong, pp 184, 220-221.*) Pathologic vertigo is generally classified as peripheral (labyrinthine) or central (brain stem or cerebellum). The clinical presentation in this case is most consistent with central vertigo. Positional (especially horizontal) nystagmus (to-and-fro oscillation of the eyes) is common in vertigo of central origin, but absent or uncommon in peripheral vertigo. The chronicity of the vertigo is characteristic of central vertigo, whereas the symptoms of peripheral vertigo generally have a finite duration and may be recurring. Tinnitus and/or deafness is often present in peripheral vertigo, but absent in central vertigo. The flocculonodular lobe, or vestibulocerebellum, is connected to the vestibular nuclei and participates in the control of balance and eye movements, particularly changes in the vestibuloocular reflex (VOR), which serves to maintain visual stability during head movement;

a lesion of this area of the cerebellum may result in vertigo and nystagmus, whereas the spinocerebellum is involved in the coordination of limb movement. Labyrinthitis and Méniére syndrome are examples of vertigo of peripheral origin. In psychogenic versus organic vertigo, nystagmus is absent during a vertiginous episode.

**95. The answer is b.** (*Ganong, pp 194-196.*) In a totally relaxed adult with eyes closed, the major component of the electroencephalogram (EEG) will be a regular pattern of 8 to 12 waves per second, called the $\alpha$-rhythm. The $\alpha$-rhythm disappears when the eyes are opened. It is most prominent in the parieto-occipital region. In deep sleep, the $\alpha$-rhythm is replaced by larger, slower waves called delta waves. In REM sleep, the EEG will show fast, irregular activity.

**96. The answer is e.** (*Ganong, pp 153-156. Widmaier, pp 208-212.*) The focal length of an ideal refractive surface is equal to the distance between the refractive surface and the image formed by a distant object. In a normal eye, the image of a distant object is formed on the retina. Therefore, the focal length is 14 mm. If the image is formed in front of the retina, the eye would be myopic (near-sighted); if the image formed behind the retina, the eye would be hyperopic (far-sighted). When an image is placed close to the eye (in ophthalmology, close means <20 ft or 6 m), the eye must accommodate (increase its refractive power) for near vision. The refractive power of a lens system in diopters is equal to the reciprocal of the focal length ($1/f$) in meters. The relationship between the refractive power $P$, or focal distance, the image distance $i$, and the object distance $o$ is given by the lens formula

$$P = 1/f = 1/o + 1/i$$

where each of the distances is given in meters. If the object distance is 0.25 m and the image distance, the distance from the cornea to the retina, is 0.014 m, the refractive power of the eye is 75 diopters (0.264/0.0035). The initial refractive power was 71 diopters (1/0.014). Therefore, to form a clear image of the object on the retina, the accommodation reflex for near vision increased the refractive power of the eye by 4 diopters.

**97. The answer is d.** (*Ganong, pp 213-216. Fauci, pp 2553, 2560-2562.*) Huntington chorea is an inherited genetic defect leading to the degeneration of neurons with the striatum (the caudate nucleus and putamen). It is progressive disease characterized by uncontrolled movements, irritability, depression, and ultimately dementia and death. Lesions of the subthalamic nucleus produce wild flinging movements called ballism; those within the anterior cerebellum produce ataxia; those within the substantia nigra produce Parkinson disease; and those within the limbic system yield emotional disorders.

**98. The answer is d.** (*Ganong, pp 226-230.*) The catecholamine, norepinephrine (and epinephrine) activates both $\alpha$- and $\beta$-adrenergic receptors. When the $\alpha_1$-adrenergic receptors are stimulated, they activate a G protein, which in turn activates phospholipase C, which hydrolyzes $PIP_2$ and produces $IP_3$ and DAG. The $IP_3$ causes the release of $Ca^2$ from the sarcoplasmic reticulum, which in turn increases muscle contraction. $\alpha_1$-Adrenergic receptors predominate on arteriolar smooth muscle, so these muscles contract when stimulated with norepinephrine. Ephedrine is both a direct and indirectly acting sympathomimetic amine. Its direct action to activate postsynaptic $\alpha$-receptors and $\beta$-receptors is weak. Ephedrine's actions are primarily due to its effects as an indirect sympathomimetic, which involves its uptake into the presynaptic nerve terminal, where it is packaged and released with norepinephrine from the sympathetic nerve terminals. The effect of adding ephedrine is to increase the number of vesicles released during each action potential and possibly to extend the duration of action of norepinephrine by prolonging its inactivation via the neuronal reuptake process. Therefore, the actions of norepinephrine are enhanced in the presence of ephedrine. There are no $\alpha$-receptors in the bronchioles, pupils, or ciliary smooth muscles in the ciliary body of the eye, so norepinephrine does not cause contraction in these areas, but rather smooth muscle relaxation caused by activation of $\beta$-receptors in these tissues. Intestinal smooth muscles have $\alpha_2$-adrenergic receptor, which mediate relaxation when bound to norepinephrine.

**99. The answer is a.** (*Ganong, pp 182-183. Fauci, pp 199-204.*) The portion of the basilar membrane vibrated by a sound depends on the frequency of the sound. High-frequency sounds produce a vibration of the basilar membrane at the base of the cochlea (near the oval and round windows); low-frequency sounds produce a vibration of the basilar membrane at the apex of the cochlea (near the helicotrema). The modiolus is the bony center of the cochlea from which the basilar membrane emerges, the spiral ganglion contains the cell bodies of the auditory nerve fibers, and the stria vascularis is the vascular bed located on the outer wall of the scala media of the cochlea responsible for endolymph secretion.

**100. The answer is e.** *(Fauci, pp 147-150, 2488. Ganong, p 206.)* The plantar reflex is a cutaneous reflex elicited by stroking the lateral surface of the sole of the foot with a noxious stimulus such as a tongue blade, beginning near the end of the heel and moving across the ball of the foot to the great toe. The normal reflex consists of plantar flexion of the toes. With upper motor neuron lesions above the S1 level of the spinal cord, a paradoxical extension of the toe is observed, associated with fanning and extension of the other toes; this is termed an extensor plantar reflex or the Babinski sign. Other signs of pyramidal tract lesions include loss of the hopping and placing reaction, the cremasteric reflex, and the abdominal scratch reflex. Damage confined to the pyramidal tract results in distal muscular weakness and loss of fine motor control. Damage to other areas of the cortical motor control system is referred to as upper motor neuron disease and produces spasticity. Damage to the basal ganglia produces a variety of signs, including dystonia (striatum), ballism (subthalamic nucleus), and tremor at rest (substantia nigra). Damaging the cerebellum causes uncoordinated movements (dysmetria, ataxia, intention tremor).

**101. The answer is d.** *(Ganong, pp 234-235.)* A variety of physiological functions, such as alertness (the sleep-wake cycle), body temperature, and secretion of hormones, exhibit cyclic activity that varies over a 24-hour period of time. These variations in activity are called circadian rhythms and are controlled by the suprachiasmatic nucleus of the hypothalamus. The paraventricular nucleus secretes oxytocin and vasopressin, the ventromedial and lateral nuclei control food intake, and the arcuate nucleus secretes gonadotropin-releasing hormone.

**102. The answer is a.** *(Ganong, pp 92-93. Fauci, pp 2611-2622. Widmaier, pp 162-166.)* Presynaptic inhibition is caused by interneurons that secrete a transmitter that increases the $Cl^-$ conductance of the presynaptic nerve ending. The increase in $Cl^-$ conductance causes a partial depolarization of the presynaptic nerve ending and a decrease in the magnitude of the action potential in the presynaptic nerve ending. Because the number of synaptic vesicles released from the presynaptic neuron is proportional to the magnitude of the action potential, fewer vesicles are released and magnitude of the postsynaptic potential is reduced. Reducing the magnitude of the postsynaptic potential decreases the probability that an action potential will be generated by the postsynaptic cell. Presynaptic inhibition does not change the membrane potential of the α-motoneuron.

**103. The answer is e.** *(McPhee and Ganong, pp 163-164. Widmaier, pp 214-215, 231.)* The loss of vision on the right half of the visual field of both eyes (right-sided homonymous hemianopia) occurs because neurons from the left half of each of the retinas do not reach the visual cortex. This would result from a lesion of the left visual pathway distal to the optic chiasm, that is, the left optic tract, where the visual information from the nasal portion of the left retina (the right hemifield of the left eye's visual field) and the temporal portion of the right retina (the right hemifield of the right eye's visual field) are carried within the same nerve tract.

**104. The answer is d.** *(Fauci, pp 164-165. McPhee and Ganong, pp 163-164. Widmaier, pp 214-215, 231.)* Compression of the optic chiasm by an enlarged pituitary gland, which may be caused by increased synthesis of thyroid-stimulating hormone (TSH) in response to decreased circulating thyroxine, damages the nasal portion of each optic nerve, which produces a loss of vision in the temporal visual field of both eyes. This defect is referred to as a bitemporal hemianopia. Bitemporal hemianopia resulting from symmetric compression of the optic chiasm may also occur with pituitary adenoma, meningioma, glioma, or aneurysm. Homonymous hemianopia (B or E), in which the loss of vision is on the same half of the visual field of both eyes, results from lesions of the contralateral optic nerve. Loss of the medial half of both visual fields (C) is called binasal hemianopia; this visual field defect is uncommon, but may occur in glaucoma, bitemporal retinal disease (eg, retinitis pigmentosa), or a tumor or aneurysm compressing both optic nerves. Total blindness of the left eye (A) would result from a complete lesion of the left optic nerve.

**105. The answer is e.** *(Ganong, pp 122, 142-147.)* Activating nociceptors on the free nerve endings of C fibers produces ischemic pain. The C fibers synapse on interneurons located within the substantia gelatinosa (laminas II and III) of the dorsal horn of the spinal cord. The pathway conveying ischemic pain to the brain is called the paleospinothalamic system. In contrast, well-localized pain sensations are carried within the neospinothalamic tract. Ischemic pain does not adapt to prolonged stimulation. Pain is produced by specific nociceptors and not by intense stimulation of other mechanical, thermal, or chemical receptors.

**106. The answer is e.** (*Ganong, pp 251-255.*) The hypothalamus regulates body temperature. Core body temperature, the temperature of the deep tissues of the body, is detected by thermoreceptors located within the anterior hypothalamus. The anterior hypothalamus also contains neurons responsible for initiating reflexes, such as vasodilation and sweating, which are designed to reduce body temperature. Heat-producing reflexes, such as shivering, and heat-maintenance reflexes, such as vasoconstriction, are initiated by neurons located within the posterior hypothalamus.

**107. The answer is a.** (*Guyton, pp 686-687.*) The Klüver-Bucy syndrome is produced in animals by removal of the amygdala from both temporal lobes. The syndrome is characterized by excessive sexual behavior and a tendency to examine objects orally. The full syndrome is rarely encountered in humans but many of its characteristics are observed in patients with bilateral temporal lobe lesions produced by encephalitis or traumatic injury.

**108. The answer is a.** (*Ganong, pp 156-160. Widmaier, pp 212-214.*) The photoreceptors (rods and cones) are unique because they are the only type of sensory cells that are depolarized at rest (ie, in the dark) and hyperpolarized in response to their adequate stimulus (ie, when exposed to light). Light causes the rods and cones to hyperpolarize by activating a G protein called transducin, which leads to the closing of $Na^+$ channels. Auditory receptors are depolarized by the flow of $K^+$ into the hair cells. Touch receptors are activated by opening channels through which both $Na^+$ and $K^+$ can flow. Depolarization is caused by the inward flow of $Na^+$. Smell and taste receptors are activated by G protein-mediated mechanisms, some of which cause the receptor cell to depolarize; other G proteins cause the release of synaptic transmitter without any change in membrane potential.

**109. The answer is b.** (*Ganong, pp 148-170. Widmaier, pp 209-212.*) The ciliary body contains the ciliary muscle, which changes the shape of the lens when your eyes focus on something, a process called accommodation. Contracting the ciliary body increases the refractive power of the eye for near vision. When the ciliary muscle contracts, it pulls the suspensory ligaments toward the cornea, which causes the lens surface to bulge, increasing its refractive power. Contraction of the ciliary muscle, which causes short-range focus, is mediated by $M_3$ cholinergic muscarinic receptors, and relaxation of the ciliary muscle, which causes long-range focus, is mediated by $\beta_2$ adrenergic receptors. The muscles of the iris control the size of the pupils, and the extraocular muscles control the position of the eye in the socket. Sympathetic activation causes dilation of the pupil (mydriasis) by stimulating $\alpha_1$ adrenergic receptors, which lead to contraction of the radial muscle in the iris of the eye. Parasympathetic stimulation causes constriction of the pupil (miosis) due to contraction of the circular muscle in the eye mediated by $M_3$ cholinergic muscarinic receptors.

**110. The answer is a.** *(Ganong, pp 171-183. Widmaier, pp 217-222.)* When sound waves pass from air to water, most of the energy contained in the sound stimulus is lost. Because the auditory receptors within the inner ear are bathed in liquid, most of the energy in the sound stimulus could be lost as the sound travels from air to water. The bones of the middle ear significantly reduce the amount of loss by amplifying the sound stimulus. Audiologists refer to this amplification phenomenon as impedance matching. Sound localization is carried out by the central nervous system (CNS), which integrates information from both ears. Frequency discrimination is a function of the basilar membrane. The stapedius and tensor tympani muscles protect the ear from loud sounds.

**111. The answer is a.** *(Fauci, pp 153-154. Ganong, pp 171-183. Widmaier, pp 222-224.)* When the hair cells are bent, $K^+$-selective channels open, $K^+$ flows into the cell, and the cell depolarizes. This unusual situation occurs because the apical surface of the hair cells, on which the stereocilia are located, is bathed in endolymph, which contains a high concentration of $K^+$. Moreover, the endolymph is positively charged with respect to the perilymph, which surrounds the basal lateral portion of the hair cell. Because the intracellular concentration of $K^+$ is similar to the extracellular concentration of $K^+$, the electrical gradient determines the direction of $K^+$ flow. Because the endolymph is positively charged and the intracellular fluid is negatively charged, $K^+$ flows into the cell.

**112. The answer is b.** (*Ganong, pp 171-172, 183-184. Widmaier, pp 222-224.*) The otolith organs provide information about the position of the head with respect to gravity. When the head is bent away from its normal upright position, otoliths (small calcium carbonate crystals within the utricle and saccule) are pulled downward by gravity. The crystals bend the stereocilia on the hair cells, causing the hair cells to depolarize. Depolarization of the hair cells stimulates the vestibular nerve fibers. Bending the head in different directions causes different otoliths to move. Therefore, the particular group of vestibular nerve fibers that is stimulated signals the direction in which the head bends.

**113. The answer is c.** (*Ganong, pp 158-159, 167.*) The light-sensitive chemical in the retinal rods is called rhodopsin. It is a combination of 11-*cis* retinal and opsin. The photoisomerization of 11-*cis* retinal to all-*trans* retinal activates rhodopsin. The subsequent separation of opsin and retinal and the reformation of 11-*cis* rhodopsin are not necessary for the activation of the visual receptors. Rhodopsin cannot absorb another photon of light, however, until it is enzymatically isomerized back to its 11-*cis* conformation.

**114. The answer is b.** (*Ganong, pp 173-184. Widmaier, pp 222-224.*) When the head rotates in one direction, the hair cells mounted on the cristae rotate along with the head. However, the flow of endolymph is delayed and as a result the cupula is moved in a direction opposite to the movement of the head. When the head moves to the right, the cupula moves toward the left; this bends the stereocilia on the hair cells in the right horizontal canal toward the kinocilium and bends the stereocilia on the hair cells in the left horizontal canal toward the kinocilium. As a result, the hair cells in the right horizontal canal depolarize and those in the left horizontal canal hyperpolarize. The depolarization of the hair cells in the right horizontal canal stimulates the right vestibular nerve, which in turn causes the eyes to deviate toward the left. The movement of the eyes toward the left as the head deviates toward the right keeps the image on the retina in focus.

**115. The answer is d.** (*Ganong, pp 153-156. Widmaier, pp 209-212.*) The increase in lens power that normally occurs when objects are placed close to the eye (the accommodation reflex) does not take place in presbyopia. The failure of the accommodation reflex occurs because the lens and lens capsule stiffen with age. There are some reports of ciliary muscle weakness accompanying presbyopia but there are none indicating that presbyopia is caused by ciliary muscle paralysis.

**116. The answer is a.** (*Ganong, pp 157-160.*) Transducin is the G protein activated by rhodopsin when light strikes the eye. Transducin activates a phosphodiesterase that hydrolyzes cGMP. When cGMP concentrations within the rods or cones decrease, sodium channels close, sodium conductance decreases, and the cell membrane potential becomes more negative (hyperpolarizes). Hyperpolarization of the cell causes a decrease in the release of neurotransmitter. Eventually the all-*trans* retinal dissociates from opsin and reduces the concentration of rhodopsin in the cell.

**117. The answer is b.** (*Ganong, p 227. Fauci, p 190. Widmaier, pp 180-184, 211.*) Parasympathetic stimulation or cholinergic muscarinic agonists used to treat glaucoma produce miosis, that is, pupillary constriction caused by contraction of the sphincter muscle of the iris. Anticholinergic agents (eg, atropine) or sympathetic stimulation produce mydriasis, that is, pupillary dilation, in which the increase in pupil size results from contraction of the radial muscle of the iris mediated by $\alpha_1$-adrenergic receptors.

**118. The answer is d.** (*Fauci, pp 198-199.*) Trauma to the chorda tympani branch of the facial nerve during third molar extractions or middle ear surgery is relatively common and can cause dysgeusia. Other mechanisms of disorders of the sense of taste, besides damage to the gustatory afferent nerves, include damage to central gustatory pathways (trauma, diabetes mellitus, hypothyroidism, stroke, CNS disorders), sensory losses (aging, Candidiadis, viral infections, many drugs, especially those that interfere with cell turnover such as antineoplastic and antithyroid agents), and transport gustatory losses (interference with access of tastant to receptor cells, such as with xerostomia, Sjögren syndrome, heavy metal intoxication, oral radiation therapy). No effective therapies exist for the sensorineural disorders of taste. Altered taste due to surgical stretch of the chorda tympani nerve usually improves within 3 to 4 months.

**119. The answer is c.** (*Ganong, pp 185-188, 250-251. Fauci, pp 196-198.*) Exposure to cigarette smoke and other airborne toxic chemicals can cause metaplasia of the olfactory neuroepithelium with resultant anosmia (absence of smell), hyposmia (decreased sense of smell), or dysosmia (distorted sense of smell). Spontaneous recovery can occur if the insult is discontinued. Vitamin A deficiency can also cause anosmia as a result of epithelial degeneration. The most common etiologies of olfactory disorders are head trauma in children and young adults (neural loss) and viral infections in older adults (sensory and transport loss). In addition, olfactory thresholds increase with age; more than 75% of people over the age of 80 have an impaired ability to identify smells. Other examples of transport losses include allergic or bacterial rhinitis, nasal polyps, nasal surgery, deviated nasal septum, and congenital abnormalities (eg, Kallman syndrome, hypogonadotropic hypogonadism with hypoosmia or anosmia, albinism). Other examples of sensory losses of smell due to injury to the receptor region include neoplasms, radiation therapy, and drugs. Currently, no clinical tests exist to differentiate these different types of olfactory losses.

**120. The answer is b.** (*Ganong, pp 51, 742.*) It has been calculated that 40% of the human genes participate to some extent in the formation of the 100 billion neurons that comprise the human central nervous system.

**121. The answer is c.** (*Ganong, pp 107-112, 238, 259, 746.*) γ-Aminobutyric acid (GABA) is the major inhibitory mediator in the brain. $GABA_A$ receptors are pentameric $Cl^-$ ion channels that are widely distributed in the CNS. The increase in $Cl^-$ conductance produced by $GABA_A$ receptors is potentiated by the anxiolytic drug, diazepam, and other benzodiazepines. Glutamate is the major excitatory transmitter in the brain. Neuropeptide Y is an excitatory neurotransmitter that has a stimulatory effect on food intake. Central nervous system actions of histamine have been implicated in arousal, sexual behavior, drinking, pain thresholds, and the sensation of itch. Antagonism of central NK-1 receptors has antidepressant activity in humans.

**122. The answer is e.** (*Fauci pp 2537-2543. McPhee and Ganong, pp 178-181. Stead, pp 324-325.*) The presence of an apolipoprotein ε4 (Apo ε4) allele on chromosome 19, especially in the homozygous 4/4 state, is an important risk factor for Alzheimer disease (AD) and cortical atrophy on CT or MRI is a diagnostic sign of AD. Also, cholinesterase inhibitors may be used to improve memory in AD by increasing available levels of acetylcholine. However, the definitive diagnosis of AD is only obtained by tissue examination on autopsy, with the presence of amyloid plaques and neurofibrillatory tangles in the neurons of the cerebral cortex, primarily in the temporal lobe, hippocampus, and nucleus basalis of Meynert (lateral septum). Short of autopsy, diagnosis is mainly clinical. Alzheimer disease is the most common cause of dementia. It is a slowly progressive dementia, and a clinical diagnosis must rule out other causes of dementia, including other major common causes such as vascular disease, Parkinson disease, alcohol dependence, alcoholism, or other drug/medication intoxication.

**123. The answer is b.** (*Fauci, pp 183-191. Stead, pp 322-323.*) Among the causes of acute vision loss, detachment of the retina is painless, and accompanied by floaters, flashing lights, and a scotoma in the peripheral visual field corresponding to the detachment. The diagnosis is confirmed by ophthalmoscopic examination of the dilated eye. Patients with a history of myopia, trauma, or prior cataract extraction are at greatest risk for retinal detachment. Another cause of sudden painless vision loss is a transient ischemic attack of the retina, also called amourosis fugax. Amourosis fugax usually results from an embolus that lodges in a retinal arteriole. Complete occlusion of the central retinal artery produces arrest of blood flow and a milky retina with a cherry red spot on the fovea. Optic neuritis is a common inflammatory disease of the optic nerve that is accompanied by eye pain, especially with eye movements. It is caused by demyelination, and often progresses to multiple sclerosis. Glaucoma and macular degeneration cause chronic vision loss. Glaucoma is the leading cause of blindness in African Americans; it is a slowly progressive, insidious optic neuropathy. Macular degeneration is the major cause of gradual, painless, bilateral central blindness in the elderly.

**124. The answer is a.** (*Ganong, pp 60-61, 742.*) Mammalian nerve fibers are classified into A, B, and C groups, and A fibers are further subdivided into $\alpha$, $\beta$, $\gamma$, and $\delta$ fibers, each of which has different histologic characteristics and functions. A$\beta$ fibers have touch, pressure, and motor functions. The dorsal root C fibers conduct some impulses generated by touch and other cutaneous receptors, as well as impulses generated by pain and temperature receptors. A$\beta$ fibers are most susceptible to pressure and C fibers are least susceptible to pressure, which explains why a limb with a transiently compressed nerve loses motor function, but not pain sensation. B fibers are preganglionic autonomic nerves; they are most susceptible to hypoxia, whereas C fibers are least susceptible to hypoxia. Local anesthetics depress transmission in the group C fibers before they affect the touch fibers in the A group. C fibers are unmyelinated, whereas A and B fibers are myelinated. In addition, C fibers generally have smaller diameters than A or B fibers. For both reasons, C fibers have lower conduction velocities than A fibers.

**125. The answer is c.** (*Ganong, pp 51-53, 60-63. Fauci, pp 2667-2670. Stead, pp 319-320.*) Guillain-Barré syndrome (GBS) is an acute, rapidly evolving demyelinating polyradiculopathy that generally manifests as an areflexic ascending motor paralysis and is autoimmune in nature. The basis for the flaccid paralysis and sensory disturbance is conduction block in the Aβ fibers; axonal conduction remains intact unless there is secondary axonal degeneration. Most cases are preceded by a viral upper respiratory infection or a GI infection. Twenty to thirty percent of all cases occurring in North America, Europe, and Australia are preceded by infection or reinfection with *Campylobacter jejuni*. A similar proportion are preceded by a herpes virus infection, often CMV or Epstein-Barr virus. The postulated immunopathogenesis of GBS associated with *C. jejuni* infection involves production of autoantibodies against gangliosides present on the surface of Schwann cells, causing widespread myelin damage. The widespread administration of the swine influenza vaccine in the United States in 1976 was associated with an increased occurrence of GBS, but influenza vaccines in use from 1992 to 1994 resulted in only one additional case of GBS per million persons vaccinated. Older-type rabies vaccines prepared in nervous system tissue are still used in developing countries and are thought to be a trigger for GBS, presumably via immunization of neural antigens. Nerve growth factor is necessary for the growth and maintenance of sympathetic neurons and some sensory neurons, not motoneurons. Experimental injection of antiserum against nerve growth factor in newborn animals produces immunosympathectomy. Oligodendrogliocytes are involved in myelin formation in the CNS, whereas Schwann cells are involved in myelin fomation in peripheral nerves.

**126. The answer is e.** (*Ganong, pp 216-217. McPhee and Ganong, pp 175-176, 186-187, 701-702. Stead, pp 318-319. Widmaier, pp 182-183, 280.*) Myasthenia gravis is an autoimmune disease in which circulating antibodies against the postsynaptic nicotinic acetylcholine receptors on the motor end plate destroy the receptors and/or prevent acetylcholine from binding.

As a result, the end-plate potential is decreased at the neuromuscular junction, causing weakness and fatigue of skeletal muscles. Approximately 75% of patients with myasthenia gravis have thymic hyperplasia and may benefit from thymectomy. Other treatments for myasthenia gravis include administration of acetylcholinesterase inhibitors, immunosuppressive agents, and plasmapheresis or intravenous immunoglobulin.

**127. The answer is c.** (*Fauci, pp 2584-2587. Ganong, pp 51-64. Widmaier, p 155.*) The conduction velocity of an action potential along an axon is proportional to the axon's diameter for both nonmyelinated and myelinated axons. For any given axon diameter, conduction velocity is greater in myelinated than in nonmyelinated fibers. Propagation via saltatory conduction in myelinated fibers is faster than propagation in nonmyelinated fibers of the same axon diameter because less charge leaks out through the myelin-covered sections of the membrane. Conduction velocities range from about 0.5 m/s for small-diameter unmyelinated fibers to about 100 m/s for large-diameter myelinated fibers. The resting membrane potential, the duration of the relative refractory period, and the magnitude of the action potential are dependent on the type and density of electrically excitable gates and the ability of the $Na^+$- $K^+$-ATPase to establish and maintain the concentration gradients. These characteristics are not related in any systematic way to the axon diameter. Bell palsy is the most common form of facial paralysis. This idiopathic disorder has a fairly abrupt onset with maximal weakness attained within about 48 hours. MRI may reveal swelling of the geniculate ganglion and facial nerve. If denervation is evident on electromyography indicating axonal degeneration, it can take up to 3 months or longer for regeneration and recovery to occur.

**128. The answer is b.** (*Fauci, pp 2549-2565. Ganong, pp 118, 202-222. Stead, pp 325-326. Widmaier, pp 307-308.*) Parkinson disease results from a reduction of dopaminergic transmission within the basal ganglia, generally due to degeneration of nigrostriatal dopaminergic neurons. The fibers going to the putamen are most severely affected. Dopaminergic neurons and receptors are steadily lost with age in the basal ganglia, but an abnormal acceleration of that process results in Parkinson disease. The diagnosis of Parkinson disease can generally be made with at least two of the cardinal signs of parkinsonism, which are, resting tremor, paucity and slowness of movement (bradykinesia), rigidity, shuffling gait, and flexed posture.

**129. The answer is b.** (*Ganong, pp 100, 603.*) Succinylcholine is a rapidly acting neuromuscular-blocking agent with a very short duration of action. Respiratory paralysis can be produced in less than 60 seconds and normal respiration typically returns within 15 minutes. Because succinylcholine can also stimulate autonomic postganglionic fibers, vagal fibers innervating the heart are stimulated. The vagal fibers release acetylcholine, which binds to muscarinic receptors on the SA node, slowing the heart. The bradycardia can be prevented by administering atropine, which blocks the muscarinic receptors on the SA node.

**130. The answer is d.** (*Ganong, p 59. Fauci, pp 274-287. Stead, pp 226-234.*) The upstroke of the action potential is caused by an inward flow of sodium ions, and therefore its magnitude depends on the extracellular sodium concentration. Decreasing the external $Na^+$ concentration decreases the size of the action potential, but has little effect on the resting membrane potential because the permeability of the membrane to $Na^+$ at rest is low. Conversely, increasing the external $K^+$ concentration decreases the resting membrane potential. Changes in external $Ca^{2+}$ concentration affect the excitability of nerve and muscle cells, but not the magnitude of the resting potential or the action potential.

**131. The answer is b.** (*Ganong, pp 223-231.*) Muscarine binds to acetylcholine muscarinic receptors on cardiac and smooth muscle. These are the same receptors activated by the release of acetylcholine by the vagus nerve. Cardiac muscarinic receptors decrease the rate of phase 4 depolarization and therefore, decrease the heart rate. A heart rate less than 60 beats/min is called bradycardia. Acetylcholine receptors on the skeletal muscle end plate are nicotinic receptors and do not respond to muscarine. Dilation of the pupils and hypertension are signs of sympathetic, not parasympathetic activity.

**132. The answer is d.** (*Ganong, pp 51-64.*) In order for propagation of an action potential to occur, the depolarization produced by one action potential must depolarize the adjacent patch of excitable membrane to the threshold level. In demyelinating diseases, such as multiple sclerosis, too much charge leaks from the membrane and as a result, not enough charge is available to bring the next patch of membrane to threshold. Increasing the duration of the action potential increases the amount of charge entering the cell, and therefore increases the probability that the next patch of excitable membrane will be depolarized to threshold. Increasing the duration of the refractory period will not affect the amount of charge entering the cell. Depolarizing the membrane and increasing potassium conductance will make it more difficult to produce an action potential. If membrane capacitance is increased, the amount of charge required to excite the next patch of membrane will be increased.

**133. The answer is c.** *(Fauci, pp 2477-2478. Ganong, pp 51-64. Widmaier, pp 144-149.)* When the permeability of a particular ion is increased, the membrane potential moves toward the equilibrium potential for that ion. The equilibrium potential for sodium (+60 mV) is much greater than the resting membrane potential. Thus, increasing the permeability for sodium causes a large depolarization. The equilibrium potentials for chloride (−80 mV) and potassium (−92 mV) are close to the resting membrane potential, so increases in their permeability have little effect on the resting membrane potential. The resting potentials of neurons and the action potentials responsible for impulse conduction are generated by ion currents and ion channels. Disorders of ion channels, that is, channelopathies, are responsible for a growing number of neurologic diseases. Mutations in $Na^+$ channels that cause an increase in sodium permeability are associated with migraine and epilepsy.

**134. The answer is b.** *(Widmaier, pp 164-175.)* Vitamin $B_{12}$ is necessary for normal neurological function because it is involved in myelin synthesis and repair. Vitamin $B_{12}$ deficiency causes damage to the white matter of the spinal cord and peripheral neuropathy. Treatment consists of vitamin $B_{12}$ administration. Although folate may be an adequate substitute for treatment of the megaloblastic anemia characteristic of vitamin $B_{12}$ deficiency, folate should not be used instead of vitamin $B_{12}$ because the neurological deficits will persist and progress.

**135. The answer is c.** *(Ganong, pp 51-64. Widmaier, pp 164-175.)* The repolarization phase of the action potential is produced by a decrease in $Na^+$ conductance caused by the inactivation of $Na^+$ channels, and the increase in $K^+$ conductance due to the activation of $K^+$ channels. Preventing the inactivation of $Na^+$ channels will decrease the downstroke velocity of the action potential. This will slow the normal repolarization phase of the action potential and thereby prolong the duration of the action potential. The relative refractory period is prolonged because of the prolonged duration of the action potential. The upstroke velocity and the magnitude depend on how rapidly and how long the sodium channels are opened. By preventing inactivation of the $Na^+$ channel, the rate of the upstroke and the magnitude of the overshoot may be increased.

**136. The answer is e.** (*Ganong, pp 30-34. Fauci, pp 2477-2478, 2691-2693.*) Electrically excitable gates are those that respond to a change in membrane potential. The most notable electrically excitable gates are those on the sodium and potassium channels that produce the nerve action potential. The potassium channel gate is opened by depolarization. Ventricular muscle sarcoplasmic reticulum releases its calcium in response to an increase in intracellular calcium. The gates opened by ACh are chemically excitable gates. In rods, sodium channels are closed when cGMP is hydrolyzed. Electrically excitable gates do not regulate the active transport of glucose.

**137. The answer is c.** (*Ganong, pp 6-8, 30-35, 51-64. McPhee and Ganong, pp 615-618. Widmaier, pp 100-107.*) The sodium-potassium pump uses the energy contained in ATP to maintain the sodium gradient across the membrane. The sodium gradient, in turn, is used to transport other substances across the membrane. For example, the Na/Ca exchanger uses the energy in the sodium gradient to help maintain the low intracellular calcium required for normal cell function. Although sodium enters the cell during an action potential, the quantity of sodium is so small that no significant change in intracellular sodium concentration occurs. Because the sodium transference is so low, the sodium equilibrium potential is not an important determinant of the resting membrane potential. Recall that transference is a measure of an ion's relative conductance:

$$T_{Na} = g_{Na} /(g_{Na} + g_K) \text{ and}$$
$$T_K = g_K/(g_{Na} + g_K)$$

where $T$ = transference and $g$ = conductance. Patients with secondary hyperaldosteronism due to malignant hypertension, renal artery stenosis, or chronic renal disease have hypernatremia, hypokalemia, and excrete large amounts of aldosterone, but have elevated plasma renin activity (PRA) in contrast to a normal PRA seen in primary hyperaldosteronism. Secondary hyperaldosteronism is common, accounting for as much as 15% of patients diagnosed with essential hypertension. The hypernatremia is mild because water is retained with $Na^+$.

**138. The answer is b.** *(Ganong, pp 111-112, 142. Fauci, pp 81-86. Stead, pp 187-188.)* Pain is the most common presenting symptom, and thus understanding pain is essential to the goals of relieving suffering, as well as preserving and restoring health. The function of the pain sensory system is to protect the body by detecting, localizing, and identifying tissue-damaging processes. Different diseases produce characteristic patterns of tissue damage; the resultant manifestations of pain and tenderness can provide important diagnostic clues and can also be used to evaluate treatment regimens. Pelvic inflammatory disease (PID) is an infection of the upper genital structures in women (uterus, ovaries, oviducts) often with involvement of neighboring organs, which is generally accompanied by lower abdominal pain with pelvic, adnexal, and cervical motion tenderness. Peripheral nerves consist of primary sensory afferent axons, motor neurons, and sympathetic postganglionic neurons. Primary sensory afferent nerves include those with large-diameter A-beta (Aβ), which normally are not involved in pain, as well as two populations of primary afferent nociceptors, the small-diameter myelinated A-delta (Aδ) and unmyelinated (C fiber) axons, which are both present in nerves to the skin and to deep somatic and visceral structures. Many Aδ and C fibers innervating viscera are completely insensitive in normal, uninjured, noninflamed tissue, but become sensitive to mechanical stimuli in the presence of inflammatory mediators. An important concept to emerge in recent years is that afferent nociceptors also have a neuroeffector function, in that they contain polypeptide mediators that are released from their nerve terminals when activated. Most notably, substance P, an 11-amino acid polypeptide found in neurons within the hypothalamus and spinal cord, is released from small Aδ and C fibers that relay information from nociceptors to neurons within the substantia gelatinosa of the spinal cord. The biologic actions of substance P include vasodilation, neurogenic edema and the accumulation of bradykinin, the release of histamine from mast cells, and the release of serotonin from platelets. Endorphins and other opioid peptides such as the enkephalins may partially inhibit the perception of pain by presynaptically inhibiting the release of substance P from nociceptor afferent fibers.

**139. The answer is a.** *(Ganong, pp 7-8. Widmaier, pp 149-159.)* The $Na^+$ equilibrium potential is approximately +60 mV and is based on the ratio of the intracellular and extracellular $Na^+$ concentrations. During an action potential, the peak of the action potential (point **A**) is close, but not equal, to the $Na^+$ equilibrium potential. The membrane potential does not reach the

Na$^+$ equilibrium potential because the Na$^+$ channels start to inactivate and the K$^+$ channels begin to activate during the upstroke of the action potential.

**140. The answer is a.** (*Ganong, pp 101-105, 227-229, 262-263, 289-290, 325-326, 344, 356-361, 641.*) Epinephrine (adrenalin) acts on both α- and β-adrenergic receptors, but has a greater affinity for β-adrenergic receptors. Activation of β$_2$-adrenergic receptors leads to relaxation of smooth muscle in the bronchi, vasculature, intestine, uterus, and bladder; to increased pancreatic insulin and glucagon secretion; and an increase in liver glycogenolysis. The bronchodilator effects of epinephrine are key in the treatment of the life-threatening effects of anaphylactic shock. Activation of β$_1$- and β$_2$-adrenergic receptors in the heart leads to an increase in the rate of SA nodal phase 4 depolarization and thus heart rate (positive chronotropic response), an increase in contractility (positive inotropic response), an increase in conduction velocity (positive dromotropic response), and an increase in cardiac excitability/irritability. The transport of Ca$^{2+}$ into skeletal muscle fibers is not affected by β-receptors. The effects of epinephrine-induced β-adrenergic receptor activation are due to G-protein-mediated activation of adenylate cyclase, which catalyzes the formation of cyclic adenosine monophosphate (cAMP) and activation of protein kinase A.

**141. The answer is b.** (*Ganong, pp 121-127, 746. Stead, pp 353-355. Widmaier, p 203.*) The Ruffini ending is a tonic receptor that produces a train of action potentials proportional to the intensity of pressure applied to the skin. The Pacinian corpuscle is a very rapidly adapting receptor that fires once or twice in response to skin deformation, but can produce a continuous train of action potentials if the stimulus is repetitively applied and withdrawn. Therefore, the Pacinian corpuscle is used to encode vibration.

**142. The answer is e.** (*Ganong, pp 199-201, 755-756.*) Narcolepsy is associated with low CSF levels of the orexins and a defect in one of the receptors for orexins (hypocretins) in the hypothalamus. Adenosine induces sleep and serotonin agonists suppress sleep. Fatal familial insomnia is a progressive prion disease, characterized by worsening insomnia, impaired autonomic and motor functions, dementia, and death.

# Musculoskeletal Physiology

## Questions

**143.** A 77-year-old woman with severe kyphoscoliosis presents with increasing dyspnea consistent with a decrease in chest wall compliance. With contraction of the external intercostal muscles during inspiration, the Golgi tendon organ (GTO) provides the central nervous system with information about which of the following?

a. The length of the muscle being moved
b. The velocity of muscle movement
c. The blood flow to the muscle being moved
d. The tension developed by the muscle being moved
e. The change in joint angle produced by the movement

**144.** A 56-year-old woman presents with a flat red rash on the face and upper trunk and an erythematous rash on the knuckles and in the shape of a V on the neck and anterior chest. She also complains of muscle weakness with difficulty getting out of a chair and combing her hair. Laboratory findings include an increased creatine phosphokinase (CPK), positive antinuclear antibody, and anti-Mi2 dermatomyositis-specific antibodies. In addition to oral prednisone, physical therapy is ordered with the goal of improving muscle strength, and thus ability to perform activities of daily living. Repetitive stimulation of a skeletal muscle fiber will cause an increase in contractile strength due to an increase in which of the following?

a. The duration of cross-bridge cycling
b. The concentration of calcium in the myoplasm
c. The magnitude of the end-plate potential
d. The number of muscle myofibrils generating tension
e. The velocity of muscle contraction

**145.** A 34-year-old woman presents with a complaint of fatigue and generalized muscle weakness. As one way to evaluate a neural versus muscular basis for her symptoms, the woman is instructed to rapidly flex her arm. During this maneuver, which of the following occurs?

a. Activity of Ia afferent fibers from the biceps (the agonist) increases.
b. Activity of Ib afferent fibers from the biceps (the agonist) decreases.
c. Activity of Ia afferent fibers from the triceps (the antagonist) increases.
d. Activity of Ib afferent fibers from the triceps (the antagonist) decreases.
e. Activity of α-motoneurons to the triceps (the antagonist) increases.

**146.** A 62-year-old man presents with a hypokinetic movement disorder characterized by bradykinesia (paucity and slowness of movement). During a normal voluntary movement, which of the following occurs?

a. Large muscle fibers are recruited before small muscle fibers.
b. Fast muscle fibers are recruited before slow muscle fibers.
c. Weak muscle fibers are recruited before strong muscle fibers.
d. Poorly perfused muscle fibers are recruited before richly perfused muscle fibers.
e. Anaerobic fibers are recruited before aerobic fibers.

**147.** A 35-year-old woman having an anxiety attack collapses. The emergency medical technician (EMT) who arrives on the scene notes that she is hyperventilating and suspects that she is suffering from tetany, a continuous contraction of skeletal muscle fibers caused by an increase in the excitability of nerves and muscle membranes. The increased membrane excitability is caused by which of the following?

a. Decreased release of inhibitory neurotransmitter from nerve terminals
b. Depolarization of the nerve and muscle membranes
c. Spontaneous release of calcium from the sarcoplasmic reticulum (SR)
d. Activation of sodium channels at more negative membrane potentials
e. Increased magnitude of the action potentials invading nerve terminals

**148.** A 32-year-old woman undergoing surgery for appendicitis develops malignant hyperthermia following halothane anesthesia. The life-threatening increase in metabolic rate and body temperature is attributed to a mutation of the ryanodine receptor in skeletal muscle, resulting in which of the following?

a. Excess calcium release from the sarcoplasmic reticulum during muscle contraction
b. Rapid repetitive firing of the presynaptic terminals of $\alpha$-motoneurons
c. Inability of skeletal muscle cells to repolarize
d. An increase in the refractory period of the $\alpha$-motoneurons
e. Production of endogenous muscle pyrogens

**149.** A 62-year-old woman presents to her primary care physician with a 2-month history of stiffness and aching in her neck, as well as bilateral shoulders and hips. After an extensive evaluation, she is diagnosed with polymyalgia rheumatica. Which of the following is most likely with polymyalgia rheumatica?

a. Creatine phosphokinase (CPK) levels are increased.
b. The erythrocyte sedimentation rate (ESR) is decreased.
c. Muscle weakness is characteristic.
d. It is usually seen in patients over age 50.
e. It does not respond to glucocorticoids.

**150.** A 47-year-old man presents with pain and swelling in the left big toe. He has been on a high-protein diet and training extensively for an iron man competition, which includes weight lifting, running, swimming, and biking. An aspirate of joint fluid demonstrates negative birefringent urate crystals and elevated 24-hour urinary uric acid levels. For maintenance therapy, which of the following agents would be best to treat the cause of his gout?

a. Aspirin
b. Allopurinol
c. Colchicine
d. Nonsteroidal anti-inflammatory drugs (NSAIDs)
e. Uricosurics

**151.** A 35-year-old woman is seen by a neurologist to evaluate her incapacitating muscle weakness. The neurologist suspects myasthenia gravis and decides to confirm his diagnosis by administering a drug that increases the force of muscle contraction in patients with myasthenia gravis. Caution is advised when administering the drug to patients with heart disease because bradycardia may develop. Which of the following most likely explains the ability of the drug to increase the force of muscle contraction in patients with myasthenia gravis?

a. Increasing the amount of acetylcholine (ACh) released by $\alpha$-motoneurons
b. Increasing the affinity of the skeletal muscle acetylcholine receptors to acetylcholine
c. Increasing the $\alpha$-motoneuron discharge rate
d. Decreasing the metabolic breakdown rate of acetylcholine
e. Decreasing the concentration of calcium in the extracellular fluid

**152.** A 5-year-old boy presents with abnormal running, jumping, and hopping. His parents have observed that he uses his arms to climb up his legs when rising from the floor. The pediatrician suspects Duchenne muscular dystrophy, and electromyography confirms a myopathy. The amount of force produced by a skeletal muscle can be increased by which of the following?

a. Increasing extracellular $Mg^{2+}$
b. Decreasing extracellular $Ca^{2+}$
c. Increasing the activity of acetylcholine esterase
d. Decreasing the interval between contractions
e. Increasing the preload beyond 2.2 mm

**153.** A 32-year-old man sees his physician after collapsing suddenly without any other physical distress. Laboratory results demonstrate an elevated serum concentration of potassium and he is diagnosed with periodic hyperkalemic paralysis, a clinical condition in which a sudden increase in extracellular potassium concentration results in muscle weakness. Which of the following is most likely to cause muscle weakness as a result of increased extracellular potassium concentration?

a. Hyperpolarization of muscle cells
b. Inactivation of sodium channels in muscle cells
c. Increased release of neurotransmitters from $\alpha$-motoneurons
d. Decreased potassium conductance in muscle cells
e. Increased duration of action potentials produced by $\alpha$-motoneurons

**154.** A 30-year-old woman is running the Boston marathon. In regard to the physiology of her different muscle tissue types, an increase in sodium conductance is associated with which of the following?

a. The plateau phase of the ventricular muscle action potential in heart
b. The downstroke of the skeletal muscle action potential
c. The upstroke of the smooth muscle action potential
d. The refractory period of the nerve cell action potential
e. The end-plate potential of the skeletal muscle fiber

**155.** A 16-year-old adolescent boy on the track team asks his pediatrician if he can take creatine on a regular basis in order to increase his muscle strength prior to a track meet. Which of the following most likely explains why he wants to take creatine?

a. Creatine increases plasma glucose concentration.
b. Creatine prevents dehydration.
c. Creatine increases muscle glycogen concentrations.
d. Creatine is converted to phosphocreatine.
e. Creatine delays the metabolism of fatty acids.

**156.** An 18-month-old boy presents with delayed dentation, short stature, difficulty and painful walking, and bowing of the legs. In vitamin D deficiency, which of the following is defective in bone?

a. Bone formation by osteoblasts
b. The composition of bone collagen
c. Calcification of the bone matrix
d. Bone resorption by osteoclasts
e. The blood supply to the haversian canals

**157.** While digesting a hamburger and fries that he eats on the way, a 32-year-old medical student walks briskly down the hallway to internal medicine grand rounds. When comparing the contractile responses in smooth and skeletal muscle, which of the following is most different?

a. The source of activator calcium
b. The role of calcium in initiating contraction
c. The mechanism of force generation
d. The source of energy used during contraction
e. The nature of the contractile proteins

**158.** A 12-year-old boy with muscular dystrophy is found to have a mutation of the gene that encodes the protein dystrophin. Genetic alterations in dystrophin lead to progressive muscular weakness because dystrophin provides structural support to the sarcolemma by binding which of the following?

a. β-Dystroglycan to laminin
b. Actin to β-dystroglycan
c. Actin to the Z lines
d. Z lines to M lines
e. Z lines to the sarcolemma

## Questions 159-160

**159.** A 24-year-old medical student is an avid bodybuilder, lifting weights approximately 2 to 3 hours/d. Which of the following best describes the action potential of skeletal muscle during his workout?

a. It spreads inward to all parts of the muscle via the T-tubules.
b. It has a prolonged plateau phase.
c. It causes the immediate uptake of $Ca^{2+}$ into the lateral sacs of the sarcoplasmic reticulum.
d. It is longer than the action potential of cardiac muscle.
e. It is not essential for contraction.

**160.** Which of the following best describes the contractile response of skeletal muscle?

a. It starts after the action potential is over.
b. It does not last as long as the action potential.
c. It produces more tension when the muscle contracts isometrically than isotonically.
d. It produces more tension when the muscle contracts isotonically than isometrically.
e. It decreases in magnitude with repeated stimulation.

**161.** A patient presents with greatly reduced exercise tolerance, including muscle pain and stiffness on exertion. The differential diagnosis includes McArdle syndrome, which results from a deficiency of which of the following enzymes?

a. Myophosphorylase
b. Hexokinase
c. Glucose-6-phosphatase
d. Galactose-1-phosphate uridyl transferase
e. Glycogen synthase

**162.** A 20-year-old man presents with stiffness in the lower back that improves with exercise. A pelvic radiograph reveals sacroiliitis. Which of the following best describes ankylosing spondylitis (AS)?

a. It is not associated with the HLA-B27 antigen.
b. It affects women more than men.
c. Peak onset is usually between ages 50 and 60 years.
d. Osteoporosis is not seen.
e. Symptoms improve with use of tumor necrosis factor $\alpha$ (TNF-$\alpha$) inhibitors.

**163.** An 87-year-old man presents with acute pain and swelling of the right knee. He is subsequently diagnosed with calcium pyrophosphate dihydrate (CPPD) deposition (pseudogout) after joint aspiration. Which of the following would be expected with CPPD deposition?

a. Aspiration reveals weakly negative birefringent crystals.
b. The temporomandibular joint (TMJ) is commonly involved.
c. There is decreased production of inorganic pyrophosphate.
d. The knee is the most commonly affected joint.
e. Rhomboid crystals are not seen in the aspirate.

# Musculoskeletal Physiology

## Answers

**143. The answer is d.** (*Ganong, pp 133-135. Widmaier, pp 300-303.*) The GTO is located in the tendon of skeletal muscles, and therefore is in series with the muscle. Each time the muscle contracts, the GTO is stretched in proportion to the tension developed by the muscle. The Ib afferent fibers (which innervate the GTO) produce a train of action potentials with a frequency that is in proportion to the deformation of the GTO. The muscle length and speed of shortening are sent to the CNS by Ia afferents that innervate the intrafusal fibers within muscle spindles.

**144. The answer is a.** (*Fauci, pp 2696-2701. Ganong, pp 65-78. Stead, pp 292-293. Widmaier, pp 258-271.*) Each time a skeletal muscle fiber is stimulated by an $\alpha$-motoneuron, enough $Ca^{2+}$ is released from its sarcoplasmic reticulum to fully activate all the troponin within the muscle. Therefore, every cross bridge can contribute to the generation of tension. However, the transmission of force from the cross bridges to the tendon does not occur until the series elastic component (SEC) of the muscle is stretched. Repetitive firing increases the amount of SEC stretch by maintaining cross-bridge cycling for a longer period of time. Repetitive firing increases neither the concentration of $Ca^{2+}$ within the myoplasm, the number of myofibrils that are activated, nor the magnitude of the end-plate potential. Because all of the cross bridges are activated each time a skeletal muscle fiber is activated, an increase in $Ca^{2+}$ concentration would have no effect on muscle strength. The skin findings, along with limitation in rising from a seated position or combing hair, are suggestive of proximal muscle weakness, characteristic of dermatomyositis.

**145. The answer is c.** (*Fauci, pp 147-150. Ganong, pp 131-134. Widmaier, p 278.*) The firing of the $\alpha$-motoneurons to the biceps muscle produces rapid flexion of the arm. Because the arm is rapidly flexed, the Ia afferent neurons innervating the muscle spindles in the biceps, which detect muscle length, will reduce their firing rate. The Ib afferents, innervating the Golgi tendon organs from the biceps, will detect the contractile activity of the biceps and increase their firing rate. The triceps are stretched during arm flexion and so their Ia afferents will increase their firing rate. Ib afferents do not respond when muscles are passively stretched, so their firing rate will not change.

**146. The answer is c.** *(Ganong, pp 73-76. Widmaier, pp 304-308.)* In general, small, weak, slow, fatigue-resistant muscle fibers are innervated by small spinal motoneurons, whereas large spinal motoneurons innervate large, fast, strong, easily fatigable muscle fibers. During most normal reflex or voluntary movements, small spinal motoneurons are recruited before large motoneurons. The slow fatigue-resistant muscle fibers have a dense capillary network for perfusion and use mitochondrial oxidative metabolism to produce adenosine triphosphate (ATP).

**147. The answer is b.** *(Ganong, pp 59, 382, 692. Widmaier, p 280.)* Membrane excitability is related to the ease with which depolarization opens $Na^+$ channels. The opening of the $Na^+$ channel in response to depolarization is, in part, related to the extracellular $Ca^{2+}$ concentration; the lower the extracellular $Ca^{2+}$ concentration, the easier it is for $Na^+$ channels to open when the membrane depolarizes. Hyperventilation (lowering arterial $CO_2$ tension) decreases extracellular $Ca^{2+}$ concentration by increasing arterial pH. When pH rises, $H^+$ is released from plasma proteins in exchange for $Ca^{2+}$, and ionized $Ca^{2+}$ concentration decreases.

**148. The answer is a.** *(Fauci, pp 118, 419. Ganong, p 255.)* The ryanodine receptor or calcium release channel on the sarcoplasmic reticulum is normally opened when skeletal muscle is activated. The flow of calcium through the open ryanodine receptor binds to troponin and initiates muscle contraction. The metabolic activity accompanying muscle contraction can warm the body. If a mutation in the ryanodine receptor causes uncontrolled release of calcium from the SR, the body temperature can rise to levels that cause brain damage.

**149. The answer is d.** *(Fauci, p 2126. Le, p 354.)* Polymyalgia rheumatica is almost always seen in patients over age 50 and can be seen in isolation or in patients with giant cell arteritis. CPK levels are not increased with the disease, and while patients may have stiffness and pain, muscle weakness is not seen. The characteristic laboratory finding in polymyalgia rheumatica is an elevated ESR, though it can be normal in some individuals. Glucocorticoids are the mainstay of treatment.

**150. The answer is b.** (*Ganong, pp 297-298. Stead, pp 298-299.*) Strenuous exercise and a high protein diet can cause overproduction of uric acid. Allopurinol, which inhibits xanthine oxidase, decreases the primary cause of gout by decreasing uric acid production. Colchicine is given in acute gout to inhibit phagocytosis of uric acid crystals by leukocytes, a process that in some way produces the joint symptoms. Nonsteroidal anti-inflammatory agents, particularly indomethacin, are also used to relieve the acute arthritic symptoms of gout. Aspirin is contraindicated in acute gout because it decreases urate excretion. Uricosurics are effective in increasing the excretion of uric acid in patients whose gout is caused by decreased urate excretion, such as chronic renal disease, diabetes ketoacidosis, use of thiazide diuretics, and ethanol ingestion.

**151. The answer is d.** (*Fauci, pp 2672-2674. Ganong, p 118. Widmaier, p 280.*) The drug used to test for myasthenia gravis is an acetylcholine esterase inhibitor. Neostigmine is an example of an acetylcholine esterase inhibitor. The drug prevents the breakdown of acetylcholine, increasing the duration of time acetylcholine remains in the synaptic cleft. Because acetylcholine can bind to the end-plate receptors for a longer time, the magnitude of the end-plate potential increases, increasing the probability of it generating an action potential. The greater the action potential force rate, the greater the source of muscle contraction. Increasing the amount of acetylcholine released by the α-motoneurons, by increasing the affinity of the skeletal muscle receptors for acetylcholine, or increasing the discharge rate of α-motoneurons could cause a similar effect. However, none of these changes would affect heart rate. The cautious use of this test in patients with heart failure results from the possibility that the decreased breakdown of acetylcholine released by the vagus nerve could decrease heart rate to dangerously low levels.

**152. The answer is d.** (*Fauci, pp 2682-2683. Ganong, p 77. Widmaier, p 280.*) When the interval between skeletal muscle contractions is small, the force produced by the two successive contractions will summate. The shorter the interval between the contractions, the greater the summation will be. Maximum summation is called tetanus. Decreasing extracellular $Ca^{2+}$ will increase the excitability of skeletal muscle fibers but does not have a direct effect on contractile force. Increasing the $Mg^{2+}$ concentration will decrease skeletal muscle excitability. Increasing the preload beyond 2.2 mm decreases the overlap between thick and thin filaments, and therefore decreases the force of contraction. Increasing the activity of acetylcholine esterase enhances the hydrolysis of ACh, and therefore decreases the likelihood that muscle contraction will be initiated.

**153. The answer is b.** *(Fauci, pp 283, 2681.)* Periodic hyperkalemic paralysis results from inactivation of the skeletal muscle membranes produced by depolarization of the skeletal muscle membrane in the presence of an increased extracellular potassium concentration. Inactivation of the sodium channels on the skeletal muscle membrane prevents action potentials from being produced, and therefore leads to muscle weakness or paralysis. Although the exact mechanism of periodic hyperkalemic paralysis is not known, it appears to be due to a mutation in the gene coding for the sodium inactivation gate.

**154. The answer is e.** *(Ganong, pp 58-59, 68-69, 78-81, 82-83, 116-118. Widmaier, pp 254-292.)* The end-plate potential in skeletal muscle is produced by an influx of sodium into the cell, which results from the increase in sodium permeability that occurs with acetylcholine binding to the nicotinic receptors on the membrane of the motor end plate. Acetylcholine binding at the motor end plate also increases the potassium conductance of the membrane. The plateau phase of ventricular muscle action potentials and the upstroke of smooth muscle action potentials are produced by an increase in calcium conductance. An increase in potassium conductance is responsible for the downstroke of the action potential. The refractory period is caused by an increase in potassium conductance and a decrease in the number of sodium channels available to produce an action potential (ie, sodium channel inactivation).

**155. The answer is d.** *(Ganong, pp 294-296.)* Phosphocreatine is rapidly converted to ATP in muscle. When the metabolic demands exceed the rate at which ATP can be generated by aerobic metabolism or glycolysis, phosphocreatine can supply the necessary ATP for a brief period of time. An increase in the concentration of phosphocreatine in muscle may increase the amount of ATP that can be produced and therefore enhance performance.

**156. The answer is c.** (*Ganong, pp 384-389. Fauci, pp 2375-2376.*) Vitamin D deficiency causes defective calcification of the bone matrix as a result of inadequate delivery of $Ca^{2+}$ and $PO_4^{3-}$ to the sites of mineralization. The disease in children is called rickets and is characterized by growth retardation, weakness and bowing of the weight-bearing bones, dental defects, and hypocalcemia, which increases parathyroid hormone and urinary phosphate losses. Several different types of inheritance lead to the vitamin D deficiency disorders, including X-linked dominant and autosomal-dominant hypophosphatemic rickets, vitamin D-dependent rickets Type I, an autosomal recessive disorder caused by inactivating mutations in the gene encoding $1\alpha$-hydroxylase enzyme, and vitamin D-dependent rickets Type II, in which there is end-organ resistance to $1,25(OH)_2D_3$, which is also usually inherited as an autosomal recessive disorder.

**157. The answer is b.** (*Ganong, pp 65-78, 82-84. Widmaier, pp 258-266, 285-290.*) The greatest difference in excitation-contraction coupling between skeletal muscle and smooth muscle involves the role of calcium in initiating contraction. In smooth muscle, calcium binds to and activates calmodulin, which, by activating myosin light chain kinase, catalyzes the phosphorylation of the 20,000-Da myosin light chain. Once the light chains are phosphorylated, myosin cross bridges bind to actin on the thin filaments, which initiates contraction. In skeletal muscle, calcium binds to troponin, which removes the tropomyosin-mediated inhibition of the actin-myosin interactions. Once the inhibition is removed, cross-bridge cycling (and contraction) begins. In both smooth and skeletal muscle, the cycling of cross bridges generates force. ATP provides the energy for the cycling of the cross bridges in both muscles. In skeletal muscle, activator calcium comes exclusively from the SR, whereas in smooth muscle calcium can come from both the SR and the extracellular fluid.

**158. The answer is b.** (*Fauci, pp 2678-2684. Ganong, pp 65-68, 77. Le, p 118.*) Dystrophin is a large protein that forms a rod, which connects the thin filaments of actin to the transmembrane protein $\beta$-dystroglycan in the sarcolemma. $\beta$-Dystroglycan is connected to laminin in the extracellular matrix by $\alpha$-dystroglycan. The dystroglycans are also associated with a complex of four transmembrane glycoproteins, called sarcoglycans. The dystrophin-glycoprotein complex adds strength to the muscle by providing a scaffolding for the fibrils and connecting them to the extracellular environment.

Muscular dystrophy is the term used for some 50 diseases that cause progressive skeletal muscle weakness. Duchenne and Becker muscular dystrophy are two types resulting from mutations in the dystrophin gene.

**159 and 160. The answers are a and c.** (*Ganong, pp 65-71. Widmaier, pp 266-271.*) Depolarization of the muscle fiber is essential for initiating muscle contraction. The action potential of skeletal muscle is transmitted to all of the fibrils along T-tubules, triggering the release of $Ca^{2+}$ from the lateral sacs of the sarcoplasmic reticulum next to the T-system. The electrical events in skeletal muscle and the ionic fluxes underlying them are similar to those in nerve. In contrast, the action potential in cardiac muscle is longer and has a prolonged plateau phase.

In isometric (same measure or length) contractions, muscle contraction increases the tension of the muscle. Isometric contraction is possible because muscles have elastic and viscous elements in series with the contractile elements, so contraction can occur without an appreciable decrease in length. In contrast, isotonic (same tension) contractions are contractions against a constant load, which decrease muscle length. Muscle fiber membrane depolarization during an action potential initiates muscle contraction via a process called excitation-contraction coupling. The duration of the contractile response of skeletal muscle (muscle twitch) exceeds the duration of the action potential, but varies with muscle fiber type. Because the muscle contractile mechanism does not have a refractory period, repeated stimulation before relaxation causes greater tension development than during a single muscle twitch, a process called summation of contractions.

**161. The answer is a.** (*Fauci, p 2460. Ganong, pp 289-290.*) In McArdle syndrome, glycogen accumulates in skeletal muscles because of a deficiency of muscle phosphorylase. Without adequate myophosphorylase, patients cannot break down their muscle glycogen to provide the energy for muscle contraction, except for normal activity or mild exercise. Thus, they have a greatly reduced exercise tolerance.

**162. The answer is e.** (*Fauci, pp 2109-2113. Le, p 353. Stead, pp 293-294.*) Ankylosing spondylitis is a chronic systemic inflammatory disorder affecting primarily the axial skeleton, but may have multiple organ involvement. The pathogenesis of AS is incompletely understood, but the response of the disease to blockade of TNF-α indicates that this cytokine plays a major role in the immunopathogenesis. The disease is associated with the HLA-B27 antigen and AS is seen more commonly in men than women, usually manifesting between ages 20 and 30. Diffuse osteoporosis is seen in the spine as the disease progresses.

**163. The answer is d.** *(Fauci, pp 2167-2168. Le, p 353.)* The knee is the most commonly affected joint in patients with CPPD deposition. The elbow, shoulder, and wrists are also affected, but involvement of the TMJ is rare. There is an increased production of inorganic pyrophosphate and joint aspiration reveals rhomboid, rod-shaped, or rectangular crystals that are weakly positive in birefringence.

# Respiratory Physiology

## Questions

**164.** A healthy 30-year-old woman is referred for a life insurance physical. History reveals that she has never smoked and vesicular breath sounds are heard at the periphery of the lung with auscultation. In the patient's spirometry tracing below, the expiratory reserve volume equals which of the following?

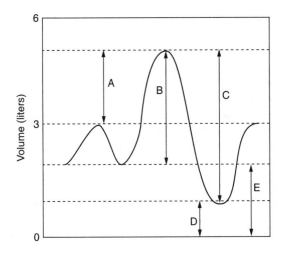

a. C
b. D
c. E
d. C + D
e. E − D

**165.** A group of third-year medical students accompanied a medical mission team to Peru. After arriving at the airport in Bolivia, they hiked to a remote mountain village in the Andes at an elevation of 18,000 ft. With a barometric pressure of 380 mm Hg at this altitude, what would be the resulting $PO_2$ of the dry inspired air?

a.   160 mm Hg
b.   100 mm Hg
c.   80 mm Hg
d.   70 mm Hg
e.   38 mm Hg

**166.** A 28-year-old man is admitted to the emergency department with multiple fractures suffered in a car accident. Arterial blood gases are ordered while the patient is breathing room air. After obtaining the arterial blood sample, the blood-gas technician draws room air into the syringe before measuring the blood-gas values. How does exposure to room air affect the measured values of $PaO_2$ and $PaCO_2$?

a.   The measured values of both $PaO_2$ and $PaCO_2$ will be higher than the patient's actual values.
b.   The measured values of both $PaO_2$ and $PaCO_2$ will be lower than the patient's actual values.
c.   The measured $PaO_2$ will be higher and the measured $PaCO_2$ will be lower than the patient's actual blood gas values.
d.   The measured $PaO_2$ will be lower and the measured $PaCO_2$ will be higher than the patient's actual blood gas values.
e.   The measured values of $PaO_2$ and $PaCO_2$ will accurately reflect the actual values.

**167.** A 68-year-old woman with pulmonary fibrosis presents with a complaint of increasing dyspnea while performing activities of daily living. She is referred for pulmonary function testing to assess the progression of her disease. Which of the following laboratory values is consistent with her diagnosis?

a.   Decreased diffusing capacity of the lung
b.   Increased residual volume
c.   Decreased $FEV_1/FVC$
d.   Increased lung compliance
e.   Increased airway resistance corrected for lung volume

**168.** A 24-year-old woman collapsed in a New York City subway station. An autopsy showed that a blood clot had traveled to her lung and caused her death. The medical examiner ultimately ruled that the blood clot was caused by the use of a birth control patch. Which of the following occurs if the blood flow to an alveolus is totally obstructed by a pulmonary thromboembolism?

a. The $\dot{V}/\dot{Q}$ ratio of the alveolus equals zero.
b. The $P_{O_2}$ of the alveolus will be equal to that in the inspired air.
c. The $P_{O_2}$ of the alveolus will be equal to the mixed venous $P_{O_2}$.
d. There will be an increase in shunting (venous admixture) in the lung.
e. There will be a decrease in alveolar dead space.

**169.** A 150-lb patient scheduled for abdominal surgery is sent for preoperative evaluation and testing. His chest x-ray is normal, and pulmonary function results on room air show:

Tidal volume = 600 mL
Respiratory rate = 12/min
Vital capacity = 5000 mL
$Pa_{O_2}$ = 90 mm Hg
$Pa_{CO_2}$ = 40 mm Hg
$P_E_{CO_2}$ = 28 mm Hg

The volume of the patient's physiological dead space, determined by applying the Bohr equation, equals which of the following?

a. 7200 mL
b. 420 mL
c. 180 mL
d. 150 mL
e. 0.3 mL

**170.** A hospitalized patient has tachypnea and significantly labored respirations requiring mechanical ventilation. Based on the pressure-volume curve of the lungs shown as curve Z in the figure below, which of the following is the most likely diagnosis for the patient?

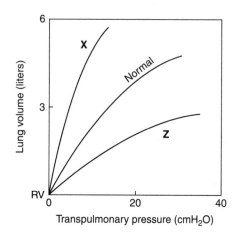

a.  Asthma
b.  Emphysema
c.  Dyspnea with aging
d.  Newborn with lecithin to sphingomyelin (L/S) ratio greater than 2
e.  Pulmonary edema

**171.** A 6'3" tall, 140-lb, 20-year-old man was watching television when he felt pain in his shoulder blades, shortness of breath, and fatigue. His father noticed how pale he was and took him to the emergency department, where a chest x-ray revealed a 55% pneumothorax of the right lung due to rupture of a bleb on the surface of the lung. What changes in lung function occur as a result of a pneumothorax?

a.  The intrapleural pressure in the affected area equals to atmospheric pressure.
b.  The chest wall on the affected side recoils inward.
c.  There is hyperinflation of the affected lung.
d.  The $\dot{V}/\dot{Q}$ ratio on the affected side increases above normal.
e.  The mediastinum shifts further to the right with each inspiration.

**172.** An 18-year-old woman with a 9-year history of wheezing on exertion is referred for pulmonary function tests. The figure below represents the spirometry tracing of a forced vital capacity. Her total lung capacity was 130% of predicted. Which of the following values will most likely be above normal?

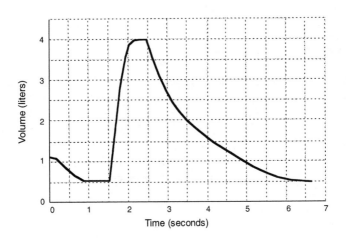

a. Vital capacity
b. Residual volume
c. Expiratory reserve volume
d. $FEV_{1.0}$/FVC
e. Maximum voluntary ventilation

**173.** A 125-lb, 40-year-old woman with a history of nasal polyps and aspirin sensitivity since childhood presents to the emergency department with status asthmaticus and hypercapnic respiratory failure. She requires immediate intubation and is placed on a mechanical ventilator on an $F_IO_2$ of 40%, a control rate of 15 breaths/min, and a tidal volume of 500 mL. Which of the following is her approximate alveolar ventilation?

a. 375 mL/min
b. 3500 mL/min
c. 5250 mL/min
d. 5625 mL/min
e. 7500 mL/min

**174.** A medical student waiting to do her first patient interview at the clinical skills center becomes very anxious and increases her rate of alveolar ventilation. If her rate of $CO_2$ production remains constant, which of the following will decrease?

a. pH
b. $Pa_{O_2}$
c. $Pa_{CO_2}$
d. $\dot{V}/\dot{Q}$
e. Alveolar-arterial $P_{O_2}$ difference

**175.** A 36-year-old man with a history of AIDS and *Pneumocystis* infection presents to the emergency department with severe respiratory distress. The patient is placed on a ventilator at a rate of 16, tidal volume of 600 mL, and $F_{I_{O_2}}$ of 1.0. An arterial blood sample taken 20 minutes later reveals a $P_{O_2}$ of 350 mm Hg, a $P_{CO_2}$ of 36 mm Hg, and a pH of 7.32. At a barometric pressure of 757 mm Hg, and assuming a normal respiratory exchange ratio (R) of 0.8, the patient's alveolar oxygen tension is approximately which of the following?

a. 105 mm Hg
b. 355 mm Hg
c. 576 mm Hg
d. 665 mm Hg
e. 712 mm Hg

**176.** A 49-year-old sedentary woman goes to her physician's office prior to starting a weight-loss exercise regimen. She is referred for an exercise stress test to evaluate cardiopulmonary function and her baseline aerobic capacity. Taking a deep inspiration to total lung capacity causes which of the following cardiopulmonary function variables to increase?

a. Alveolar surface tension
b. Airway resistance
c. Elastic recoil of the lung
d. Intrapleural pressure
e. Lung compliance

**177.** A 27-year-old man develops adult respiratory distress syndrome (ARDS) after near-drowning. Conventional mechanical ventilation on 100% $O_2$ together with inhaled nitric oxide do not provide sufficient oxygenation. Porcine surfactant is instilled via fiberoptic bronchoscope, and the $Paco_2$, fraction of inspired oxygen ($F_1O_2$), and shunting improve impressively. The improvements in respiratory function occurred because surfactant increased which of the following?

a. Bronchiolar smooth muscle tone
b. The pressure gradient needed to inflate the alveoli
c. Lung compliance
d. Alveolar surface tension
e. The work of breathing

**178.** In the maximal expiratory flow-volume curves below, curve A would be typical of which of the following clinical presentations?

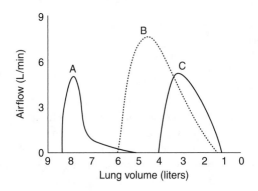

a. A 75-year-old man who has smoked two packs of cigarettes per day for 60 years. His breath sounds are decreased bilaterally, and his chest x-ray shows flattening of the diaphragm.
b. A 68-year-old man presents with a dry cough that has persisted for 3 months. His chest x-ray shows opacities in the lower and middle lung fields. The man states he was exposed to asbestos for approximately 10 years when he worked in a factory in his thirties.
c. A 57-year-old woman with pulmonary fibrosis who presents to the emergency room with shortness of breath.
d. An 84-year-old woman with a history of myocardial infarction who reports shortness of breath that worsens in the recumbent position.
e. A healthy, 22-year-old man getting his Army enlistment physical. He has never smoked, but is tired that morning, and does not use much effort while exhaling.

**179.** A 30-year-old woman is admitted to the emergency department with dyspnea, tachycardia, confusion, and other signs of hypoxia. The following laboratory data were obtained while the patient was breathing room air:

$Pa_{O_2}$ = 67 mm Hg
$Pa_{CO_2}$ = 60 mm Hg
pH = 7.27
$[HCO_3^-]$ = 26 meq/L
[Hb] = 15 g%
$Sa_{O_2}$ = 90%
$Pv_{O_2}$ = 30 mm Hg
$Sv_{O_2}$ = 55%
$\dot{V}_{O_2}$ = 350 mL/min
$Ca_{O_2}$-$Cv_{O_2}$ = 7 mL $O_2$/100 mL

Which of the following is the most appropriate classification of the patient's hypoxia?

a. Hypoxic hypoxia (hypoxemia)
b. Anemic hypoxia
c. Stagnant (hypoperfusion) hypoxia
d. Histotoxic hypoxia
e. Carbon monoxide poisoning

**180.** A 14-year-old adolescent girl presents with a lump in the neck. Fine needle aspiration biopsy reveals acinic cell carcinoma of the parotid gland. During the parotidectomy, there is compression injury of the glossopharyngeal nerve. As a result, which of the following respiratory reflexes will be impaired?

a. Aortic chemoreceptor reflex
b. Carotid body chemoreceptor reflex
c. Hering-Breuer inflation reflex
d. Irritant airway reflex
e. Juxta pulmonary capillary (J) receptor reflex

**181.** A 68-year-old woman convalescing from surgery developed a fever, hypoxemia, and shortness of breath. She was given 100% $O_2$ for 30 minutes, and the laboratory results were as follows:

$Pa_{O_2}$ = 95 mm Hg
$Pa_{CO_2}$ = 33 mm Hg
pH = 7.46
$[HCO_3^-]$ = 22 mEq/L
[Hb] = 15 g%
$Sa_{O_2}$ = 95%

The response to 100% $O_2$ reveals that the patient has which of the following?

a. Alveolar hypoventilation
b. Diffusion impairment
c. $\dot{V}/\dot{Q}$ inequality with low $\dot{V}/\dot{Q}$ units
d. Right-to-left shunting
e. Carbon monoxide poisoning

**182.** A 59-year-old man with right lower lobar pneumonia begins experiencing increasing respiratory distress. The patient is moved to the ICU, intubated, and placed on a mechanical ventilator. With the patient positioned on his left side, which of the following variables will be lower in the left lung compared to the right lung?

a. Alveolar ventilation per unit volume
b. Lung compliance
c. $Pa_{CO_2}$
d. Pulmonary blood flow
e. $\dot{V}/\dot{Q}$ ratio

**183.** A 26-year-old man training for a marathon reaches a workload that exceeds his anaerobic threshold. If he continues running at or above this workload, which of the following will increase?

a. Alveolar ventilation
b. Arterial pH
c. $Pa_{CO_2}$
d. Plasma $[HCO_3^-]$
e. Firing of the central chemoreceptors

**184.** A 67-year-old man who is a candidate for cardiac transplantation undergoes cardiac catheterization to assess his hemodynamic status. Findings include:

Pulmonary artery pressure = 35 mm Hg
Cardiac output = 4 L/min
Left atrial pressure = 15 mm Hg
Right atrial pressure = 10 mm Hg

Which of the following values is his pulmonary vascular resistance?

a.  0.16 L/min/mm Hg
b.  0.2 L/min/mm Hg
c.  5 mm Hg/L/min
d.  6.25 mm Hg/L/min

**185.** A 36-year-old woman is found comatose at her home and is life-flighted to the nearest regional medical center. Blood gases reveal a normal $Pao_2$ but a lower-than-normal arterial $O_2$ saturation. Which of the following conditions is most consistent with the findings?

a.  Anemia
b.  Carbon monoxide poisoning
c.  Hypoventilation
d.  Low $\dot{V}/\dot{Q}$ ratio
e.  Right-to-left shunt

**186.** A 10-year-old girl presents in the pediatrician's office with a nonproductive cough, wheezing, and shortness of breath. Her mother reports that these symptoms have been episodic over the past two years, but this time her daughter has been getting worse over the past several days. Using a screening pulmonary function machine in the office, the girl first generated curve #1. Subsequent to administration of an inhaled bronchodilator, she generated curve #2. What is the most likely explanation for the increased flow measured in curve #2?

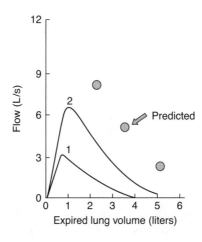

a. Increased patient effort
b. Mast cell degranulation in bronchial smooth muscle
c. Activation of $\alpha$-adrenergic receptors in bronchial smooth muscle
d. Increased parasympathetic nerve discharge to bronchial smooth muscle
e. Stimulation of $\beta_2$-adrenergic receptors in bronchial smooth muscle

**187.** A 58-year-old woman experiences an acute exacerbation of asthma, which causes her breathing to become labored and faster. As a result, which of the following changes in airflow is expected?

a. Flow in the trachea and upper airways will become more laminar.
b. The pressure gradient required for airflow will increase.
c. The resistance to airflow will decrease.
d. The resistance to airflow will increase linearly with the decrease in airway radius.
e. Reynolds number will decrease.

**188.** A 54-year-old man with severe asbestosis reports worsening of his dyspnea. Pulmonary function tests are ordered and the patient is instructed to take in a maximal inspiration and then to exhale as hard and fast as he can to generate a maximal expiratory flow-volume (MEFV) curve. As a result, the patient generates curve C shown below:

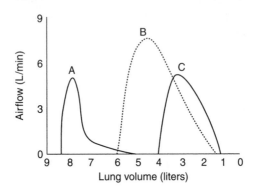

The patient's MEFV curve is consistent with which of the following sets of values?

|   | FVC (liters) | FVC (% predicted) | FEV$_1$ (liters) | FEV$_1$ (% predicted) | FEV$_1$/FVC |
|---|---|---|---|---|---|
| a. | 4.2 | 85 | 3.4 | 90 | 81 |
| b. | 4.2 | 85 | 2.1 | 32 | 50 |
| c. | 3.1 | 48 | 2.8 | 50 | 90 |
| d. | 3.1 | 48 | 2.0 | 40 | 65 |
| e. | 1.5 | 25 | 1.0 | 20 | 67 |

**189.** Noninvasive color Doppler ultrasound studies are ordered on a term infant and a preterm infant of 28-weeks' gestation. Which of the following is likely to have a lower value in the preterm infant compared to the term infant?

a. Pulmonary artery pressure
b. Pulmonary blood flow
c. Pulmonary vascular resistance
d. Pulmonary capillary hydrostatic pressure
e. Blood flow from the pulmonary artery through the ductus arteriosus

**190.** A 35-year-old woman with gestational diabetes develops hypertension and preeclampsia, requiring the preterm delivery of her fetus of 30-weeks' gestation. The mother is given two doses of betamethasone, 12 mg, intramuscularly, 24 hours apart. Which of the following is the purpose of the antenatal steroid therapy?

a. Increase fetal $P_{O_2}$
b. Increase blood flow to the fetal lungs
c. Shift the fetal oxyhemoglobin dissociation curve to the right
d. Increase blood flow from the right atrium into the left atrium across the foramen ovale
e. Increase the lecithin/sphingomyelin ratio in the amniotic fluid

**191.** A 62-year-old man with congestive heart failure (CHF) develops increasing shortness of breath in the recumbent position. A chest x-ray reveals cardiomegaly, horizontal lines perpendicular to the lateral lung surface indicative of increased opacity in the pulmonary septa, and lung consolidation. Pulmonary edema in CHF is promoted by which of the following?

a. Decreased pulmonary interstitial oncotic pressure
b. Increased pulmonary capillary hydrostatic pressure
c. Increased pulmonary capillary oncotic pressure
d. Increased pulmonary interstitial hydrostatic pressure
e. Decreased pulmonary capillary permeability

**192.** A 76-year-old patient with emphysema presents for his annual pulmonary function testing to assess the progression of his disease. As a result of alveolar septal departitioning in emphysema, there is a decrease in which of the following?

a. Airway resistance
b. Alveolar dead space
c. Diffusing capacity
d. Lung compliance
e. Total lung capacity

**193.** A patient with a myocardial infarction develops progressive dyspnea and hypoxemia suggestive of cardiogenic shock. She is transferred to the medical intensive care unit and a Swan-Ganz catheter is inserted. The patient is found to have a pulmonary artery wedge pressure of 30 mm Hg, which is indicative of a decrease in which of the following?

a. Left atrial pressure
b. Left ventricular end-diastolic pressure
c. Left ventricular preload
d. Net fluid absorption into the pulmonary capillaries
e. Pulmonary capillary hydrostatic pressure

**194.** A 68-year-old man with chronic obstructive pulmonary disease entered the emergency department complaining of shortness of breath. His respirations were 35 per minute and labored. He had a productive cough and rales were heard over all lung fields. The patient had a rather ashen complexion and his nail beds gave clear evidence of cyanosis. An arterial blood sample was obtained and a chest x-ray was ordered. The patient was then placed on an $O_2$ mask delivering 40% $O_2$. One-half hour later, the physician was called to the bedside by the nurse who found the patient unresponsive. The patient's complexion had changed to a flushed pink with no trace of cyanosis. His respirations were quiet at a rate of 6 per minute and a tidal volume of 300 mL. Repeat arterial blood gases showed that his arterial $Pco_2$ had increased from 55 to 70 mm Hg, and his $Pao_2$ increased from 55 to 70 mm Hg. Oxygen therapy most likely resulted in which of the following?

a. Alveolar hypoventilation
b. Hypoxic pulmonary vasoconstriction
c. Increased firing of carotid body chemoreceptors
d. Elimination of the hypercapnic drive
e. Oxygen toxicity

**195.** A scientist doing experiments with sodium cyanide started experiencing headache, dizziness, clumsiness, decreased visual acuity, and nausea. The medical student doing research in the laboratory was not certain if this was unusual behavior for the professor, but thought it best to take him to the emergency department to be evaluated for possible hypoxia. Blood values obtained on the professor while he was breathing room air were as follows:

| | |
|---|---|
| Hb: 16 g/dL | $Sao_2$: 97.5% |
| $Pao_2$: 102 mm Hg | $Pvo_2$: 65 mm Hg |
| $Paco_2$: 27 mm Hg | $Svo_2$: 90% |
| pH: 7.57 | Cardiac output: 5.6 L/min |
| $[HCO_3^-]$: 23 mEq/L | |

The professor's hypoxia is most likely the result of which of the following?

a. Hypoxemia
b. Impaired hemoglobin oxygen transport
c. Impaired oxygen delivery
d. Impaired oxygen utilization
e. Impaired diffusion across the alveolar-capillary membrane

**196.** A 42-week gestation infant is delivered by cesarean section. Which of the following occurs with the baby's first diaphragmatic respiration?

a. $Pao_2$ increases
b. Pulmonary vascular resistance increases
c. Pulmonary capillary hydrostatic pressure increases
d. Systemic vascular resistance decreases
e. All of the fetal vascular channels functionally close

**197.** A 29-year-old woman is admitted to the hospital because of increasing dyspnea and swelling of both feet. An examination of her chest shows a severe pectus excavatum with only 2 cm of space between the vertebral bodies and the sternum. Pulmonary function tests show FVC and $FEV_1$/FVC values that were 15% and 100%, respectively, of predicted. Which of the following laboratory measurements will most likely be below normal in this patient?

a. Elastic recoil of the chest wall
b. Arterial $Pco_2$
c. Hemoglobin concentration
d. Plasma bicarbonate concentration
e. Arterial pH

**198.** An 18-year-old male college freshman living in a dormitory contracts meningitis, which causes a centrally mediated increase in his respiratory rate. The pacemaker neurons responsible for respiratory rhythmogenesis are located in which of the following regions of the brain?

a. Apneustic center in the pons
b. Central chemoreceptors in the medulla
c. Inspiratory neurons in the dorsal respiratory group
d. Pontine respiratory groups
e. Pre-Bötzinger complex in the ventral respiratory group

**199.** A 56-year-old man presents to the emergency department with severe abdominal pain and a temperature of 103°F. The patient is in severe respiratory distress. Moderate amounts of pulmonary edema fluid are aspirated during suctioning. The patient is placed on a ventilator with an $F_IO_2$ of 0.5 and an arterial blood gas sample reveals a $Po_2$ of 160 mm Hg and a $Pco_2$ of 40 mm Hg. His alveolar oxygen tension, at a barometric pressure of 747 mm Hg and a respiratory exchange ratio (R) of 0.8, is approximately what?

a. 100 mm Hg
b. 200 mm Hg
c. 300 mm Hg
d. 400 mm Hg
e. 500 mm Hg

**200.** A 68-year-old man who has chronic obstructive pulmonary disease (COPD) presents to his pulmonologist with fatigue, dyspnea at rest, and peripheral edema. His blood gases on room air are $Pao_2$ = 60 mm Hg, $Paco_2$ = 60 mm Hg, and pH = 7.36. His alveolar-arterial (A-a) $O_2$ gradient, at a barometric pressure of 760 mm Hg and a respiratory exchange ratio (R) of 0.8, is approximately what?

a. 5 mm Hg
b. 10 mm Hg
c. 15 mm Hg
d. 20 mm Hg
e. 25 mm Hg

**201.** A 45-year-old man presents at the doctor's office with severe back pain that he attributes to an injury from operating a jackhammer for his job as a cement worker. An MRI of the spine confirms a herniated disk. The patient reports that he smokes 1 to 2 packs of cigarettes a day for the past 30 years, so the neurosurgeon requests pulmonary function studies prior to the patient's back surgery. During a forced expiration, the patient generates an intrapleural pressure of 20 mm Hg. The patient's equal pressure point will move closer to the mouth and forced expiratory volume will increase if there is an increase in which of the following?

a. Inspired lung volume
b. Lung compliance
c. Airway resistance
d. Expiratory effort
e. Airway smooth muscle tone

**202.** A healthy, 24-year-old man is prescribed sustained-release bupropion (Zyban) for smoking cessation. Twenty-one days after therapy he presents to his family physician with intermittent fever and a generalized rash, at which point the bupropion therapy is discontinued. A month later he develops a dry, intermittent cough and dyspnea. Which of the following pulmonary function test results is consistent with a diagnosis of allergic bronchospasm?

a. An increased forced vital capacity
b. A decreased $FEV_1/FVC$
c. An increased diffusing capacity
d. A decreased residual volume
e. An increased lung compliance

**203.** A 5-month-old infant is admitted to the hospital for evaluation because of repeated episodes of sleep apnea. During a ventilatory response test, his ventilation did not increase when $Pa_{CO_2}$ was increased, but decreased during hyperoxia. Which of the following is the most likely cause of this infant's apnea?

a. Bronchospasm
b. Diaphragmatic fatigue
c. Decreased irritant receptor sensitivity
d. Peripheral chemoreceptor hypersensitivity
e. Dysfunctional central chemoreceptors

**204.** A 66-year-old woman presents with a chief complaint of shortness of breath accompanying alternating chills and spiking fever. She has an increase in heart rate and respiratory rate. The right lower lobe is dull to percussion and increased vocal fremitus and bronchovesicular breathing are auscultated over this region. Ventilation-perfusion ($\dot{V}/\dot{Q}$) abnormalities occurring in a patient with lobar pneumonia will generally cause a decrease in which of the following?

a. Alveolar ventilation
b. Arterial carbon dioxide tension
c. Arterial pH
d. Anion gap
e. A-a gradient for oxygen

**205.** A 72-year-old man with congestive heart failure, paroxysmal nocturnal dyspnea, and orthopnea is referred for pulmonary function testing in the supine and upright positions. Which of the following is higher at the apex of the lung than at the base when a person is upright?

a. Ventilation
b. Blood flow
c. $\dot{V}/\dot{Q}$ ratio
d. $Paco_2$
e. Lung compliance

**206.** A 58-year-old factory worker, who has worked in the insulation industry for over 30 years, develops progressive shortness of breath. His wife has tried to get him to go to the doctor, and he finally relents with the appearance of hemoptysis. A chest x-ray is consistent with an alveolitis from asbestos inhalation. Which of the following is the major route for removal of small particles from the alveoli?

a. Bulk flow
b. Diffusion
c. Expectoration
d. Phagocytosis
e. Ciliary transport

**207.** A 65-year-old smoker develops a squamous cell bronchogenic carcinoma, which metastasizes to the tracheobronchial and parasternal lymph nodes. The chest x-ray is consistent with accumulation of fluid in the pulmonary interstitial space. Flow of fluid through the lymphatic vessels will be decreased if there is an increase in which of the following?

a. Capillary pressure
b. Capillary permeability
c. Interstitial protein concentration
d. Capillary oncotic pressure
e. Central venous pressure

**208.** The wife of a recently married 24-year-old medical student reports that even though her husband doesn't snore, he stops breathing for periods of 1 to 2 minutes while he is sleeping. His physician refers him for a polysomnography study and pulmonary function testing, including ventilatory response curves. The tests confirm the apneic episodes during sleep and show depressed ventilatory responsiveness of the peripheral and central chemoreceptors. Both the peripheral and the central chemoreceptors mediate increased ventilation in response to which of the following?

a. Acute hypercapnia
b. Acute metabolic acidosis
c. Chronic hypercapnia
d. Chronic hypertension
e. Chronic hypoxemia

**209.** A 57-year-old woman presents with dyspnea on exertion. Pulmonary function studies with plethysmography demonstrate an increase in the work of breathing, and the oxygen consumption is higher than normal at rest. Which of the following will decrease the oxygen consumption of the respiratory muscles?

a. A decrease in lung compliance
b. A decrease in airway resistance
c. A decrease in the diffusing capacity of the lung
d. An increase in the rate of respiration
e. An increase in tidal volume

**210.** An 18-year-old man is life-flighted to a Level 1 trauma center after being thrown from his motorcycle. It is determined that he has a brain transection above the pons. How will this lesion affect the control of breathing in this patient?

a. All breathing movements will cease.
b. The central chemoreceptors will no longer be able to exert any control over ventilation.
c. The peripheral chemoreceptors will no longer be able to exert any control over ventilation.
d. The Hering-Breuer reflex will be abolished.
e. The limbic system will no longer be able to exert any control over ventilation.

**211.** A 48-year-old coal miner complains of shortness of breath and a productive cough. The history reveals that he has smoked 1 to 2 packs of cigarettes per day since he was 16 years old. Pulmonary function studies are ordered, including an esophageal balloon study to measure intrapleural pressures. Normally, intrapleural pressure is negative throughout a tidal inspiration and expiration because of which of the following?

a. The lungs have the tendency to recoil outward throughout a tidal breath.
b. The chest wall has the tendency to recoil inward throughout a tidal breath.
c. The intact pleura causes the lungs and chest wall to recoil away from each other throughout a tidal breath.
d. The intact pleura causes the lungs and chest wall to recoil in the same direction throughout a tidal breath.
e. There is always a small leak in the visceral pleura causing some air to escape into the pleural space during a tidal breath.

**212.** A 57-year-old man undergoes total knee replacement for severe degenerative joint disease. Four days after surgery, he develops an acute onset of shortness of breath and right-sided pleuritic chest pain. He is now in moderate distress with a respiratory rate of 28 breaths/min, tidal volume of 450 mL, heart rate of 120 bpm, and blood pressure of 125/85 mm Hg. Arterial blood gases on room air at a barometric pressure = 760 mm Hg and R = 0.8 were $Pa_{O_2}$ = 60 mm Hg, $Sa_{O_2}$ = 90%, $Pa_{CO_2}$ = 30 mm Hg, pH = 7.50, $[HCO_3^-]$ = 22 mEq/L, and $P_E_{CO_2}$ = 10 mm Hg. The right lower extremity is healing well, but is red, tender, warm to touch, and has 2+ pitting edema. The most likely cause of these postoperative findings is:

a. Atelectasis
b. Pneumonia
c. Pneumothorax
d. Pulmonary embolism
e. Sepsis

**213.** A 28-year-old male oboe player in the symphony is referred to a pulmonologist due to increasing exertional dyspnea while playing. A complete pulmonary function study is ordered, and the patient is instructed to swallow an esophageal balloon for estimating changes in intrapleural pressures at various lung volumes. The figure below illustrates the change in the patient's intrapleural pressure during a single tidal breath.

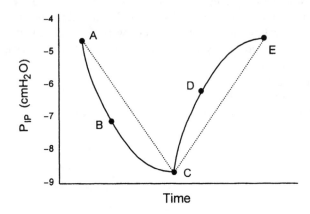

At which point on the diagram is inspiratory airflow the greatest?

a. A
b. B
c. C
d. D
e. E

**214.** A 40-year-old woman is admitted to the intensive care unit with hypotension and shortness of breath. Arterial blood gases reveal a $PaCO_2$ of 10 mm Hg and a bicarbonate concentration of 12 mEq/L. These findings are indicative of which of the following acid-base states?

a. Normal
b. Respiratory acidosis
c. Metabolic acidosis
d. Respiratory alkalosis
e. Metabolic alkalosis

## Questions 215 and 216

A 32-year-old man is hospitalized with severe respiratory disease following aspiration pneumonia. Inhaled nitric oxide is administered and he is placed in a prone position to improve oxygenation. Values obtained after the administration of nitric oxide are:

Mean pulmonary capillary oxygen content = 19 mL/dL
Arterial oxygen content = 18 mL/dL
Mixed venous oxygen content = 14 mL/dL
Cardiac output = 6 L/min

**215.** Which of the following is the patient's shunt fraction (the ratio of shunted to total pulmonary blood flow)?

a. 10%
b. 20%
c. 30%
d. 40%
e. 50%

**216.** What is the patient's oxygen consumption?

a. 200 mL/min
b. 210 mL/min
c. 220 mL/min
d. 230 mL/min
e. 240 mL/min

**217.** A 37-year-old woman is admitted to the hospital with severe kyphoscoliosis and respiratory muscle weakness. Which of the following physiological variables is most likely decreased in this patient?

a. Airway resistance
b. Alveolar surface tension
c. Arterial carbon dioxide tension
d. Chest wall compliance
e. $FEV_{1.0}/FVC$

**218.** An 83-year-old woman is found unresponsive by her son approximately 3 hours after she returned to her hospital room following gall bladder surgery. The nurse reported that the patient had asked for her pain meds and said she was going to rest for a while. Arterial blood gases reveal hypercapnia and hypoxemia. Which of the following is the most likely cause of the high arterial $Pco_2$?

a. Decreased metabolic activity
b. Decreased alveolar dead space
c. Hypoventilation
d. Hypoxemia
e. $\dot{V}/\dot{Q}$ inequality

**219.** A 29-year-old man with AIDS presents with a painful, red, swollen area on top of his shin, which is warm to the touch. He has a fever, tachypnea, and tachycardia, and is hospitalized and started on IV antibiotics. His condition progresses rapidly to septicemia and septic shock. He is transported to the ICU, intubated, and started on mechanical ventilation. A Swan-Ganz catheter is inserted to monitor pulmonary hemodynamics and lung fluid balance. Which of the following conditions will cause a decrease in pulmonary vascular resistance?

a. Alveolar hypoxia
b. Decreased pH in the pulmonary artery
c. Increased cardiac output
d. Inflation of the lungs to total lung capacity
e. Sympathetic stimulation of the pulmonary vessels

**220.** A healthy 32-year-old woman undergoes pulmonary exercise stress testing prior to starting a training regimen in preparation for her first marathon. Normally, during moderate aerobic exercise, which of the following occurs?

a. $Pao_2$ increases
b. $Paco_2$ decreases
c. Arterial pH decreases
d. Alveolar ventilation increases
e. Blood lactate level increases

**221.** A 56-year-old woman presents to her physician complaining of fatigue, headaches, and dyspnea on exertion. She states that she sometimes gets blue lips and fingers when she tries to exercise. Pulmonary function tests reveal an increase, rather than a decrease, in the diffusing capacity of the lung. Which of the following conditions best accounts for an increase in the diffusing capacity?

a. Congestive heart failure
b. COPD
c. Fibrotic lung disease
d. Polycythemia
e. Pulmonary embolism

**222.** A 49-year-old farmer develops a headache and becomes dizzy after working on a tractor in his barn. His wife suspects carbon monoxide poisoning and brings him to the emergency department where he complains of dizziness, lightheadedness, headache, and nausea. The patient's skin is red, he does not appear to be in respiratory distress, and denies dyspnea. Blood levels of carboxyhemoglobin are elevated. Which of the following best explains the absence of respiratory signs and symptoms associated with carbon monoxide poisoning?

a. Blood flow to the carotid body is decreased.
b. Arterial oxygen content is normal.
c. Cerebrospinal fluid pH is normal.
d. Central chemoreceptors are depressed.
e. Arterial oxygen tension is normal.

**223.** A 68-year-old patient with shortness of breath is referred for pulmonary function testing, including lung volumes, flow-volume curves, and lung compliance. Which one of the following statements best characterizes lung compliance?

a. It is equivalent to $\Delta P/\Delta V$.
b. It is inversely related to the elastic recoil properties of the lung.
c. It decreases with advancing age.
d. It increases when there is a deficiency of surfactant.
e. It increases in patients with pulmonary edema.

**224.** A 36-year-old man visits his doctor because his wife has long complained of his snoring, but recently observed that his breathing stops for a couple of minutes at a time while he is sleeping. He undergoes polysomnography and ventilatory response testing to ascertain the extent and cause of his sleep apnea. The activity of the central chemoreceptors is stimulated by which of the following?

a. An increase in the $P_{CO_2}$ of blood flowing through the brain
b. A decrease in the $P_{O_2}$ of blood flowing through the brain
c. An increase in the pH of the CSF
d. A decrease in the metabolic rate of the surrounding brain tissue
e. Hypoxemia, hypercapnia, and metabolic acidosis

**225.** A patient complains of paroxysmal episodes of not being able to catch her breath. When no abnormalities are detected with conventional pulmonary function screening, the pulmonologist orders a methacholine challenge test. Which of the following will increase as a result of stimulating cholinergic receptors on the bronchial smooth muscle?

a. Lung compliance
b. Airway diameter
c. Elastic work of breathing
d. Resistive work of breathing
e. Anatomic dead space

**226.** A 28-year-old woman on oral contraceptives develops tachypnea and reports dyspnea. A ventilation/perfusion scan is ordered to check for pulmonary thromboemboli. Which of the following best explains why, as she takes in a normal inspiration, more air goes to the alveoli at the base of the lung than to the alveoli at the apex of the lung?

a. The alveoli at the base of the lung have more surfactant.
b. The alveoli at the base of the lung are more compliant.
c. The alveoli at the base of the lung have higher $\dot{V}/\dot{Q}$ ratios.
d. There is a more negative intrapleural pressure at the base of the lung.
e. There is more blood flow to the base of the lung.

**227.** A 21-year-old woman presents with cough and shortness of breath. The physician conducts a pulmonary function screening test in his office, and the patient generates the maximum flow-volume curve shown to the right of the normal curve in the diagram below. These findings are consistent with which of the following conditions?

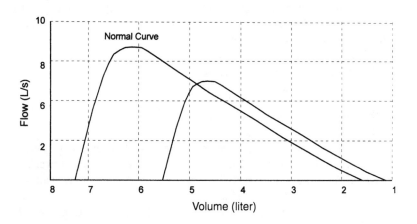

a. Asthma
b. Chronic bronchitis
c. Cystic fibrosis
d. Decreased effort
e. Sarcoidosis

**228.** A 56-year-old man presents for his annual physical examination. His BMI has increased from 28 to 33 over the past year and the fat deposition is mainly around the abdomen. His blood pressure has increased from 125/85 to 140/95 mm Hg since the last visit. Other physical findings are unremarkable and he and his spouse state that he does not snore. Past medical history and social history are insignificant except for his sedentary lifestyle. Exercise stress testing is ordered prior to placing the patient on a regular exercise regimen. Aerobic exercise causes which of the following changes in pulmonary physiology?

a. The overall $\dot{V}/\dot{Q}$ ratio of the lungs decreases.
b. Diffusing capacity of the lungs increases.
c. Mean pulmonary artery pressure decreases.
d. Pulmonary blood flow decreases.
e. Pulmonary vascular resistance increases.

**229.** A 43-year-old woman develops shortness of breath following a cholecystectomy. Bronchial breath sounds and crackles are heard over all lung fields and the lungs are dull on percussion. A chest x-ray demonstrates a pattern of diffuse opacification characteristic of atelectasis. Intrapulmonary shunting will cause which of the following changes in arterial blood gas values?

| | pH | $Paco_2$ | $Pao_2$ |
|---|---|---|---|
| A. | ↑ | ↓ | ↑ |
| B. | ↑ | ↓ | ↓ |
| C. | ↓ | ↓ | ↓ |
| D. | ↓ | ↑ | ↓ |

a. A
b. B
c. C
d. D

**230.** A 49-year-old coal miner presents with dyspnea, a nonproductive cough, and decreased exercise tolerance. Lung function tests reveal: total lung capacity = 3.34 L (56% of predicted), residual volume = 0.88 L (54% of predicted), and forced vital capacity = 1.38 L (30% of predicted). His arterial $P_{O_2}$ is 68 mm Hg. Which of the following values will be approximately normal?

a. Diffusing capacity
b. $FEV_1/FVC$ ratio
c. Functional residual capacity
d. Lung compliance
e. $\dot{V}/\dot{Q}$ ratio

**231.** A 43-year-old woman with a history of asthma presents to the emergency department with an acute asthma attack after her bronchodilator inhaler ran out the day before. Airway resistance is greater

a. With laminar flow than with turbulent flow
b. At lower values for Reynolds number
c. During inspiration compared to expiration
d. At low lung volumes compared to high lung volumes
e. In the total cross section of the small airways compared to the total cross section of the central airways

**232.** A 78-year-old woman presents to her family physician's office with a chief complaint of fatigue and shortness of breath. The doctor indicates that he wants her to go to the hospital to get some pulmonary function tests, but there is one he is able to do in the office. A spirometer can be used to directly measure which of the following?

a. Functional residual capacity
b. Peak flow rate
c. Residual volume
d. Total lung capacity
e. Vital capacity

**233.** A patient with Wegener glomerulonephritis presents with sinusitis and hemoptysis. His chest radiograph shows several large cavitary pulmonary nodules, consistent with ventilation-perfusion imbalance with low $\dot{V}/\dot{Q}$ units. Which of the following will be greater than normal in a patient with a low $\dot{V}/\dot{Q}$ ratio?

a. $Paco_2$
b. $Pao_2$
c. A-a gradient
d. Oxygen dissolved in blood
e. Oxygen combined with hemoglobin

**234.** An 18-year-old woman presents to her primary care physician with an increased frequency of asthma exacerbations over the previous year. At the time of her visit, her physical examination and flow-volume loop are normal. At which point on the flow-volume loop pictured below will airflow remain constant despite an increased respiratory effort?

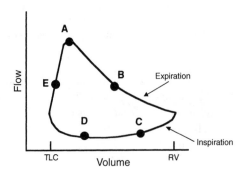

a. A
b. B
c. C
d. D
e. E

# Respiratory Physiology

## *Answers*

**164. The answer is e.** (*Fauci, p 1586. Ganong, pp 651-652. Levitzky, pp 54-57.*) Expiratory reserve volume (ERV) is the maximal volume of gas that can be exhaled in excess of a passive, tidal expiration. The ERV is not labeled in the diagram, but can be calculated from the difference between the functional residual capacity (FRC) and the residual volume (RV), designated as E and D, respectively. The FRC is the volume of gas remaining in the lungs following a passive, tidal exhalation. The RV is the volume of gas remaining in the lungs following a maximal expiration. The inspiratory reserve volume (IRV) is designated by A, the inspiratory capacity (IC) by B, and the vital capacity (VC) by C in the figure.

**165. The answer is c.** (*Ganong, pp 647-648, 684-685. Levitzky, pp 71-73, 234-235.*) According to Dalton law, the partial pressure of a gas is the product of the fractional composition of the gas and the total pressure of the gaseous mixture. Oxygen constitutes approximately 21% of dry atmospheric air. Therefore, the partial pressure of $O_2$ in dry atmospheric air equals the fractional concentration of oxygen ($F_IO_2$) times the atmospheric (barometric) pressure. At sea level, the barometric pressure is 760 mm Hg, yielding a $P_IO_2$ of 160 mm Hg. At high altitude, the barometric pressure decreases in proportion to the decreased weight of the air above it. At an elevation of 18,000 ft in the Peruvian Andes, the barometric pressure is 380 mm Hg, yielding a $P_IO_2$ of 80 mm Hg. Once inside the respiratory tract, the inspired air becomes warmed and humidified. The partial pressure of $H_2O$ vapor is temperature-, rather than concentration-dependent, and at body temperature (37°C) is 47 mm Hg. The presence of $H_2O$ vapor reduces the partial pressure of the other gases in the atmosphere, and the $PH_2O$ must be subtracted from the total barometric pressure before multiplying by the fractional concentration of a gas to yield the partial pressure of the gas. Thus, at sea level, the humidified $P_IO_2$ in the conducting airways is 0.21 (760-47) or 150 mm Hg, whereas, at 18,000 ft, the humidified, tracheal $Po_2$ would be 0.21 (380-47) or 70 mm Hg.

**166. The answer is c.** (*Ganong, pp 647-648. Levitzky, pp 71-73.*) Room air contains 21% $O_2$ and 0.04% $CO_2$, yielding a $P_IO_2$ of 160 mm Hg and a $P_Ico_2$

of 0.3 mm Hg. Thus, if a sample of arterial blood is equilibrated with room air, the measured $Pa_{O_2}$ will have an inaccurately high reading and the $Pa_{CO_2}$ will have an inaccurately low reading. For this reason, collecting an "anaerobic" blood sample is critical in blood gas analysis. Also, once the sample is obtained, the syringe should be placed in a container of crushed ice to prevent any metabolism by the red blood cells, which can also affect the accuracy of the readings. In addition to being certain that an air bubble is not left in the syringe, it is best to use a glass rather than a plastic syringe because the arterial pressure will pump the blood sample into a glass syringe without requiring aspiration, and glass is more impermeable to the diffusion of gases than plastic. A plastic syringe is permissible if one is drawing the blood sample from an arterial line rather than doing an arterial "stick" and if the sample is promptly analyzed.

**167. The answer is a.** (*Fauci, pp 1586-1592, 1643-1651. Ganong, pp 660-661. Levitzky, pp 44-46, 58, 137-141, 265, 550. Stead, pp 255-257.*) In pulmonary fibrosis, the diffusing capacity of the lung is decreased due to an increase in the thickness of the diffusional barrier, as predicted by Fick law of diffusion. Pulmonary fibrosis causes "stiff" lungs, and is characterized by a decrease in lung compliance and an increase in lung elastic recoil. This results in pulmonary function findings typical of a restrictive impairment, including a decrease in all lung volumes and capacities and a ratio of the forced expiratory volume exhaled in one second ($FEV_{1.0}$) to the total forced vital capacity (FVC) that is normal or increased. Although airway resistance is increased at lower lung volumes, the airway resistance in restrictive disorders is normal when corrected for lung volume. An increased airway resistance is the hallmark of an obstructive impairment.

**168. The answer is b.** (*Fauci, pp 731-735, 1588-1592, 1651-1657. Levitzky, pp 114-117. Stead, pp 272-273.*) A pulmonary thromboembolism results in areas of the lung that are ventilated, but not perfused, yielding $\dot{V}/\dot{Q}$ ratios of infinity and an increase in alveolar dead space. When the $\dot{V}/\dot{Q}$ ratio equals ∞, the $P_{A_{O_2}}$ of the affected alveoli will be the same as that in the humidified inspired air because atmospheric air enters the alveoli via the process of ventilation but no gas exchange takes place because the alveoli are not perfused. Areas of the lung that are perfused but not ventilated constitute areas of shunting (venous admixture), characterized as a $\dot{V}/\dot{Q}$ ratio equal to 0, and having $P_{A_{O_2}}$ values that equilibrate with the mixed venous blood.

**169. The answer is c.** (*Ganong, pp 658-660. Levitzky, pp 67-71.*) Physiological dead space is the volume of the respiratory tract that is ventilated but not perfused by the pulmonary circulation. Bohr equation for determination of the ratio of the physiologic deadspace ($V_D$) to the tidal volume ($V_T$) is

$$V_D/V_T = \text{Paco}_2 - \text{P}_\text{E}\text{CO}_2/\text{Paco}_2$$
$$V_D/V_T = 40 - 28/40 = 0.3$$
$$V_D/V_T \times V_T = V_D$$
$$0.3 \times 600 \text{ mL} = 180 \text{ mL}$$

Physiologic deadspace volume = anatomic + alveolar deadspace

Anatomic dead space can be measured by Fowler technique, but is often estimated as 1 mL per pound of body weight. Because there is normally no alveolar deadspace, physiologic deadspace volume approximates anatomic deadspace volume in persons with normal lung function.

**170. The answer is e.** (*Ganong, pp 654-658. Levitzky, pp 20-28.*) Lung compliance is defined as the ease with which the lungs are expanded, and is calculated as the change in volume per change in pressure ($\Delta V/\Delta P$), which is the slope of the pressure-volume curve of the lung. Thus, curve Z is the pressure-volume curve of an individual with a decrease in lung compliance. The abnormal accumulation of fluid in the lungs (pulmonary edema) causes a restrictive pulmonary impairment characterized by a decreased lung compliance. An L/S ratio ≥2 indicates normal biochemical maturation of the lung, with normal surfactant production and lung compliance (normal curve). If the L/S ratio is less than 2, such as may occur in preterm infants, there is an increased incidence of respiratory distress syndrome of the newborn, a restrictive impairment that would be characterized by curve Z. Aging and emphysema are characterized by an increase in lung compliance (curve X), which increases airway resistance. The increase in airway resistance in asthma is not associated with an increase (or decrease) in lung compliance.

**171. The answer is a.** (*Fauci, pp 1560-1561. Ganong, p 688. Levitzky, pp 12-14, 113-117. Stead, pp 273-274.*) When air enters the pleural space due to interruption of the pleural surface through either the rupture of the lung or a hole in the chest wall, the pressure in the pleural space becomes atmospheric, the lung on the affected side collapses because of the lung's tendency to recoil inward, and the chest wall on the affected side recoils outward. Because the intrapleural pressure is atmospheric, the mediastinum shifts farther to the normal side with each inspiration. With collapse of the lung, the $\dot{V}/\dot{Q}$ ratio on the affected side decreases.

**172. The answer is b.** *(Fauci, p 1586-1588, 1596-1607. Ganong, pp 651-652, 688-689. Levitzky, pp 41-46, 58-59, 265. Stead, pp 255-256, 263-265.)* During a forced vital capacity (FVC), the patient is asked to breathe in as much air as possible (up to the total lung capacity), and then exhale all of the gas in her lung as fast as possible, which, in this case is 3.5 L. The $FEV_{1.0}$ is the volume of gas expelled from the lung during the first second, which, in this case, is 2 L. The ratio of the $FEV_{1.0}$ to the FVC in this patient is 2 L/3.5 L, which equals 0.57. Normally, $FEV_{1.0}/FVC$ should be ≥0.8. The decreased $FEV_{1.0}/FVC$ is indicative of an obstructive impairment. Obstructive lung diseases, such as asthma, are characterized by a greater-than-normal total lung capacity (TLC), residual volume (RV), and functional residual capacity (FRC). The inspiratory and expiratory reserves (inspiratory capacity and expiratory volume) are decreased, as is the vital capacity and the maximum voluntary ventilation.

**173. The answer is d.** *(Fauci, p 1606. Ganong, pp 658-660. Levitzky, pp 65-67.)* Alveolar ventilation ($\dot{V}_A$) equals the tidal volume ($V_T$) minus the deadspace volume ($V_D$) times the breathing frequency ($f$). The dead space volume can be estimated as 1 mL/lb of body weight.

$$\dot{V}_A = (V_T - V_D) \times f$$
$$\dot{V}_A = (500 \text{ mL} - 125 \text{ mL}) \times 15 \text{ breaths/min}$$
$$\dot{V}_A = 5625 \text{ mL/min}$$

**174. The answer is c.** *(Levitzky, pp 73-75.)* Because the dead space air does not participate in gas exchange, the entire output of $CO_2$ in the expired gas comes from the alveolar gas. Accordingly, alveolar (and arterial) $P_{CO_2}$ can be expressed in terms of $CO_2$ output and alveolar ventilation according to the equation:

$$P_A CO_2 = Pa CO_2 = \dot{V}_{CO_2}/\dot{V}_A$$

Thus, an increase in alveolar ventilation at a constant rate of carbon dioxide production will lower $P_A CO_2$ and $P_A CO_2$. Hyperventilation increases $P_{AO_2}$

and Pao$_2$, with no change in the alveolar-arterial Po$_2$ difference. The $\dot{V}/\dot{Q}$ will be normal or increased.

**175. The answer is d.** *(Fauci, pp 1137-1138, 1170 -1172, 1267-1269, 1590-1592. Ganong, p 660. Levitzky, p 75. Stead, pp 202-204.)* The alveolar air equation is used to calculate the P$_a$O$_2$.

$$P_AO_2 = P_IO_2 - (Paco_2/R)$$

Given the barometric pressure of 757 mm Hg, F$_I$O$_2$ = 1.0 (100% O$_2$), Paco$_2$ = 36 mm Hg, and R = 0.8, then

$$P_AO_2 = (1.0)(757 - 47) - (36/0.8)$$
$$= 710 - 45 = 665 \text{ mm Hg}$$

*Pneumocystis* is an opportunistic fungal pulmonary pathogen that is an important cause of pneumonia (pneumocystosis) in immunocompromised hosts. HIV patients with a CD4+ cell count below 200/μL have an increased risk of developing *Pneumocystis* pneumonia. According to new, and still evolving nomenclature, *Pneumocystis carinii* is the name of the organism derived from rats, and *Pneumocystis jiroveci* is the name of the organism derived from humans.

**176. The answer is c.** *(Levitzky, pp 11-53.)* As lung volume increases toward total lung capacity (TLC), the compliance of the lungs (slope of pressure-volume curve) decreases and elastic recoil of the lung increases, that is, the lungs resist further expansion. Intrapleural pressure decreases, becoming more subatmospheric during inspiration, approaching −30 cm H$_2$O at TLC. The more subatmospheric (negative compared to zero reference atmospheric pressure) increases radial traction and the transmural pressure across the intrathoracic airways (P$_{in}$ − P$_{out}$) increases, which increases airway radius, and decreases airway resistance according to Poiseuille law. Alveolar surface tension varies inversely with alveolar radius, decreasing at higher alveolar volumes during inspiration.

**177. The answer is c.** *(Fauci, pp 1680-1684. Ganong, pp 654-655. Levitzky, pp 26-28. Stead, p 270.)* Pulmonary surfactant increases lung compliance by lowering alveolar surface tension. As a result, the pressure gradient needed to inflate the alveoli decreases, as does the work of breathing. Although surfactant replacement therapy has proven to be beneficial in respiratory distress syndrome of the newborn, clinical trials of surfactant therapy in ARDS has had disappointing outcomes.

**178. The answer is a.** *(Fauci, pp 1583-1588, 1635-1642. Levitzky, pp 44-46. Stead, pp 255-256.)* Cigarette smoking is the major cause of chronic obstructive pulmonary disease (COPD). In obstructive lung diseases, the increase in airway resistance causes a decrease in expiratory flow rates and "air-trapping," which results in an increased residual volume, and thus total lung capacity. This hyperinflation pushes the diaphragm into a flattened position. Asbestosis and pulmonary fibrosis are restrictive lung diseases, in which curve C would be the typical maximal expiratory flow-volume (MEFV) curve. Decreased effort would decrease flow rates during the effort-dependent portion of a MEFV curve, but not during the effort-independent portion.

**179. The answer is a.** *(Ganong, pp 683-691. Levitzky, pp 181-184.)* Alveolar hypoventilation (as evidenced by the higher-than-normal value of $Paco_2$) is a type of hypoxic hypoxia or hypoxemia (as evidenced by the decreased $Pao_2$). Anemic hypoxia is characterized by a decreased concentration of hemoglobin (anemia) or a reduction in the saturation of hemoglobin with oxygen ($Sao_2$) expected for a given $Pao_2$, as would occur in carbon monoxide poisoning or methemoglobinemia. Stagnant hypoxia is characterized by a decreased cardiac output; in this patient, cardiac output, calculated as

$$(\dot{V}o_2/Cao_2 - Cvo_2)$$

is 5 L/min, which is normal. In histotoxic hypoxia, oxygen extraction is impaired, and thus $Cao_2 - Cvo_2$ would be less than normal and $Svo_2$ would be greater than normal.

**180. The answer is b.** *(Fauci, pp 220, 548-551, 1220-1221. Ganong, pp 672-675, 678-679. Levitzky, pp 195-201.)* The afferent pathway from the carotid body chemoreceptors is Hering nerve, a branch of cranial nerve IX, the glossopharyngeal nerve. The vagus nerve constitutes the afferent pathway from the aortic chemoreceptors, the J receptors, the irritant airway receptors, and the rapidly adapting stretch receptors mediating the Hering-Breuer inflation reflex.

**181. The answer is d.** (*Ganong, pp 683-691. Levitzky, pp 181-184.*) The classification of the causes of hypoxemia (low $Pao_2$) are (1) reduced $P_{A}O_2$ (alveolar hypoventilation or reduced $P_1O_2$ found at high altitude or with breathing low concentrations of oxygen), (2) diffusion impairment, (3) ventilation/perfusion inequality, and (4) right-to-left shunting (venous admixture). Left-to-right shunting does not cause hypoxemia. Administration of 100% $O_2$ corrects the hypoxemia caused by alveolar hypoventilation, diffusion impairment, or ventilation/perfusion inequality, but not that due to right-to-left shunting (venous admixture). Alveolar hypoventilation would have an increased $Paco_2$. In carbon monoxide poisoning, the $Sao_2$ would be lower than normal. On 100% $O_2$, the $Pao_2$ should be $\geq 500$ mm Hg and the A-a $Po_2$ difference should be $\leq 100$ mm Hg. This patient's $Pao_2$ is only 95 mm Hg on 100% $O_2$, indicating the presence of right-to-left shunting, that is, areas of the lung that are perfused but not ventilated ($\dot{V}/\dot{Q}$ ratio = 0). Postoperative complications such as pneumonia, pulmonary edema, and atelectasis are all causes of intrapulmonary right-to-left shunts.

**182. The answer is e.** (*Fauci, p 1589-1592. Ganong, pp 662-663. Levitzky, pp 125-127.*) Even in normal individuals, the dependent lung has a greater ventilation per unit volume and a greater pulmonary blood flow, but because the effects of gravity (hydrostatic pressure) are greater for blood than air because blood is more dense, the increase in perfusion exceeds the increase in ventilation, and the $\dot{V}/\dot{Q}$ ratio decreases. An area with a lower $\dot{V}/\dot{Q}$ has less gas exchange, and thus $Paco_2$ increases and $Pao_2$ decreases. These changes are exacerbated in pneumonia, which causes an increase in the number of low $\dot{V}/\dot{Q}$ areas in the lung. The greater hydrostatic pressure in the dependent lung causes an increased (less negative) intrapleural pressure, which decreases lung volume, and places the pressure-volume curve of the lung on a steeper slope (increased compliance). In patients with unilateral pneumonia, simply positioning the unaffected lung downward may result in improved ventilation-perfusion matching and an increase in $Pao_2$ of 10 to 15 mm Hg.

**183. The answer is a.** (*Ganong, pp 681-683. Levitzky, pp 208-212.*) During exercise, minute ventilation and alveolar ventilation increase linearly with carbon dioxide production up to a level of about 60% of the maximal workload. Above that level, called the anaerobic threshold, muscle lactate spills into the circulation causing a metabolic acidosis, characterized by a decrease in pH and $[HCO_3^-]$. The increased $[H^+]$ stimulates the peripheral (not central) chemoreceptors to increase alveolar ventilation proportionally more than the increase in carbon dioxide production, resulting in a decrease in $Paco_2$.

**184. The answer is c.** *(Ganong, p 650. Levitzky, pp 90-91.)* Pulmonary vascular resistance (PVR) is calculated as:

$$PVR = \Delta P/\dot{Q} = \text{Mean PAP} - \text{mean LAP/pulmonary blood flow}$$
$$= 35 - 15 \text{ mm Hg/4 L/min} = 5 \text{ mm Hg/L/min}$$

**185. The answer is b.** *(Fauci, pp 229-231. Ganong, pp 683-692. Levitzky, pp 153-156, 181-184. Stead, p 253.)* Hemoglobin has 210× greater affinity for carbon monoxide than for oxygen. Thus, in carbon monoxide poisoning, the amount of dissolved oxygen, as reflected by the $Pao_2$ may be normal, but the saturation of hemoglobin with oxygen will be lower than expected for a given $Pao_2$. $\dot{V}/\dot{Q}$ mismatch with low $\dot{V}/\dot{Q}$ units, hypoventilation, and right-to-left shunting are all causes of hypoxemia (decreased $Pao_2$). In anemia, hemoglobin concentration is reduced, but the saturation of hemoglobin $O_2$ is normal.

**186. The answer is e.** *(Fauci, pp 1596-1605. Ganong, p 654. Levitzky, pp 32-36, 44-48.)* Reversibility of airway obstruction is assessed by the change in expiratory flow rate before and after administration of a bronchodilator. The mechanism of action of many bronchodilator drugs is stimulation of $\beta_2$-adrenergic receptors, which leads to an increase in expiratory airflow due to a decrease in airway resistance resulting from an increase in airway radius as predicted by Poiseuille law. In contrast, stimulation of $\alpha$-adrenergic receptors on, or parasympathetic nerves to, bronchial smooth muscle, as well as mast cell degranulation, all cause bronchoconstriction, which would decrease expiratory flow rates. An increased effort would increase expiratory airflow on the effort-dependent portion of the maximal expiratory flow-volume curve, but not the effort-independent portion.

**187. The answer is b.** *(Ganong, pp 582-585. Levitzky, pp 32-35.)* An increased velocity of airflow will increase turbulent airflow, as predicted by an increased Reynolds number. Resistance to turbulent airflow exceeds that for laminar airflow, and thus the pressure gradient required for airflow increases when flow is turbulent. Because the velocity of airflow is greatest in the trachea and large airways, the predisposition to turbulent airflow is greater in the central than in the peripheral airways. Airway resistance varies inversely with the fourth power of airway radius, according to Poiseuille law.

**188. The answer is c.** *(Fauci, pp 1586-1589, 1612-1614. Levitzky, pp 44-46. Stead, pp 255-257.)* Curve C is the maximal expiratory flow-volume (MEFV) curve typical of a restrictive impairment. In restrictive parenchymal diseases, lung compliance is decreased and lung elastic recoil is increased, causing all lung volumes and capacities to be lower than normal (which eliminates choices a and b) and the $FEV_{1.0}$/FVC ratio to be normal or increased above the normal value of 0.7 (which eliminates choices d and e).

**189. The answer is b.** *(Ganong, pp 627-629.)* In the fetal circulation, pulmonary vascular resistance is increased compared to the term infant or the adult circulation because of (a) the increased muscular media of the pulmonary vessels and (b) the pulmonary vascular $Po_2$ of only approximately 25 mm Hg, which causes hypoxic pulmonary vasoconstriction. As a result, pulmonary artery pressure (PAP), as well as the pulmonary capillary hydrostatic pressure, is greater and pulmonary blood flow is less in the preterm than in the term infant. The greater PAP increases the pressure gradient from the pulmonary artery to the aorta, which increases the flow through the ductus arteriosus in the preterm infant.

**190. The answer is e.** *(Ganong, pp 656-657.)* Maturation of surfactant production in fetal lungs is accelerated by glucocorticoid hormones, which increases the lecithin to sphingomyelin (L/S) ratio of the amniotic fluid. Lecithin (phosphatidylcholine) and sphingomyelin are choline phospholipids found in a variety of tissues. Lecithin is a major component of surfactant and its synthesis increases as the fetus matures and the lungs are prepared for expansion. Surfactant, a lipoprotein mixture, prevents alveolar collapse by permitting the surface tension of the alveolar lining to vary during inspiration and expiration. Thus, measurement of the L/S ratio in amniotic fluid provides an index of fetal lung maturity.

**191. The answer is b.** *(Fauci, pp 224, 233-234, 1446, 1706. Ganong, pp 592-594, 662. Levitzky, pp 107-110. Stead, pp 25-26.)* In congestive heart failure, left ventricular dysfunction increases left ventricular end-diastolic pressure, which raises left atrial pressure, pulmonary venous pressure, and pulmonary capillary pressure, which is the hydrostatic pressure tending to drive fluid movement out of the pulmonary capillaries, according to Starling law. Thus, pulmonary edema, generally limited to the interstitium of the lungs, is a hallmark of congestive heart failure. All of the other responses would act to decrease fluid movement out of the capillary, in accordance with Starling law.

**192. The answer is c.** *(Ganong, pp 654-655, 660-661, 689. Levitzky, pp 22-23, 37-58, 137-140.)* Destruction of the alveolar septa in emphysema causes a loss of pulmonary capillaries, which decreases the surface area available for diffusion, and therefore decreases the rate of diffusion in accordance with Fick law. Alveolar septal departitioning with destruction of pulmonary capillaries results in enlargement of the air spaces distal to the terminal bronchioles and an increase in alveolar dead space, that is, alveoli that are ventilated but not perfused. Elastic fibers are also found in the alveolar septa. In emphysema, the destruction of elastic fibers decreases lung elastic recoil, and increases lung compliance. The loss of elastic recoil increases intrapleural pressures, which decreases transmural pressure across the noncartilaginous airways (less radial traction), which decreases airway caliber and increases airway resistance in accordance with Poiseuille law. In addition, the loss of elastic recoil impairs the ability to oppose dynamic compression of the airways. As a result, dynamic compression occurs closer to the alveoli during forced expirations, resulting in air trapping and an increase in residual volume and total lung capacity.

**193. The answer is d.** *(Fauci, pp 1702-1707. Ganong, pp 592-594, 662. Levitzky, pp 107-110. Stead, pp 25-26.)* Pulmonary artery wedge pressure (PAWP) measured with a Swan-Ganz catheter is an index of the pulmonary capillary hydrostatic pressure. Normal PAWP is ≤12 mm Hg. Thus, an elevated PAWP of 30 mm Hg will drive fluid movement out of the pulmonary capillaries, according to Starling law, thereby decreasing net fluid reabsorption into the pulmonary capillaries. Because of the paucity of smooth muscle in the pulmonary vasculature, pulmonary vascular resistance is distributed evenly across the arterioles, capillaries, and venules and there is a steady decline in pressures across the pulmonary circulation, with no large pressure drop across any element, such as seen in the systemic arterioles. As a result, PAWP is also an index of the pressures downstream in the left atrium and in the left ventricle at the end of diastole; that is, PAWP is an index of left ventricular preload.

**194. The answer is a.** *(Fauci, p 1641. Ganong, pp 684, 691. Levitzky, pp 156, 181-182, 202-209. Stead, pp 262-263.)* The hypercapnic drive for breathing is attenuated in COPD patients with chronic hypercapnia because compensated respiratory acidosis in the cerebrospinal fluid eliminates the direct stimulus to the central chemoreceptors. Because alveolar ventilation also causes hypoxemia, the decrease in $Pa_{O_2}$ stimulating the peripheral chemoreceptors (hypoxic drive) becomes the primary drive to breathe in chronic hypercapnia. Although supplemental oxygen is the only pharmacologic therapy demonstrated to decrease mortality in patients with COPD, administration of too high of an oxygen concentration can raise $Pa_{O_2}$ above the threshold necessary for adequate firing of the peripheral chemoreceptors, which will "knock out" the hypoxic drive and cause an $O_2$-induced hypoventilation, as evidenced by a further rise in $Pa_{CO_2}$. The potential for $O_2$-induced hypoventilation should not be a deterrent to oxygen therapy when indicated in patients with COPD, as supplemental oxygen is the only therapy for COPD shown to extend life, in addition to improving IQ, exercise tolerance, and cor pulmonale.

**195. The answer is d.** *(Fauci, pp 229-231. Ganong, pp 683-691. Levitzky, pp 181-184.)* Cyanide impairs oxidative phosphorylation, which impairs the ability of the tissues to utilize oxygen causing hypoxia. In histotoxic hypoxia, oxygen extraction ($Ca_{O_2}$-$Cv_{O_2}$) is impaired, as evidenced by greater-than-normal values of $Pv_{O_2}$ (normal = 40 mm Hg) and $Sv_{O_2}$ (normal = 75%). The patient is not hypoxemic and does not have a diffusion defect because $Pa_{O_2}$ is not lower than normal (80 to 100 mm Hg). Hemoglobin oxygen transport is not impaired because both hemoglobin concentration and hemoglobin saturation with oxygen are normal. Oxygen delivery is not impaired because both cardiac output and arterial oxygen content are normal.

**196. The answer is a.** *(Ganong, pp 628-629.)* With the first diaphragmatic respiration in extrauterine life, the lungs replace the placenta as the organ of gas exchange and the infant's Pao$_2$ increases, which attenuates the hypoxic pulmonary vasoconstriction present in the fetus, causing pulmonary vascular resistance and pressures to decrease. The increased Pao$_2$ constricts the systemic vessels, and, coupled with elimination of the placental circulation, which contributes 40% of the cardiac output in the fetus, results in a rise in systemic vascular resistance. Five of the six vascular channels functionally close at birth, but the ductus arteriosus remains open normally for approximately 48 hours (though ductal flow is reversed from that in fetal life).

**197. The answer is e.** (*Fauci, pp 1586-1588, 2468. Levitzky, pp 20-23, 41-42. Stead, pp 255-257.*) The low FVC (forced vital capacity) with a normal FEV$_1$/FVC ratio is indicative of a severe restrictive impairment, consistent with the presentation of pectus excavatum, an abnormal formation of the rib cage where the breastbone caves in, resulting in a sunken chest appearance. As a result, hypoventilation (increased Paco$_2$) and respiratory acidosis (decreased pH) would ensue. To compensate for the respiratory acidosis, arterial bicarbonate concentration would increase. The decreased chest wall compliance in pectus excavatum would increase the elastic recoil of the chest wall.

**198. The answer is e.** (*Ganong, pp 192-193, 671-673. Levitzky, pp 189-195, 207-209.*) The main components of the respiratory control pattern generator for the automatic control of breathing are located in the medulla. The basic respiratory rhythm is initiated by a small group of synaptically coupled pacemaker cells in the pre-Bötzinger complex on either side of the medulla between the nucleus ambiguus and the lateral reticular nucleus in an area called the ventral respiratory group. This basic rhythm can be modified by many factors, including higher centers in the cerebral cortex and hypothalamus and input from the reticular activating system and pontine respiratory centers.

**199. The answer is c.** (*Levitzky, pp 75, 264.*) The alveolar oxygen tension is calculated using the modified alveolar gas equation:

$$P_{A}O_2 = P_{I}O_2 - Paco_2/R$$
$$P_{A}O_2 = [0.5 \times (747 - 47 \text{ mm Hg})] - 40 \text{ mm Hg}/0.8$$
$$P_{A}O_2 = 350 \text{ mm Hg} - 50 \text{ mm Hg} = 300 \text{ mm Hg}$$

**200. The answer is c.** *(Levitzky, pp 75, 181-182, 264.)* The A-a $O_2$ gradient is the partial pressure difference between the alveolar gas and arterial blood. The $Pa_{O_2}$ has been measured. The alveolar oxygen tension must be calculated using the modified alveolar gas equation

$$P_{A}O_2 = P_{I}O_2 - Pa_{CO_2}/R$$
$$P_{A}O_2 = [0.21 \times (760 - 47 \text{ mm Hg})] - 60 \text{ mm Hg}/0.8$$
$$P_{A}O_2 = 150 \text{ mm Hg} - 75 \text{ mm Hg} = 75 \text{ mm Hg}$$
$$(A\text{-}a) \ O_2 \text{ gradient} = 75 \text{ mm Hg} - 60 \text{ mm Hg} = 15 \text{ mm Hg}$$

The patient's low arterial oxygen tension (hypoxemia; hypoxic hypoxia) results from a low $P_{A}O_2$ due to hypoventilation (as evidenced by the elevated $Pa_{CO_2}$), and thus the (A-a) $O_2$ gradient is within the normal range.

**201. The answer is a.** *(Levitzky, pp 37-40.)* The equal pressure point is the point at which the pressure inside the airways equals the intrapleural pressure. The intra-airway pressure closest to the alveoli equals the sum of the recoil pressure (exerted by the alveoli) and the intrapleural pressure (produced by the muscles of expiration). The equal pressure point moves further away from the lungs if the recoil force is increased and moves closer to the lungs when the intrapleural pressure is increased. Increasing the lung volume expands the alveoli, making their recoil force greater and the intrapleural pressure less (more negative). This moves the equal pressure point toward the mouth. If airway resistance increases by increasing airway smooth muscle tone or increasing lung compliance, then a greater expiratory effort and consequently a greater intrapleural pressure will be necessary to expel the gas from the lungs. The higher intrapleural pressure when airway resistance is increased will cause the equal pressure point to be reached closer to the alveoli, decreasing the volume of gas exhaled, and increasing residual volume due to air trapping behind the compressed airways.

**202. The answer is b.** *(Levitzky, pp 32-48.)* Bronchospasm increases the resistance to airflow, which makes it more difficult to expel gas rapidly from the lung during expiration, so although both $FEV_1$ and vital capacity decrease, the percent of gas expelled in 1 second as a function of the total amount that can be expelled (the $FEV_1/FVC$ ratio) also decreases dramatically. Obstructive disease also produces air trapping, which increases the residual volume, functional residual capacity, and total lung capacity.

**203. The answer is e.** (*Ganong, pp 672-678, 693-694. Levitzky, pp 199-200, 202-211.*) The central chemoreceptors play the major role in providing the normal drive to breathe. They respond to changes in [$H^+$] in the cerebrospinal fluid (CSF), which are brought about by changes in arterial $Pco_2$. The failure of $CO_2$ to significantly increase ventilation indicates that the central chemoreceptors are not functioning properly. The peripheral chemoreceptors are stimulated by hypoxia, hypercapnia, and acidemia, and thus are functioning appropriately because ventilation decreased when $Po_2$ was increased (hyperoxia) and increased slightly in response to an increase in arterial $Pco_2$. Obstructive sleep apnea is caused by upper airway obstruction due to hypotonic pharyngeal or genioglossus muscles or too much fat around the pharynx, but not because of obstruction of the tracheobronchial tree by bronchospasm. Diaphragmatic fatigue can cause hypoventilation, but is not associated with apneic episodes, perhaps because of the increased contribution of the accessory muscles of respiration. The reflex effect of stimulation of the irritant receptors by mechanical or chemical irritation of the airways is bronchoconstriction and cough.

**204. The answer is b.** (*Fauci, pp 1584-1585. Ganong, pp 662, 672-677, 686-688. Levitzky, pp 113-116, 174-175, 180-183, 210-211.*) $\dot{V}/\dot{Q}$ mismatches will cause arterial oxygen levels ($Pao_2$) to decrease. A decreased $Pao_2$ will stimulate the peripheral chemoreceptors, which, in turn, will increase alveolar ventilation and decrease $Paco_2$. The decreased $Paco_2$ will cause a respiratory alkalosis (increasing pH). Hypoxemia may also cause lactate levels to rise, increasing the anion gap (and blunting the rise in pH). The fall in $Pao_2$ causes the A-a gradient to rise.

**205. The answer is c.** (*Ganong, pp 643-644, 662-663, 686-688. Levitzky, pp 125-128. Stead, pp 25-27.*) The alveoli at the apex of the lung are larger than those at the base so their compliance is less. Because the compliance is reduced, less inspired gas goes to the apex than to the base. Also, because the apex is above the heart, less blood flows through the apex than through the base. However, the reduction in airflow is less than the reduction in blood flow, so that the $\dot{V}/\dot{Q}$ ratio at the top of the lung is greater than it is at the bottom. The increased $\dot{V}/\dot{Q}$ ratio at the apex makes $P_ACO_2$ lower and $P_AO_2$ higher at the apex than they are at the base.

**206. The answer is d.** (*Ganong, pp 664-665. Levitzky, pp 216-222. Stead, pp 276-277.*) The lung has a variety of mechanisms to remove particulate matter from the inspired gas. Large particles become deposited in the mucus layer that lies within the bronchi. The mucus is swept up and out of the bronchioles by the ciliated epithelial cells that line the bronchioles. Smaller particles remain suspended in the inspired gas and reach the alveoli. Alveolar macrophages remove these particles by phagocytosis. The macrophages are usually removed from the lung through the lymphatic or blood circulation.

**207. The answer is d.** (*Ganong, pp 592-594.*) Lymph flow is proportional to the amount of fluid filtered out of the capillaries. The amount of fluid filtered out of the capillaries depends on the Starling forces and capillary permeability. Increasing capillary oncotic pressure directly decreases filtration by increasing the hydrostatic (osmotic) force drawing water into the capillary. Increasing capillary pressure, capillary permeability, and interstitial protein concentration (oncotic pressure) all directly increase lymph flow. When venous pressure is increased, the capillary hydrostatic pressure is increased and, again, capillary filtration is increased. Lymph flow is normally approximately 2 to 3 L per day.

**208. The answer is a.** (*Fauci, pp 1665-1668. Ganong, pp 662, 672-677, 686-688. Levitzky, pp 205-209.*) Both the central chemoreceptors, located on or near the ventral surface of the medulla, and the peripheral chemoreceptors, in the carotid and aortic bodies, cause an increase in ventilation in response to an acute increase in $Paco_2$. The peripheral chemoreceptors also cause an increase in ventilation in response to a decrease in arterial pH and a decrease in $Pao_2$. The central chemoreceptors are unresponsive to hypoxemia (acute or chronic). In addition, the central chemoreceptors do not mediate the increase in ventilation in response to a decrease in arterial pH because the blood-brain barrier is relatively impermeable to hydrogen ions. Neither the central chemoreceptors nor the carotid bodies are stimulated by an increase in arterial blood pressure; hypertension may elicit apnea as a result of baroreceptor stimulation.

**209. The answer is b.** (*Ganong, pp 657-658. Levitzky, pp 49-51.*) Respiratory muscles consume oxygen in proportion to the work of breathing. The work of breathing is equal to the product of the change in volume for each breath and the change in pressure necessary to overcome the resistive work of breathing and the elastic work of breathing. Resistive work includes work to overcome tissue as well as airway resistance; thus a decreased airway resistance will decrease the work of breathing and the oxygen consumption of the respiratory muscles. A decreased lung compliance would increase the elastic work of breathing. An increase in respiratory rate or tidal volume increases the work of breathing.

**210. The answer is e.** (*Ganong, pp 671-679. Levitzky, pp 189-198.*) Transection of the brainstem above the pons would prevent any voluntary changes in ventilation by cutting the pathways from the higher centers. Breathing would continue because the pontine-medullary centers that control rhythmic ventilation would be intact. Inputs to the brainstem from the central and peripheral chemoreceptors that stimulate ventilation and from lung stretch receptors that inhibit inspiration (Hering-Breuer reflex) would also be intact and these reflexes would be maintained.

**211. The answer is c.** (*Ganong, pp 655-665. Levitzky, pp 12-23, 29-32.*) When the pleura, and hence the lung-chest wall system, are intact, the inward elastic recoil of the lung opposing the outward elastic recoil of the chest wall results in a subatmospheric (negative) pressure within the pleural space. When one reaches lung volumes in excess of approximately 70% of the total lung capacity, the chest wall recoil is also inward.

**212. The answer is d.** (*Fauci, 731-735, 1651-1657.*) All of these are postoperative complications, but the presentation is most closely associated with the development of a pulmonary thromboembolism secondary to venous stasis in the extremity. The patient's deadspace-to-tidal volume ratio is 0.67 in contrast to a normal value in the range from 0.2 to 0.4. The increase in deadspace ventilation indicates that there is an increase in the volume of the respiratory track that is ventilated, but not perfused. Pulmonary embolism is a deadspace-producing disease, whereas, pneumonia, atelectasis, and pneumothorax are all shunt-producing diseases, that is, they increase the volume of the respiratory track that is perfused but not ventilated.

**213. The answer is b.** (*Ganong, pp 651-655. Levitzky, pp 17-20.*) During inspiration (curve **ABC**), the respiratory muscles pull the chest wall out and diaphragm down and intrapleural pressure ($P_{IP}$) becomes more negative (subatmospheric). The muscles must overcome the elastic recoil forces of the lungs and the resistance of the airways to airflow. The $P_{IP}$ necessary to overcome the elastic forces of the lung is depicted by dashed line **AC**. The $P_{IP}$ necessary to overcome the airway resistance is the difference between dashed line **AC** and curve **ABC**. The maximum airflow occurs at point **B**, where the difference between the two is the greatest.

**214. The answer is d.** *(Ganong, pp 732-734. Levitzky, pp 164-181.)* The arterial pH can be calculated using the Henderson-Hasselbalch equation.

$$pH = 6.1 + \log [HCO_3^-]/(Pa_{CO_2} \times 0.03 \text{ mmol/L/mm Hg})$$
$$pH = 6.1 + \log 12 \text{ mmol/L}/(10 \text{ mm Hg} \times 0.03 \text{ mmol/L/mm Hg})$$
$$pH = 6.1 + \log 40 = 6.1 + 1.6 = 7.7$$

The patient has an alkalemia due to hyperventilation and therefore is suffering from a respiratory alkalosis. In an acute respiratory alkalosis, the bicarbonate typically decreases by 2 mM for each 10 mm Hg decrease in $Pa_{CO_2}$; in a chronic respiratory alkalosis, the bicarbonate typically decreases 4 mM for each 10 mm Hg decrease in $Pa_{CO_2}$. In this case, the $Pa_{CO_2}$ has decreased by 30 mm Hg. Because bicarbonate has decreased by 12 mM, the diagnosis is consistent with a chronic respiratory alkalosis.

**215 and 216. The answers are 215-b, 216-e.** *(Ganong, pp 570-571. Levitzky, pp 120-122, 263.)* The fraction of the pulmonary blood flowing bypassing the lung (the shunt, $\dot{Q}_s$) compared to the total pulmonary blood flow ($\dot{Q}_T$) is calculated using the equation

$$\dot{Q}_s/\dot{Q}_T = C_cO_2 - C_aO_2 / C_cO_2 - C_vO_2$$
$$= \frac{19 \text{ mL/dL} - 18 \text{ mL/dL}}{19 \text{ mL/dL} - 14 \text{ mL/dL}}$$
$$= 0.2$$

where $C_c$ is the end pulmonary capillary blood oxygen content, $Ca_{O_2}$ is the arterial oxygen content, and $C_vO_2$ is the mixed venous oxygen content. At a resting cardiac output, the normal amount of shunting is 3% to 5% of the cardiac output. In this case, there is a 20% shunt.

The oxygen consumption can be calculated if the cardiac output (CO) and the difference between the arterial and venous oxygen content are known using the Fick equation:

$$\dot{V}_{O_2} = CO \times (C_aO_2 - C_vO_2)$$
$$\dot{V}_{O_2} = 6 \text{ L/min} \times (18 \text{ mL/dL} - 14 \text{ mL/dL})$$
$$\dot{V}_{O_2} = 240 \text{ mL/min}$$

**217. The answer is d.** *(Fauci, pp 221-223, 1586-1589, 1661-1664. Levitzky, pp 23, 171-173. Stead, pp 255-257.)* Kyphoscoliosis is a deformity of the spine involving both lateral displacement (scoliosis) and anteroposterior angulation (kyphosis), which decrease the compliance of the chest wall. Decreased chest wall compliance and respiratory muscle weakness cause inadequate alveolar ventilation, which leads to an accumulation of carbon dioxide and a decrease in arterial pH (respiratory acidosis). Restrictive impairments are characterized by a decrease in all lung volumes and capacities, but a normal or increased ratio of $FEV_{1.0}$ to FVC.

**218. The answer is c.** *(Fauci pp 209-210, 1589-1592. Levitzky, pp 65-67, 73-75, 171-172.)* A decrease in alveolar ventilation results in an increased $Paco_2$. Alveolar hypoventilation in this patient is likely due to shallow breathing from abdominal pain or depressed respirations secondary to pain medication. A decrease in metabolic activity would decrease the rate of production of carbon dioxide ($Vco_2$), which would decrease $Paco_2$, assuming that alveolar ventilation does not change. $\dot{V}/\dot{Q}$ inequality causes hypoxemia, and thus reflex hyperventilation. At a constant tidal volume and respiratory rate, a decrease in the deadspace volume would increase alveolar ventilation, and thus lower the $Paco_2$.

**219. The answer is c.** *(Fauci, pp 798-803, 1695-1702. Ganong, pp 661-664. Levitzky, pp 90-102, 105-107.)* Increasing cardiac output causes pulmonary vascular resistance (PVR) to passively decrease due to two mechanisms—distention of perfused vessels and recruitment of more parallel vascular beds. Cardiac output is often elevated in septic shock, which differentiates it from hypovolemic and cardiogenic shock. Decreasing alveolar $Po_2$ causes hypoxic pulmonary vasoconstriction and a rise in PVR. Increasing alveolar $Pco_2$ or pulmonary artery $H^+$ concentration also causes PVR to rise. The sympathetic nervous system exerts little effect on PVR under physiologic conditions, but stimulation of sympathetic nerves will constrict the pulmonary vessels, causing increased PVR. At high lung volumes, the pulmonary capillaries ("alveolar" vessels) are stretched and compressed causing an increased PVR; this is true with spontaneous respirations and occurs even more so with positive pressure ventilation.

**220. The answer is d.** *(Ganong, pp 74-75, 681-683. Levitzky, pp 228-233).* During moderate aerobic exercise, oxygen consumption and $CO_2$ production increase, but alveolar ventilation increases in proportion. Thus, $Paco_2$ (and $Pao_2$) do not change. Arterial pH and blood lactate concentration are also normal during moderate aerobic exercise, but during anaerobic exercise, which is reached at workloads that exceed approximately 60% of the maximal workload (called the anaerobic threshold), there is increased production of muscle lactic acid, which spills over into the circulation, causing an increase in the concentration of blood lactate and a decrease in the pH of the blood.

**221. The answer is d.** (*Fauci, pp 362-363, 1589-1592. Ganong, pp 660-661. Levitzky, pp 130-140.*) The diffusing capacity is the volume of gas transported across the lung per minute per mm Hg partial pressure difference. Diffusing capacity is measured by measuring the transfer of oxygen or carbon monoxide across the alveolar-capillary membrane. Because the partial pressure of oxygen and carbon monoxide is affected by their chemical reactions with hemoglobin, as well as their transfer through the membrane, the diffusing capacity of the lung is determined both by the diffusing capacity of the membrane itself, as well as by the reaction with hemoglobin. Increases in the diffusing capacity can be produced by increasing the concentration of hemoglobin within the blood (polycythemia). The approach to the patient with polycythemia includes determination of not only hematocrit, but also red cell mass, erythropoietin levels, arterial oxygen saturation, and hemoglobin's affinity for oxygen in order to distinguish among the various causes. The diffusing capacity of the membrane can be calculated by rearranging Fick law of diffusion, and is related to the ratio of the surface area available for diffusion and the thickness of the alveolar-capillary interface. The area available for diffusion is decreased by alveolar-septal departitioning in emphysema and by obstruction of the pulmonary vascular bed by pulmonary emboli. The thickness of the diffusional barrier is increased by interstitial fibrosis and by interstitial or alveolar edema found in congestive heart failure.

**222. The answer is e.** (*Fauci, pp 160, 164, 188, 229, 290, 642, 673, 902, 1590, 1618, 1723-1724, 2553. Ganong, pp 690-691. Levitzky, pp 153-154, 183. Stead, p 253.*) The decrease in arterial oxygen saturation caused by carbon monoxide poisoning reduces the oxyhemoglobin and thus total arterial oxygen contents but does not reduce the amount of oxygen dissolved in the plasma, which determines the arterial oxygen tension. Carbon monoxide is odorless and tasteless and dyspnea and respiratory distress are late signs, which is the reason that it is so important to install carbon monoxide detectors in homes and businesses. Respiratory distress becomes manifest with severe tissue hypoxia and anaerobic glycolysis, which leads to lactic acidosis. The decrease in arterial pH stimulates ventilation via the peripheral chemoreceptors. The resultant hyperventilation decreases arterial (and CSF) $Pco_2$, causing CSF pH to rise. Carboxyhemoglobin has a cherry-red color.

**223. The answer is b.** (*Ganong, pp 654-657. Levitzky, pp 20-28.*) Lung compliance is an index of lung distensibility or the ease with which the lungs are expanded; thus, compliance is the inverse of elastic recoil. Compliance is defined as the ratio of change of lung volume to the change in pressure required to inflate the lung ($\Delta V/\Delta P$). Compliance decreases in patients with pulmonary edema or surfactant deficiency and increases when there is a loss of elastic fibers in the lungs, such as occurs in patients with emphysema and with aging.

**224. The answer is a.** (*Fauci, pp 1665-1668. Ganong, pp 675-678. Levitzky, pp 207-209.*) The central chemoreceptors, located at or near the ventral surface of the medulla, are stimulated to increase ventilation by a decrease in the pH of their extra-cellular fluid (ECF). The pH of this ECF is affected by the $Pco_2$ of the blood supply to the medullary chemoreceptor area, as well as by the $CO_2$ and lactic acid production of the surrounding brain tissue. The central chemoreceptors are not stimulated by decreases in $Pao_2$ or blood oxygen content but rather can be depressed by long-term or severe decreases in oxygen supply.

**225. The answer is d.** (*Fauci, p 1602. Ganong, pp 649-650, 654, 657-659. Levitzky, pp 32-36, 49-50.*) Methacholine is a cholinergic agonist, which causes constriction of bronchial smooth muscle. Bronchoconstriction reduces airway radius, which increases airway resistance, and thus the resistive work of breathing. Methacholine-induced bronchoconstriction decreases the anatomic dead space but has no significant effect on the lung compliance, and thus does not affect the elastic work of breathing.

**226. The answer is b.** (*Ganong, pp 658. Levitzky, pp 125-127.*) During inspiration, when all alveoli are subjected to essentially the same alveolar pressure, more air will go to the more compliant alveoli in the base of the lung. Because the lungs are essentially "hanging" in the chest, the force of gravity on the lungs causes the intrapleural pressure to increase (become less negative) at the base of the lungs compared to the apex (more negative intrapleural pressure). This also causes the alveoli at the apex of the lung to be larger than those at the base of the lung. Larger alveoli are already more inflated and are less compliant than smaller alveoli. Because of the effect of gravity on blood, more blood flow will go to the base of the lung. Ventilation is about three 3 times greater at the base of the lung, but flow is about 10 times greater at the base than at the apex of the lung; therefore, the $\dot{V}/\dot{Q}$ ratio is lower at the base than at the apex in a normal lung.

**227. The answer is e.** (*Fauci, pp 1586-1589, 2135-2142. Levitzky, pp 44-46. Stead, pp 255-257, 289-290.*) A restrictive impairment in which lung elastic recoil is increased and lung compliance is decreased, such as occurs in sarcoidosis, shifts the normal maximal expiratory flow-volume curve down and to the right. Maximum expiratory flows are also decreased in conditions that increase airway resistance, for example, asthma, emphysema, and cystic fibrosis, and when muscular effort is decreased, for example, fatigue, but lung volumes would be increased in the obstructive impairments and normal if fatigue was an isolated factor.

**228. The answer is b.** (*Fauci, p 456. Levitzky, pp 86-98, 130-132, 228-234.*) The lungs and heart are in series, so the entire cardiac output flows through the lungs. The increased pulmonary blood flow during exercise increases the surface area for diffusion, and therefore increases the diffusing capacity in accordance with Fick law of diffusion. The increased perfusion of the lungs is accompanied by an even greater increase in ventilation, so the $\dot{V}/\dot{Q}$ ratio of the whole lung, as well as most areas of the lung, increases during exercise. The increase in blood flow through the pulmonary circulation during exercise increases the diameter of the pulmonary vessels and therefore decreases their resistance. Systolic, diastolic, and mean pulmonary artery pressure increase slightly during exercise because of the increased pulmonary blood flow and blood volume.

**229. The answer is b.** (*Fauci, pp 1584-1585, 1675-1676. Levitzky, pp 181-184.*) Type III respiratory failure occurs as a result of lung atelectasis, which commonly occurs in the perioperative period. Following general anesthesia, decreases in functional residual capacity lead to collapse of dependent lung units. This leads to intrapulmonary shunting (areas that are perfused but not ventilated). When the $\dot{V}/\dot{Q}$ ratio is 0, there is no gas exchange and arterial oxygen tension decreases. The hypoxemia stimulates the peripheral chemoreceptors to increase respiratory drive, causing a respiratory alkalosis. Perioperative atelectasis can be treated by frequent changes in position, chest physiotherapy, aggressive control of incisional or abdominal pain, and intermittent positive-pressure breathing. Typical chest examination findings in atelectasis with a patent airway include bronchial, rather than the normal vesicular, breath sounds heard at the lung bases and the presence of crackles, an adventitious (abnormal) breath sound in which there are discontinuous, typically inspiratory sounds on inspiration created by the alveoli and small airways opening and closing with respiration.

**230. The answer is b.** *(Fauci, pp 1586-1588. Levitzky, pp 41-46. Stead, pp 255-257.)* The reduced lung volumes indicate a restrictive lung disease. Although the amount of gas that can be expelled from the lung in 1 second will be less than normal, the increased recoil force of the lung will produce an $FEV_1/FVC$ ratio that is close to normal. All lung volumes and capacities are decreased in patients with restrictive lung disease. The diffusing capacity will be reduced because the small lung volumes reduce the surface area available for gas exchange, and the fibrotic changes in the lungs increase the thickness of the diffusion barrier. The presence of $\dot{V}/\dot{Q}$ abnormalities is indicated by the hypoxemia and need for supplemental oxygen.

**231. The answer is d.** *(Levitzky, pp 32-40.)* As lung volume decreases, intrapleural pressure increases in accordance with Boyle's law. The greater intrapleural pressure decreases the radial traction on the airways, thereby decreasing airway diameter and increasing airway resistance. During a forced expiration or at residual volume, the intrapleural pressure actually becomes positive, compressing the airways and increasing their resistance. The vagus nerve constricts airway smooth muscle. Resistances in parallel add as reciprocals. Thus, the large number of small, peripheral airways increases the number of airways arranged in parallel, and lowers the total resistance of the peripheral airways compared to the total cross-section of the central airways.

**232. The answer is e.** *(Ganong, pp 651-652. Levitzky, pp 41, 54-59.)* A spirometer is an instrument that records the volume of air moved into and out of the lungs during breathing, and therefore can only be used to measure lung volumes and capacities that can be exchanged with the environment. Spirometry can be used to measure the vital capacity, which is the maximal amount of gas that can be expired following a maximal inspiration. Spirometry cannot be used to meaure the volume of the gas that remains in the lungs following a maximal expiration (residual volume), and thus cannot directly measure the lung capacities that contain the residual volume, that is, the functional residual capacity and the total lung capacity. The peak flow rate is the maximal rate at which the volume of gas is exhaled. The measurement of flow rate requires a pneumotach, an instrument that integrates exhaled volume to derive the flow rate, or by a peak flow meter that patients can use at home, which are calibrated to record exhaled flow rates.

**233. The answer is c.** *(Fauci, pp 1643-1644, 1650, 2119-2124. Levitzky, pp 113-116, 122-127, 181-184.)* Areas with low $\dot{V}/\dot{Q}$ ratios produce hypoxemia or a decreased $Pa_{O_2}$, which leads to (a) a decrease in the dissolved oxygen content of the blood and (b) a decrease in $Pa_{CO_2}$, due to stimulation of the peripheral chemoreceptors. At lower $Pa_{O_2}$ levels, arterial oxygen saturation is decreased, which decreases the oxyhemoglobin content. Because the mixed alveolar $P_{O_2}$ is normal and the arterial $P_{O_2}$ is less than normal, the A-a gradient is greater than normal.

**234. The answer is b.** *(Levitzky, pp 44-46.)* A maximal expiratory flow-volume curve is generated during a forced vital capacity maneuver. Only the initial expiratory flow is effort-dependent. That is, increasing expiratory effort will increase expiratory flow at points E and A (peak flow), but not at point B, which is referred to as the effort-independent portion of the maximal expiratory flow-volume curve. The inability to increase flow rates during the effort-independent portion is caused by compression of the noncartilaginous airways by the positive intrapleural pressures that are generated during a forced expiration when the expiratory muscles are actively contracted, a phenomenon called dynamic compression of the airways. No effort limitation occurs during inspiration (points C and D) because increased inspiratory efforts make the intrapleural pressure more negative, which expands the airways, lowering their resistance.

# Cardiovascular Physiology

## Questions

**235.** A 42-year-old woman with mitral prolapse is admitted to the hospital for evaluation of her cardiac function. Which of the following values is the best index of the preload on her heart?

a. Blood volume
b. Central venous pressure
c. Pulmonary capillary wedge pressure
d. Left ventricular end-diastolic volume
e. Left ventricular end-diastolic pressure

**236.** A patient presents to the emergency department with intermittent chest pain. The ECG and blood tests are negative for myocardial infarction, but the echocardiogram shows thickening of the left ventricular muscle and narrowing of the aortic valve. Medications to reduce afterload are prescribed. Which of the following values would provide the best measure of the effectiveness of the medication in reducing left ventricular afterload in this patient?

a. Left ventricular end-diastolic pressure
b. Left ventricular mean systolic pressure
c. Pulmonary capillary wedge pressure
d. Total peripheral resistance
e. Mean arterial blood pressure

**237.** A 55-year-old man reports several recent episodes of syncope. An electrocardiogram is performed. Which of the following arrhythmias is most commonly associated with syncope?

a. Sinus arrhythmia
b. First-degree heart block
c. Second-degree heart block
d. Third-degree heart block
e. Multifocal atrial tachycardia (MAT)

**238.** During a routine physical examination, a 32-year-old woman is found to have second-degree heart block. Which of the following ECG recordings was obtained from the patient during her physical examination?

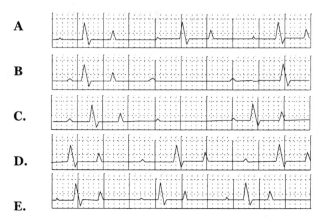

a.  A
b.  B
c.  C
d.  D
e.  E

**239.** The following 6-lead frontal ECG was performed as part of an annual physical examination. Which of the following is the mean electrical axis of the patient?

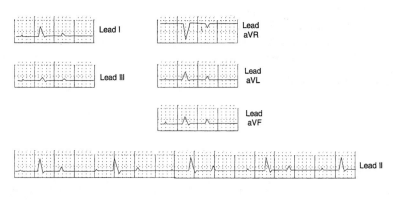

a. −10°
b. +10°
c. +20°
d. +40°
e. +70°

**240.** The spouse of a 58-year-old man calls 911 because her husband complains of chest pain radiating down his left arm. He is transported to the emergency department, where an electrocardiogram and cardiac enzymes indicate a recent myocardial infarction. The man is sent for a cardiac catheterization, including coronary angiography and hemodynamic recordings throughout the cardiac cycle. No valvular defects were present. During ventricular ejection, the pressure difference smallest in magnitude is between which of the following?

a. Pulmonary artery and left atrium
b. Right ventricle and right atrium
c. Left ventricle and aorta
d. Left ventricle and left atrium
e. Aorta and capillaries

**241.** An 82-year-old woman was admitted to the hospital with ascites, peripheral edema, and shortness of breath. Cardiac catheterization was ordered and the following values were obtained:

Pulmonary vein $O_2$ content = 20 mL/100 mL
Pulmonary artery $O_2$ content = 12 mL/100 mL
Oxygen consumption ($VO_2$) = 280 mL/min
Stroke volume = 40 mL

What is the woman's cardiac output?

a. 2.86 L/min
b. 3.5 L/min
c. 7.0 L/min
d. 8.0 L/min
e. 9.24 L/min

**242.** A 66-year-old man is referred to a cardiologist for evaluation. Physical examination reveals a diastolic murmur prominent over the left sternal border, a decrease in diastolic pressure, and an increase in pulse pressure. Which of the following is the most likely diagnosis?

a. Aortic regurgitation
b. Pulmonic stenosis
c. Mitral valve prolapse
d. Pulmonary regurgitation
e. Aortic stenosis

**243.** A patient undergoes cardiac transplantation for severe idiopathic cardiomyopathy. Upon release from the hospital, the patient is referred to a cardiac rehabilitation program. The exercise technologist starts the patient on a walking regimen. In transplant patients, stroke volume may increase during exercise by which of the following mechanisms?

a. An increase in heart rate
b. An increase in arterial blood pressure
c. A decrease in venous compliance
d. A decrease in myocardial contractility
e. An increase in total peripheral resistance

**244.** A patient complaining of an irregular heart beat is referred for a cardiac electrophysiological (EP) study. Propagation of the action potential through the heart is fastest in which of the following?

a. SA node
b. Atrial muscle
c. AV node
d. Purkinje fibers
e. Ventricular muscle

**245.** A 75-year-old woman presents with fatigue, edema, and shortness of breath. Her physician prescribes a diuretic and a positive inotropic agent. Which of the following changes is primarily responsible for the improvement in her condition?

a. A reduction in heart rate
b. A reduction in heart size
c. An increase in ventricular end-diastolic pressure
d. An increase in wall thickness
e. An increase in cardiac excitability

**246.** A 37-year-old woman undergoes a CT scan of the abdomen, which reveals a large peritoneal mass. A subsequent magnetic resonance angiography study showed that the abdominal aorta was constricted to one-half of its resting diameter. As a result, resistance to blood flow through the vessel would be which of the following?

a. Decreased in half
b. Decreased 16-fold
c. Increased by 50%
d. Doubled
e. Increased 16-fold

**247.** A 52-year-old man presents with black tarry stools and hypotension. An endoscopy is ordered and reveals a bleeding ulcer in the antrum of the stomach. Baroreflex-induced compensation for the mild hemorrhage will cause which of the following values to be lower than it was before the hemorrhage?

a. Venous capacitance
b. Ventricular contractility
c. Total peripheral resistance
d. Heart rate
e. Coronary blood flow

**248.** A 22-year-old woman is hospitalized with a history of respiratory distress, fever, and fatigue. ST-segment and T-wave abnormalities suggest myocarditis, which is attributed to an acute viral origin. Over the next several days, significant peripheral edema develops. The edema is most likely caused by which of the following?

a. Decreased capillary permeability
b. Decreased arterial pressure
c. Increased plasma protein concentration
d. Increased lymphatic flow
e. Increased central venous pressure

**249.** A patient undergoes cardiac catheterization to assess his left ventricular function prior to thoracic surgery. What is his ejection fraction percentage, as determined from the left ventricular pressure-volume curve illustrated below?

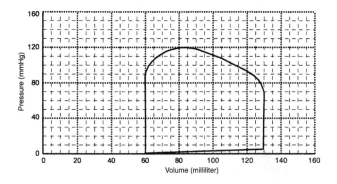

a. 34%
b. 44%
c. 54%
d. 64%
e. 74%

**250.** A 38-year-old man has a murmur that ceases with the onset of the second heart sound. The second heart sound occurs at the onset of which phase of the cardiac cycle?

a. Isovolumetric contraction
b. Rapid ejection
c. Systole
d. Isovolumetric relaxation
e. Rapid ventricular filling

**251.** A 58-year-old woman with idiopathic pulmonary hypertension presents with right ventricular hypertrophy and cor pulmonale. Her electrocardiogram shows positive QRS complexes in leads $V_1$, III, and aVF, and equiphasic QRS complexes in lead aVR. Which of the following is her mean QRS vector?

a. $-120°$
b. $-150°$
c. $+120°$
d. $+90°$
e. $+60°$

**252.** A 57-year-old man complains of palpitation that he notices is relieved by pressing on his eyeball. His electrocardiogram is shown below. Which of the following is most likely to accompany this condition?

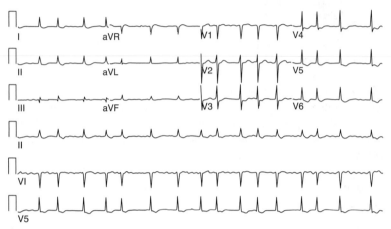

*(Reproduced, with permission, from Crawford MH. Current Diagnosis & Treatment: Cardiology, 3rd ed. New York: McGraw-Hill; 2009:260.)*

a. An increased venous A wave
b. An increased left atrial pressure
c. A decreased heart rate
d. An increased stroke volume
e. An increased mean arterial blood pressure

**253.** A 24-year-old woman undergoes an annual physical examination for participation on the varsity track team at her college. While auscultating her heart sounds, the sports medicine physician instructs the woman to take in a deep inspiration. During this maneuver, he detects splitting of the second heart sound. Which of the following is the mechanism underlying this finding?

a. A decrease in heart rate
b. An increased left ventricular stroke volume
c. Delayed closing of the aortic valve
d. Delayed opening of the mitral valve
e. Delayed closing of the pulmonic valve

**254.** A 55-year-old woman presents for her annual physical examination. Upon auscultation, a third heart sound is heard. The differential diagnosis of this finding includes which of the following?

a. Anemia
b. Tricuspid stenosis
c. Mitral stenosis
d. Right bundle branch block

**255.** A 23-year-old woman presents with fatigue and is found to have a systolic murmur and higher than normal cardiac output. The differential diagnosis based on these findings includes which of the following?

a. Hypertension
b. Third-degree heart block
c. Anemia
d. Aortic regurgitation
e. Cardiac tamponade

**256.** Ventricular pressure-volume curves are determined in two different patients, as illustrated below. Which of the following is greater in patient #1?

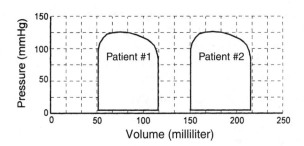

a. Preload
b. Afterload
c. Stroke volume
d. Cardiac work
e. Cardiac efficiency

**257.** Physical examination of a 41-year-old narcotic abuser reveals an early systolic murmur. The physician also notes a 7-cm distance between the height of the blood in his right internal jugular vein and sternal angle (normal = 3 cm). Which of the following conditions is most likely responsible for the physical findings?

a. Mitral stenosis
b. Tricuspid regurgitation
c. Atherosclerosis
d. Aortic regurgitation
e. Tachycardia

**258.** A 42-year-old woman with lightheadedness and recurrent syncope is taken to the emergency department where she is given atropine. Her symptoms are relieved by an increase in which of the following?

a. Heart rate
b. PR interval
c. Ventricular contractility
d. Ejection fraction
e. Stroke volume

**259.** A 50-year-old woman complains of intermittent chest discomfort that occurs most frequently when she drinks lots of coffee to stay up to meet deadlines at work. She is referred to cardiology for an exercise stress test to rule out cardiac ischemia as the cause for her angina. The test will be considered positive if which of the following occurs?

a. Mean arterial blood pressure increases
b. ST-segment depression occurs
c. Tachycardia develops
d. A diastolic murmur is heard
e. The QRS complex widens

**260.** A 64-year-old woman is postoperative day one after a lumbar laminectomy. She suddenly stands up after being supine since the operation. As a result, which of the following hemodynamic variables will increase?

a. End-diastolic volume
b. Renal blood flow
c. Venous return
d. Pulse pressure
e. Ejection fraction

**261.** A newborn baby is cyanotic upon delivery. The cyanosis is not relieved by breathing 100% oxygen. A diagnosis of persistent fetal circulation is made based on which of the following?

a. Mitral regurgitation
b. Left ventricular hypertrophy
c. Pulmonary vasoconstriction and hypertension
d. Systemic hypertension
e. Aortic coarctation

**262.** A 19-year-old man severs an artery in a motorcycle accident. A bystander applies a tourniquet to stop the bleeding. When the paramedics arrive, the blood pressure of the injured man was only slightly hypotensive and his pupils were reactive. The greatest percentage of the redistributed blood volume came from which of the following?

a. Heart
b. Aorta
c. Arteries and arterioles
d. Capillaries
e. Venules and veins

**263.** An 84-year-old woman presents with paroxysmal dizziness, syncope, confusion, and fatigue. Her heart rate did not change when the patient was instructed to perform a Valsalva maneuver. A 24-hour Holter monitor revealed periodic episodes of sinus bradycardia. Phase-4 depolarization of SA nodal cells is caused by which of the following?

a. An increase in the flow of sodium into the cell
b. A decrease in the flow of potassium out of the cell
c. An increase in the activity of the Na/Ca exchanger
d. A decrease in the flow of chloride out of the cell
e. A decrease in the activity of the Na-K pump

**264.** During auscultation of a patient with long-standing hypertension, the physician notes that the splitting of the second heart sound is reversed with P2 occurring before A2. Which of the following is a common electro-cardiographic finding accompanying paradoxical splitting of the second heart sound?

a. Sinus bradycardia
b. Sinus tachycardia
c. Sinus arrhythmia
d. Left bundle branch block
e. Right bundle branch block

**265.** An 83-year-old woman with long-standing hypertension presents after a near-syncopal episode upon standing. Her blood pressure is taken sitting and then standing. Systolic pressure decreased slightly and pulse pressure increased in the standing position. Which of the following can lead to an increased pulse pressure?

a. An increased heart rate
b. A decreased stroke volume
c. An increase in total peripheral resistance
d. A decrease in aortic compliance
e. A decrease in venous capacitance

**266.** A 75-year-old woman makes an appointment to see her physician because of exertional dyspnea and an episode of syncope while dancing with her husband at their granddaughter's wedding. A systolic ejection murmur is auscultated that radiates to the carotid arteries. Her signs and symptoms are most likely due to which of the following?

a. Aortic regurgitation
b. Pulmonic regurgitation
c. Aortic stenosis
d. Mitral stenosis
e. Tricuspid stenosis

**267.** A cardiac catheterization is performed on a 39-year-old man who presents with angina. The left ventricular pressure-volume curve shows a decreased stroke volume and ejection fraction. Which of the following mechanisms may compromise stroke volume following myocardial infarction?

a. An increase in central venous pressure
b. An increase in heart rate
c. A decrease in systemic blood pressure
d. A decrease in total peripheral resistance
e. A positive inotropic response

**268.** A 42-year-old athlete becomes alarmed when he notices a series of heart palpitations several hours after he exercises. After examining the patient's ECG, the physician notes a sinus rhythm with occasional PVCs (premature ventricular complexes). The physician tells his patient that the palpitations are due to interpolated beats and that they are not a cause for alarm. Benign PVCs may occur because the athlete has which of the following?

a. A prolonged PR interval
b. Bradycardia
c. ST-segment depression
d. An alternative bundle of Kent
e. Inverted atrial P waves

**269.** A 56-year-old man was admitted to the hospital with angina and diaphoresis. A myocardial infarction is suspected, and a 12-lead electrocardiogram (ECG) is ordered and shown below. The ECG is most effective in detecting a decrease in which of the following?

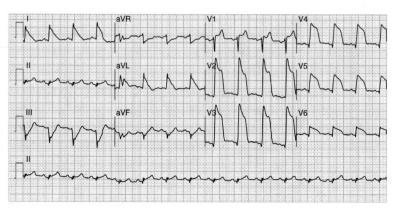

(Reproduced, with permission, from Fauci AS, Braunwald E, Kasper DL, et al. Harrison's Principles of Internal Medicine, 17th ed. New York: McGraw-Hill, 2008:e19-5.)

a. Ventricular contractility
b. Mean blood pressure
c. Total peripheral resistance
d. Ejection fraction
e. Coronary blood flow

**270.** A 48-year-old sedentary, obese man with four-vessel coronary occlusive disease has a massive myocardial infarction while shoveling snow. In the blizzard conditions, it takes the ambulance over an hour to reach the man's home. When the paramedics arrive, the patient's radial pulse is rapid and thready, he has pink froth coming from his mouth, and he is nonresponsive. Increasing which of the following would lead to an increased stroke volume in cardiogenic shock?

a. Heart rate
b. Venous compliance
c. Ventricular contractility
d. Total peripheral resistance
e. Pulmonary capillary wedge pressure

**271.** A patient comes to his physician complaining that he is no longer able to exercise as long as he used to. The physician auscultates crepitant rales and a third heart sound; blood pressure is normal. He sends the patient to cardiology to rule out heart failure. Which of the following is most consistent with a diagnosis of left heart failure?

a. A decreased heart rate
b. An increased left ventricular wall stress
c. An increased left ventricular ejection fraction
d. A decreased left ventricular energy consumption
e. A decreased pulmonary arterial wedge pressure

**272.** A pacemaker is inserted in a patient in order to shorten the PR interval detected on their ECG. Which of the following events normally occurs during the PR interval?

a. The ventricle is contracting.
b. The cardiac action potential passes through the AV node.
c. There is no change in the voltage tracing on the ECG.
d. The mitral and aortic valves are both closed.
e. The second heart sound is heard.

**273.** A 47-year-old woman is brought to the emergency department because she fainted at the gym during her daily aerobic workout. A prominent systolic murmur is heard and a presumptive diagnosis of aortic stenosis is made. Which of the following is consistent with that diagnosis?

a. A decreased pulse pressure
b. An increased arterial pressure
c. A decreased left ventricular diastolic pressure
d. An increased ejection fraction
e. A decreased cardiac oxygen consumption

**274.** The phases of the ventricular muscle action potential are represented by the lettered points on the diagram below. At which point on the ventricular action potential is membrane potential most dependent on calcium permeability?

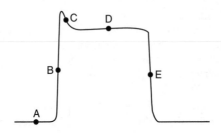

a. Point A
b. Point B
c. Point C
d. Point D
e. Point E

**275.** During which interval on the ECG below does the aortic valve close?

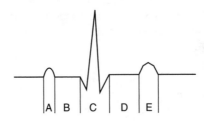

a. A
b. B
c. C
d. D
e. E

**276.** A patient with an inferior MI develops a stable bradycardia of 50 beats/min. The cardiologist orders an ECG to evaluate whether there is sinus node dysfunction or an atrioventricular conduction disturbance. The diagnosis of a first-degree heart block is made in which of the following cases?

a. The PR interval of the ECG is increased.
b. The P wave of the ECG is never followed by a QRS complex.
c. The P wave of the ECG is sometimes followed by a QRS complex.
d. The T wave of the ECG is inverted.
e. The ST segment of the ECG is elevated.

**277.** In the hemodynamic pressure tracings below, rapid ventricular filling begins at which point on the figure below?

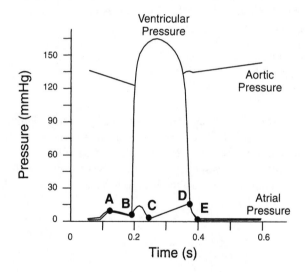

a. A
b. B
c. C
d. D
e. E

**278.** A 67-year-old man who has difficulty breathing when he exercises makes an appointment to see his physician. Auscultation reveals a holosystolic murmur leading to the diagnosis of mitral regurgitation. Which of the following findings is most likely to be present?

a. A decreased arterial pressure
b. An increased pulse pressure
c. An increased v wave
d. A decreased cardiac output
e. A decreased left ventricular preload

**279.** A 43-year-old man comes to his physician complaining of exhaustion and shortness of breath. After completing the physical examination, the physician suspects the patient may be suffering from cardiac tamponade. Which of the following observations led to the physician's putative diagnosis?

a. Hypertension
b. Bradycardia
c. Third heart sound
d. Pulsus paradoxus
e. Expiratory rales

**280.** A 74-year-old black man with a past medical history significant for two previous myocardial infarctions is given digitalis because of congestive heart failure (ejection fraction is 25% by echocardiography). Which of the shifts in the Starling curves shown below are consistent with the changes in ventricular function before and after digitalis in a patient with heart failure?

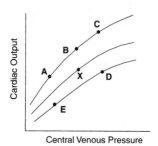

a. X → A
b. D → X
c. E → D
d. C → B
e. X → C

**281.** An EMT arrives at the scene of an automobile accident, and finds a hemorrhaging, unconscious young woman. Which of the following is a sign of hemorrhagic shock?

a. Metabolic alkalosis
b. Warm skin
c. Polyuria
d. Bradycardia
e. Low hematocrit

**282.** A 37-year-old patient is brought to the emergency department in shock. Which of the following is a reason to direct treatment toward anaphylactic shock rather than hypovolemic shock?

a. Cardiac output is higher than normal.
b. Ventricular contractility is greater than normal.
c. Total peripheral resistance is greater than normal.
d. Serum creatinine is elevated.
e. Heart rate is greater than normal.

**283.** During a routine physical examination, a 35-year-old man is found to have a blood pressure of 170/105 mm Hg. History reveals episodes of headache accompanied by palpitations, diaphoresis, and anxiety. A diagnosis of pheochromocytoma is made after documentation of catecholamine excess in lab work and an MRI reveals a right adrenal mass. Which of the following should be administered preoperatively to control blood pressure in this patient?

a. An α-adrenergic agonist
b. A β-adrenergic agonist
c. An α-adrenergic antagonist
d. A glycoprotein IIb/IIIa antagonist

**284.** Cardiac function and venous function curves were generated in a patient undergoing several maneuvers to evaluate his cardiac and cardio-vascular reserves. Starting from the control point, to which point did the curves shift when the person was given a transfusion of saline?

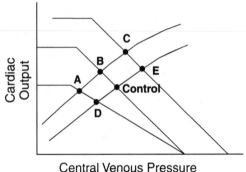

a.  A
b.  B
c.  C
d.  D
e.  E

**285.** A 40-year-old woman with metabolic syndrome is prescribed a low-calorie diet and 30 minutes of daily aerobic exercise. Sympathetic stimulation during exercise has which of the following cardiac effects?

a.  An increase in the duration of systole
b.  An increase in the duration of diastole
c.  An increase in the activity of the sarcoplasmic reticulum (SR) calcium pump
d.  A decrease in the concentration of $Ca^{2+}$ during systole

**286.** A 23-year-old collegiate dance squad member adopts a sedentary lifestyle once she starts medical school. After the Gross Anatomy course, she decides to restore her state of physical fitness by resuming a regular exercise routine. The cardiovascular responses to isotonic exercise include an increase in which of the following?
a. Stroke volume
b. Diastolic pressure
c. Venous compliance
d. Pulmonary arterial resistance
e. Total peripheral resistance

**287.** The following diagram illustrates the relative resistance of three vessels. Which of the following is the ratio of the flow in vessel X to the flow in vessel Y?

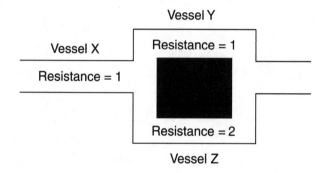

a. 1:1
b. 3:2
c. 2:1
d. 3:1
e. 4:3

**288.** A 2-year-old boy is mauled by a black bear while hiking with his family in the Appalachian mountains. A claw-puncture wound to the skull compressed the underlying brain tissue. Which of the following occurs in response to an increased intracranial pressure?

a. Blood pressure and heart rate increase.
b. Blood pressure and heart rate decrease.
c. Blood pressure increases and heart rate decreases.
d. Blood pressure decreases and heart rate increases.
e. Blood pressure and heart rate remain constant.

**289.** A 75-year-old woman presents to her primary care physician's office in follow-up for her hypertension of 25 years. She is currently on losartan. Her EKG is shown below. Considering the history presented, this patient's left ventricular wall stress will be decreased by an increase in which of the following?

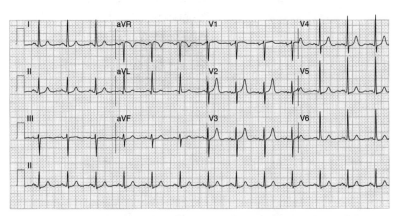

*(Reproduced, with permission, from Fauci AS, Braunwald E, Kasper DL, et al. Harrison's Principles of Internal Medicine, 17th ed. New York: McGraw-Hill, 2008:e19-28.)*

a. Mean arterial pressure
b. Total peripheral resistance
c. Left ventricular end-diastolic volume
d. Contractility of the left atrium
e. The thickness of the free wall of the left ventricle

**290.** During which interval on the ECG below does the bundle of His depolarize?

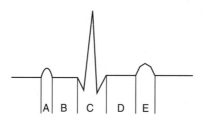

a. A
b. B
c. C
d. D
e. E

**291.** A 48-year-old man develops chest pain while running. His wife takes him to the emergency department, where the following ECG is obtained. The electrocardiographic changes are consistent with a diagnosis of which of the following?

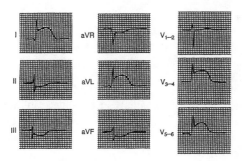

a. Hyperkalemia
b. Hypokalemia
c. Anterior infarction
d. Posterior infarction
e. Ventricular premature beat

**292.** A 47-year-old black man with type II diabetes reports for his 6-month check-up. His doctor prescribes a daily 30-minute routine of walking at a brisk pace. During aerobic exercise, blood flow remains relatively constant within which of the following?

a. Brain
b. Heart
c. Skin
d. Skeletal muscles
e. Kidneys

**293.** A 56-year-old man presents with complaints of fatigue and headaches. During the physical examination, he is found to have a wide pulse pressure. Which of the following conditions causes pulse pressure to increase?

a. Tachycardia
b. Hypertension
c. Hemorrhage
d. Aortic stenosis
e. Heart failure

**294.** A 22-year-old man ruptures his spleen in a motorcycle accident. A reduction in blood pressure would cause a decrease in which of the following?

a. Heart rate
b. Myocardial contractility
c. Total peripheral resistance
d. Venous compliance
e. Cardiac output

**295.** An 18-year-old man sits quietly in his physician's office prior to a routine physical examination for clearance to play college baseball. Which of the following organs has the highest arteriovenous $O_2$ difference under these normal resting conditions?

a. Brain
b. Heart
c. Skeletal muscle
d. Kidney
e. Liver

**296.** The graph below illustrates the pressure-volume curves for the arterial and venous systems. Which of the following is the approximate ratio of the arterial compliance to the venous compliance?

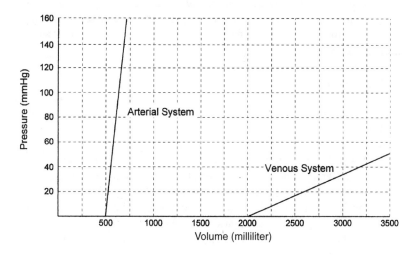

a.  15:1
b.  10:1
c.  1:1
d.  1:10
e.  1:20

**297.** A 63-year-old woman presents to the emergency room with complaints of dyspnea, an elevated jugular venous pulse, and bilateral lower extremity edema. She is diagnosed with congestive heart failure and is prescribed captopril. Which of the following best describes the use of an angiotensin-converting enzyme inhibitor?

a.  Afterload is increased.
b.  Survival is decreased.
c.  Bradykinin is reduced.
d.  A nonproductive cough can develop.
e.  Arteriolar vasoconstriction is augmented.

**298.** A 29-year-old woman presents at the obstetrics/gynecology office with breast tenderness. She's concerned she may have a lump because her mother had breast cancer, and reports that she cannot be pregnant because she just finished her menstrual period about 2 weeks ago. An assay for human chorionic gonadotropin (hCG) in her urine is positive, confirming pregnancy. In the developing fetus, which vessel has the greatest partial pressure of oxygen?

a. Umbilical vein
b. Umbilical arteries
c. Aorta
d. Ductus arteriosus
e. Ductus venosus

**299.** A 6-year-old girl undergoes a routine physical examination for entry into the first grade. She is found to be tachycardic, and has a wide pulse pressure. A thrill and a continuous murmur with late systolic accentuation at the upper left sternal edge are detected upon auscultation. Echocardiography reveals a patent ductus arteriosus. Which of the following best describes the function of the ductus arteriosus in the fetal circulation?

a. It delivers oxygenated blood from the placenta to the left ventricle.
b. It is located in the septum between the left and right atrium.
c. It diverts oxygenated blood away from the lungs to the aorta.
d. It allows blood to flow from the aorta to the pulmonary artery.
e. It is a high resistance conduit, which helps to maintain normal fetal blood pressure.

**300.** A 63-year-old woman presented with acute onset of right eye pain. Ophthalmic and neurologic examinations were normal except for a loud right carotid bruit. The eye pain ceased following carotid endarterectomy. The bruit was most likely caused by which of the following?

a. A high velocity of blood within the carotid artery
b. An increase in blood viscosity
c. Widening of the carotid artery
d. An increase in hematocrit
e. Lengthening of the carotid artery

**301.** A 57-year-old woman is undergoing a femoral popliteal bypass for her peripheral vascular disease. The vascular surgeon wishes to induce a localized arteriolar constriction to help control hemostasis. An increase in the local concentration of which of the following agents will cause systemic vasoconstriction?

a.   Nitric oxide
b.   Angiotensin II
c.   Atrial natriuretic peptide
d.   A $\beta_2$-adrenergic agonist
e.   Adenosine

**302.** A patient is referred to the heart station for exercise stress testing. Baseline and exercise levels of cardiac and venous function are measured and plotted on the graphs below. The point marked "Control" represents baseline cardiovascular function in the resting state in the supine position. During treadmill exercise, there will be a shift from the resting state to which of the following points?

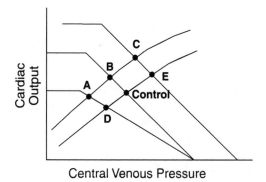

a.   A
b.   B
c.   C
d.   D
e.   E

**303.** In the pressure-volume loop below, systole begins at which of the following points?

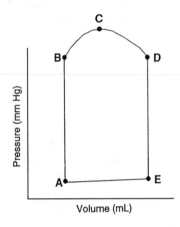

a. A
b. B
c. C
d. D
e. E

**304.** A 27-year-old woman gave birth without complications 48 hours ago to a term 7-lb 6-oz boy. Which of the following best describes the functional closure of the ductus arteriosus?

a. It is independent of gestational age.
b. It occurs due to hypoxic pulmonary vasoconstriction.
c. It precedes closure of the foramen ovale.
d. It causes blood to flow from the aorta into the pulmonary artery.
e. It is the final event required for conversion of the transitional circulation in the newborn to the adult circulatory pattern.

**305.** A 32-year-old man is diagnosed with primary hypertension. His physician recommends a drug for hypertension that acts by decreasing vascular smooth muscle contractile activity without affecting ventricular contractility. Which of the following is the most likely site of action for the drug?

a. β-Adrenergic receptors
b. Calmodulin
c. Troponin
d. Tropomyosin
e. Protein kinase A

**306.** A 64-year-old man was admitted to the hospital with edema and congestive heart failure. He was found to have diastolic dysfunction characterized by inadequate filling of the heart during diastole. The decrease in ventricular filling is due to a decrease in ventricular muscle compliance. Which of the following proteins determines the normal stiffness of ventricular muscle?

a. Calmodulin
b. Troponin
c. Tropomyosin
d. Titin
e. Myosin light chain kinase

**307.** A 62-year-old man with a history of diabetes mellitus and hypertension arrives in the emergency room with substernal chest pain for the last hour. He is given intravenous nitroglycerin to help reduce the pain. Which of the following would be expected with the use of nitrates?

a. Arterial blood pressure is increased.
b. Venous return to the heart is increased.
c. Left ventricular wall stress is increased.
d. Myocardial oxygen demand is decreased.
e. Coronary blood flow is decreased.

**308.** During a clinical elective, a second-year medical student auscultates the heart of a patient, which reveals normal $S_1$ and $S_2$ heart sounds with no murmurs. In correlating his physical examination with the cardiac cycle, when does the highest coronary blood flow per gram of left ventricular myocardium occur?

a. When aortic pressure is highest
b. When left ventricular pressure is highest
c. When aortic blood flow is highest
d. At the beginning of isovolumic contraction
e. At the beginning of diastole

**309.** A 59-year-old man with an ejection fraction of 15%, who is being treated with medications for his heart failure, is asked whether he would like to participate in a trial for an experimental drug. The drug being tested is designed to decrease the expression of phospholamban on ventricular muscle cells. Which of the following would be increased by decreasing phospholamban?

a. The activity of the sodium-potassium pump
b. The diastolic stiffness of the ventricular muscle cells
c. The activity of the L-type calcium channels
d. The duration of the ventricular muscle action potential
e. The concentration of calcium within the SR

**310.** A 22-year-old man with no history of congenital heart disease has a normal physical examination prior to entering the military. Which of the following characteristics is most similar in the systemic and pulmonary circulations of this patient?

a. Preload
b. Afterload
c. Peak systolic pressure
d. Blood volume
e. Stroke work

# Cardiovascular Physiology

## *Answers*

**235. The answer is d.** (*Ganong, pp 571-574.*) Preload is the degree to which the myocardium is stretched before it contracts, that is, the length of the sarcomere at the end of diastole. In vivo, the variable most directly related to sarcomere length during end-diastole is left ventricular end-diastolic volume. Although blood volume, central venous pressure, pulmonary capillary wedge pressure, and left ventricular end-diastolic pressure can all influence preload, they all exert their influence through changes in end-diastolic volume.

**236. The answer is b.** (*Ganong, pp 571-576.*) Afterload is the tension at which the load is lifted during the contraction of a sarcomere. According to the law of Laplace ($T = P \times r/w$), the tension ($T$) is proportional to the pressure ($P$) and radius ($r$) and inversely proportional to the thickness of the ventricle wall ($w$) during systole. The mean left ventricular systolic pressure would therefore be the best index of afterload in vivo. Mean arterial blood pressure (MAP) is normally the same as ventricular pressure and therefore a good index of afterload. However, in a patient with aortic stenosis, the ventricular pressure is higher than the aortic pressure. Although the total peripheral resistance (TPR) can influence afterload by causing changes in mean arterial blood pressure, changes in TPR do not always cause corresponding changes in afterload. For example, during aerobic exercise, afterload (MAP) is often increased, whereas TPR is reduced and following a hemorrhage, TPR is high, whereas afterload (MAP) is low. Pulmonary capillary wedge pressure and left ventricular end-diastolic pressure are estimates of the volume of blood in the ventricle during diastole and are indices of preload.

**237. The answer is d.** (*Fauci, pp 139-143. Ganong, pp 554-556, 640. Stead, pp 44-46.*) Syncope (fainting) is a transient loss of consciousness caused by an inadequate blood flow to the brain. Transient decreases in cerebral blood flow are usually due to one of three general mechanisms: disorders of vascular tone or blood volume, cardiovascular disorders, or cerebrovascular disease. Approximately one-fourth of syncopal episodes are of cardiac origin and are due to either transient obstruction of blood flow through the heart or sudden decreases in cardiac output due to cardiac arrhythmias, such as bradycardia, heart block, or sinus arrest (neurocardiogenic syncope). Third-degree (complete) heart block results when conduction of the action potential from the atria to the ventricles is completely interrupted. Under these conditions, pacemaker cells within the His-Purkinje system or the ventricular muscle cause the ventricles to beat at a low rate (idioventricular rhythm) independently of the atria. Third-degree heart block is caused by conduction system disturbances, inferior wall MI, and digitalis toxicity. When the conduction disturbance is due to disease in the AV node, the idioventricular rhythm is normally about 45 beats/min. When the conduction disturbance is below the AV node (infranodal block) due to disease in the bundle of His, firing of more peripheral ventricular pacemakers can decrease heart rate to below 30 beats/min with periods of asystole that may last a minute or more. The resultant cerebral ischemia causes dizziness and fainting (Stokes-Adams syndrome). Sinus arrhythmia is a change of the heart rate produced by the normal variation in the rate of phase 4 depolarization of the SA nodal pacemaker cells between inspiration and expiration. First-degree heart block is defined as a higher-than-normal PR interval (> 0.2 seconds). Second-degree heart block occurs when the action potential fails to reach the ventricles some, but not all, of the time. Multifocal atrial tachycardia is a heart rate above 100 beats/min with at least three different P-wave morphologies and varying PR intervals.

**238. The answer is c.** (*Ganong, pp 554-556. Stead, pp 6-8, 44-45.*) Conduction abnormalities can produce first-degree, second-degree, or third-degree heart block. In a second-degree heart block, a P wave is not always followed by a QRS complex as in trace C, where the second P wave is not followed by a QRS complex. In a first-degree heart block, trace D, the interval between the beginning of the P wave and the beginning of the QRS complex (the PR interval) is longer than normal (> 0.2 seconds). In a third-degree heart block, conduction between the atria and ventricles is completely blocked so the atrial beats (represented by the P waves) and the ventricular beats (represented by the QRS complex) are completely dissociated.

**239. The answer is d.** (*Ganong, p 553. Stead, pp 6-7.*) The mean electrical axis (MEA) represents the average direction traveled by the ventricular muscle action potentials as they propagate through the heart. The propagation path and the mass of tissue through which the action potentials travel influence the MEA. Normally the MEA ranges from −30° to +100°. The MEA is approximately perpendicular to the axis of the limb lead with the smallest QRS-wave magnitude. In this case, the smallest deflection is in lead III. Therefore, the MEA lies along lead aVR. Because the QRS complex is negative in aVR, the MEA is approximately +30 degrees. Because the QRS complex is greater in lead II than in lead I, the MEA is between +60 degrees and +30 degrees.

**240. The answer is c.** (*Ganong, pp 565-568.*) The pressure gradient between regions of the cardiovascular system is directly proportional to the resistance of the intervening structures. During ventricular ejection, the aortic valves are open and do not offer any significant resistance to blood flow. Therefore, there is very little, if any, pressure difference between the left ventricle and the aorta. Because the tricuspid valve is closed during ventricular ejection, there is an appreciable pressure difference between the right ventricle and the left atrium, although this pressure difference is opposite in direction to the flow of blood through the circulatory system. Although pulmonary vascular resistance is relatively small compared with systemic vascular resistance, it nonetheless produces a pressure drop between the right ventricle and the left atrium. Because most of the resistance in the systemic vasculature occurs at the level of the arterioles, there is a large pressure gradient between the aorta and the capillaries.

**241. The answer is b.** (*Ganong, pp 570-571.*) Cardiac output can be measured by using the Fick principle, which asserts that the rate of uptake of a substance by the body (eg, $O_2$ consumption in milliliters per minute) is equal to the difference between its concentrations (milliliters per liter of blood) in arterial and venous blood multiplied by the rate of blood flow (cardiac output). This principle is restricted to situations in which arterial blood is the only source of the substance measured. If oxygen consumption by the body at steady state is measured over a period of time and the difference in arterial $O_2$ and venous $O_2$ measured by sampling arterial blood and pulmonary arterial blood (which is fully mixed venous blood), cardiac output is obtained from the expression.

$$CO = \dot{V}O_2/a\text{-}vO_2$$

$$CO = \frac{280 \text{ mL/min}}{20 \text{ mL/100 mL} - 12 \text{ mL/100 mL}}$$

$$CO = \frac{280 \text{ mL/min}}{8 \text{ mL/100 mL}}$$

$$CO = 280 \text{ mL/min} \times 100 \text{ mL/8 mL}$$

$$= 3500 \text{ mL/min}$$

$$= 3.5 \text{ L/min}$$

**242. The answer is a.** (*Ganong, pp 569-570, 587.*) Blood leaks from the aorta into the left ventricle during diastole in patients with regurgitant aortic valves producing a diastolic murmur. The rapid flow of blood into the left ventricle during diastole also causes an increase in end-diastolic volume (preload), which results in a larger stroke volume and therefore a larger pulse pressure. Typically, mean blood pressure remains the same so the larger pulse pressure is accompanied by an increased systolic and decreased diastolic presure. If too much of the stroke volume flows back into the heart during diastole, mean blood pressure will fall and the baroreceptor reflex will cause an increase in heart rate.

**243. The answer is c.** (*Ganong, pp 571-576, 632-635.*) Cardiac output increases during exercise primarily due to sympathetically mediated increases in heart rate. Patients with transplanted hearts are able to increase their cardiac output during exercise in the absence of cardiac innervation through increases in stroke volume brought about by operation of the Frank-Starling mechanism. Stroke volume increases with an increase in preload (Frank-Starling mechanism), a decrease in afterload, or an increase in contractility. Preload is the volume of blood within the ventricles at the end of diastole. Decreasing venous compliance forces more blood into the ventricle, resulting in an increased preload and an increased stroke volume. Increasing afterload (aortic pressure or total peripheral resistance) and decreasing contractility decrease stroke volume. An increase in heart rate may result in a decreased filling time and therefore a decrease in preload and stroke volume.

**244. The answer is d.** (*Ganong, pp 549-550.*) The most rapid conduction of the action potential occurs through the Purkinje fibers. The slowest conduction occurs in the AV node. Pacemaker cells located within the SA node initiate the cardiac action potential normally. The action potential propagates from the SA node into the atrial muscle fibers. It then passes through the AV node and the His-Purkinje network to the ventricular muscle fibers. The rapid conduction of the action potential through the His-Purkinje network ensures rapid and synchronous activation of the entire ventricular muscle. The slow conduction through the AV node produces a delay between atrial and ventricular systole, allowing the ventricle to receive the blood ejected by the atria before it contracts.

**245. The answer is b.** *(Fauci, pp 1443-1453. Ganong, pp 643-644, 726.)* In heart failure, the inability to pump enough blood to satisfy the energy requirements of the tissues leads to an increase in end-diastolic volume and end-diastolic pressure, which can lead to pulmonary edema, hence the term congestive heart failure. In addition, the large end-diastolic volume increases the wall stress that must be developed by the heart with each beat, and this increases the myocardial requirement for oxygen. Administration of a positive inotropic drug such as digoxin increases the stroke volume, which increases the cardiac output to the tissues. The greater ejection fraction lowers the end-diastolic volume, which decreases heart size and thus wall stress, according to the Laplace law. As a result, myocardial oxygen demand is lowered.

**246. The answer is e.** *(Ganong, pp 584-585.)* According to the Poiseuille law, resistance is inversely proportional to the fourth power of the radius $[R \infty (1/r^4)]$. Therefore, if the radius of a blood vessel is decreased by a factor of 2, the resistance to blood flow would increase by a factor of $2^4$, or by 16 times.

**247. The answer is a.** *(Ganong, pp 605-607, 636-639.)* The fall in blood volume and pressure produced by hemorrhage elicits the baroreceptor reflex. The reflex increases the activity of the sympathetic nervous system and decreases the activity of the parasympathetic nerves innervating the heart. Sympathetic stimulation of the smooth muscle surrounding the venous vessels decreases their compliance, causing end-diastolic volume (EDV) to increase. The EDV does not increase above the levels observed prior to the hemorrhage, however. Heart rate, ventricular contractility, and total peripheral resistance are all increased above their prehemorrhage levels by sympathetic stimulation. The coronary blood flow increases to meet the increased energy requirements of the heart beating at a higher rate with increased contractility.

**248. The answer is e.** *(Ganong, pp 592-594.)* Net filtration from systemic capillaries is dependent on the Starling forces and capillary permeability. The equation is

$$\text{Net filtration} = K_f \left[ (P_{\text{capillary}} - P_{\text{tissue}}) - (\pi_{\text{capillary}} - \pi_{\text{tissue}}) \right],$$

where $K_f$ is the filtration coefficient of the membrane, and is directly proportional to capillary permeability, $P_{\text{capillary}}$ and $P_{\text{tissue}}$ are the hydrostatic pressures in the capillary and tissue (interstitial space), respectively, and $\pi_{\text{capillary}}$ and $\pi_{\text{tissue}}$ are the osmotic (colloid oncotic) pressures in the capillary and interstitial space, respectively. Increasing central venous pressure increases the capillary hydrostatic pressure ($P_{\text{capillary}}$), which increases the filtration of fluid from the systemic capillaries, leading to edema. All of the other choices will cause a decrease in filtration.

**249. The answer is c.** *(Ganong, pp 565, 643. Widmaier, p 380.)* The ejection fraction (EF) is equal to the stroke volume (SV) divided by the end-diastolic volume (EDV) and the stroke volume (SV) is equal to the end-diastolic volume (EDV) minus the end-systolic volume (ESV).

$$EF = SV/EDV = EDV - ESV/EDV$$

In this case, the end-diastolic volume is 130 mL and the end-systolic volume is 60 mL. Therefore, the ejection fraction is 70 mL/130 mL or 0.54 (54%).

**250. The answer is d.** *(Ganong, pp 565-567. Widmaier, pp 373-378.)* Closure of the semilunar valves (aortic and pulmonic valves) marks the beginning of the isovolumetric relaxation phase of the cardiac cycle. During this brief period (approximately 0.06 seconds), the ventricles are closed and myocardial relaxation, which began during protodiastole, continues. Intraventricular pressure falls rapidly, although ventricular volume changes little. When intraventricular pressure falls below atrial pressure, the mitral and tricuspid valves open and rapid filling of the ventricles begins.

**251. The answer is c.** *(Fauci, pp 1388-1393. Ganong, pp 551-553.)* The ECG leads are configured so that a positive (upright) deflection is recorded in a lead if the wave of depolarization spreads toward the positive pole of that lead, and a negative deflection if the wave spreads toward the negative pole. If the mean orientation of the depolarization vector is at right angles to a given lead axis, a biphasic (equally positive and negative) deflection will be recorded. Therefore, the equiphasic QRS complex in lead aVR indicates that the mean QRS vector is 90° away from +210°. If the QRS complex is positive in leads III and aVF, the mean electrical axis must move toward +120° and +90°, respectively. Thus, the mean QRS vector must be +120°. Right axis deviation (mean QRS vector to the right of 110°) is characteristic of the right ventricular strain or hypertrophy associated with pulmonary hypertension. The positive QRS complex in lead $V_1$ is also characteristic of right axis deviation.

**252. The answer is b.** *(Fauci, pp 1384, 1427-1428. Ganong, pp 556-557, 569, 573.)* The ECG shows the irregular rhythm of atrial fibrillation. Atrial fibrillation is an arrhythmia in which the electrical activity of the atrium becomes disorganized and therefore unable to produce a coordinated atrial contraction. The absence of an atrial pulse reduces the emptying of the atria during diastole and results in an enlarged left atrium and increased left atrial pressure. The venous A wave represents atrial contraction and disappears due to the absence of an atrial beat. Decreased filling of the heart results in a decrease in stroke volume. Heart rate increases because the continuous electrical activity of the atria initiates a high rate of ventricular activity. Systemic blood pressure typically falls because of inadequate filling of the ventricles and the resulting decrease in stroke volume. The oculocardiac reflex is a decrease in heart rate that occurs when pressure is applied to the eyeball via connections between the ophthalmic branch of the trigeminal nerve (afferents) and the vagus nerve (efferents) to the SA node.

**253. The answer is e.** *(Fauci, p 1385. Ganong, pp 566-569.)* The second heart sound ($S_2$) is associated with the closing of the aortic and pulmonic valves. The aortic valve normally closes slightly before the pulmonic valve, resulting in a splitting of the second heart sound into two components. During inspiration, the preload on the right heart is increased, resulting in a larger stroke volume. This causes the delay in the closing of the pulmonic valve and a prolongation of the interval between the two components of the second heart sound. Closure of the mitral valve and tricuspid valves is associated with the first heart sound ($S_1$). Heart rate is higher during inspiration than during expiration.

**254. The answer is a.** *(Fauci, pp 1469-1470, 1481-1482, Ganong, pp 567-569. Stead, pp 27-29.)* The third heart sound ($S_3$) is associated with rapid ventricular filling of the left ventricle. $S_3$ is usually a normal finding in children and young adults. It is usually abnormal in adults over the age of 40 and is heard with high output states such as anemia, valvular disease such as mitral regurgitation, and in states of impaired ventricular function such as in dilated cardiomyopathy.

**255. The answer is c.** *(Fauci, pp 1475-1477. Ganong, pp 569-570, 582-583.)* The magnitude of the cardiac output is regulated to maintain an adequate blood pressure and to deliver an adequate supply of oxygen to the tissues. In anemia, a greater cardiac output is required to supply oxygen to the tissues because the oxygen-carrying capacity of the blood is reduced. The reduced blood viscosity increases the velocity and thus the turbulence of the blood flow, which makes systolic murmurs common in anemic patients. In aortic regurgitation, the stroke volume will be increased, but a portion of the blood ejected by the heart will return to the heart during diastole (diastolic murmur). Thus, the output delivered to the tissues does not increase despite the fact that the blood ejected by the heart has increased. In hypertension, third-degree heart block, and cardiac tamponade (decreased filling of the heart due to accumulation of fluid within the pericardium), cardiac output will be normal or reduced.

**256. The answer is e.** *(Ganong, pp 570-576.)* Efficiency is defined as work divided by energy consumption. The heart represented by pressure-volume curve 1 in the diagram has a lower end-diastolic volume and therefore ejects blood at a lower wall stress than the heart represented by pressure-volume curve 2. Cardiac energy consumption is directly related to wall stress. Because both hearts eject the same amount of blood (stroke volume) at the same pressure, they perform the same amount of work.

**257. The answer is b.** *(Fauci, pp 1384, 1386-1387, 1479. Ganong, pp 569-570.)* Early systolic murmurs begin with the first heart sound and end in midsystole. The higher-than-normal height of the jugular blood column (jugular venous pulse or JVP) reflects an increased right atrial pressure. The combination of an early systolic murmur and high right atrial pressure is indicative of tricuspid regurgitation. This lesion is common in narcotic abusers with infective endocarditis. Mitral stenosis and aortic regurgitation produce diastolic murmurs.

**258. The answer is a.** *(Fauci, pp 1419, 1422. Ganong, pp 100-101.)* Although the cause of her syncope is not given in the history, it is presumably produced by an abnormally slow heart rate due to increased release of acetylcholine by the vagus nerve or by acetylcholine agonists such as muscarine, which is found in certain mushrooms. Atropine blocks the acetylcholine receptors on the SA and AV node, leading to an increased heart rate.

**259. The answer is b.** *(Fauci, pp 1393-1394, 1404, 1515-1521.)* A stress test is conducted by asking a patient to increase his or her exercise intensity while monitoring blood pressure and the electrical activity of the heart. Ischemia occurs if the myocardial oxygen demand brought about by the increased exercise intensity is not matched by an increase in myocardial blood flow. An ischemic episode is indicated by ST-segment depression. Mean arterial blood pressure and heart rate normally rise during exercise. The presence of a diastolic murmur or conduction abnormalities in the ECG are not diagnostic of ischemic heart disease. The exercise test will also be terminated if dizziness, dyspnea, or ventricular tachycardia develop or if blood pressure falls.

**260. The answer is e.** *(Ganong, pp 630-631. Widmaier, pp 414-415.)* When a person rises suddenly, blood pools in the dependent portions of the body, causing decreases in venous return, left ventricular end-diastolic volume, stroke volume, and pulse pressure. The reduced stroke volume leads to a drop in cardiac output and therefore a drop in blood pressure. Decreased blood pressure produces the baroreceptor reflex, leading to an increase in sympathetic activity, which increases total peripheral resistance, cardiac contractility, heart rate, and ejection fraction. These changes in the cardiovascular system return blood pressure toward normal.

**261. The answer is c.** *(Ganong, pp 627-629.)* Persistent fetal circulation (or persistent pulmonary hypertension) occurs when the normal reduction of pulmonary vascular resistance does not occur at birth. In utero, pulmonary artery pressure and pulmonary vascular resistance are high and pulmonary blood flow is low, constituting only approximately 5% to 10% of the cardiac output. Of the venous return to the right atrium, about one-third flows into the left atrium through the foramen ovale and the remaining two-thirds flows into the right ventricle and is pumped into the main pulmonary artery. Almost all of this blood (90%) flows from right-to-left into the aorta through the ductus arteriosus. At birth, initiation of extrauterine respiration raises alveolar $PO_2$, causing a decrease in pulmonary vascular resistance accompanied by a decrease in pulmonary artery pressure and an increase in pulmonary blood flow. The increased pulmonary venous return to the left atrium raises left atrial pressure above right atrial pressure, causing functional closure of the foramen ovale. The ventilation-induced increase in arterial $PO_2$ constricts the systemic vessels, which, along with the elimination of the placental circulation that comprised 40% of the fetal cardiac output, increases systemic vascular resistance and aortic pressure rises above pulmonary artery pressure. As a consequence, blood flows across the ductus arteriosus from aorta to pulmonary artery (left-to-right). If the transition to extrauterine respiration is impaired, and the infant has arterial hypoxia despite administration of 100% $O_2$, then pulmonary vascular resistance and pulmonary artery pressure remain high, causing the persistence of the right-to-left flow of blood across the ductus arteriosus, which exacerbates the hypoxemia, and causes cyanosis.

**262. The answer is e.** (*Ganong, pp 577-580, 637-639. Widmaier, pp 399-400, 413-414.*) The total circulating blood volume is approximately 70 mL/kg, about two-thirds of which is found in the systemic veins and venules. A significant volume of blood (15%) is found in the pulmonary circulation. The large volume of blood found on the venous side of the circulation is used to adjust circulating blood volume. For example during hemorrhage, contraction of the veins and venules of the skin increases the amount of blood available for perfusion of the heart and brain.

**263. The answer is a.** (*Ganong, pp 78-81, 547-549. Le,p 250. Widmaier, pp 369-370.*) Phase-4 depolarization is caused by the activation of a $Na^+$ channel. The channel is activated when the membrane hyperpolarizes in contrast to the Na channel responsible for the action potential, which is activated when the cell depolarizes. Potassium conductance decreases during phase-4 depolarization and thus the flow of potassium out of the cell is diminished; however, this change in potassium current is not responsible for phase-4 depolarization. Chloride conductance does not change during phase-4. The Na/Ca exchanger maintains low intracellular calcium at rest and may reverse its direction and pump calcium into the cell during phase 2 of the cardiac action potential. However, neither the Na/Ca exchanger nor the Na-K pump is involved in phase-4 depolarization.

**264. The answer is d.** *(Fauci, pp 1385-1388. Ganong, pp 554-556, 566-570.)* Normal splitting of the second heart sound occurs because the aortic valve (A2) closes before the pulmonic valve (P2). The splitting will be reversed by any condition that delays the closing of the aortic valve. The most common cause of reversed splitting is left bundle branch block in which activation of the left ventricle is delayed. A right bundle branch block would prolong P2, thus causing increased physiological splitting. Similarly, during inspiration, there will be prolongation of the normal splitting of the second heart sound, not reversed splitting. Sinus arrhythmia refers to the increased heart rate during inspiration, which is accompanied by an increased venous return and thus an increased right ventricular preload, which prolongs the duration of right ventricular ejection, and thus delays closure of the pulmonic valve during inspiration. Increases or decreases in heart rate do not alter the normal pattern of valvular closure.

**265. The answer is d.** *(Ganong, pp 587-592. Widmaier, pp 384-387.)* Pulse pressure is the difference between the systolic and diastolic pressure that occurs during the cardiac cycle. It is determined by the change in volume in the aorta during systole and the compliance of the aorta. A decrease in aortic compliance (ie, an increase in the stiffness of the aorta) will increase pulse pressure. When mean arterial pressure increases, the average volume of blood in the aorta is higher than normal. The increased volume decreases aortic compliance. Assuming that the stroke volume remains normal, the decreased compliance will result in an increased pulse pressure. If heart rate increases, stroke volume and therefore pulse pressure will decrease. An increase in total peripheral resistance will prevent blood from flowing out of the aorta during systole and therefore decrease pulse pressure. In aortic stenosis, the rate at which blood is ejected from the ventricle is decreased. The decreased ejection rate provides time for blood to flow from the aorta to the periphery during systole. Therefore, the increase in aortic volume during systole and the pulse pressure are decreased.

**266. The answer is c.** *(Fauci, pp 1472-1475. Le, p 248. Stead, pp 37-38.)* Patients with aortic stenosis are usually asymptomatic until the aortic valve orifice becomes significantly narrowed. The systolic murmur auscultated is due to the turbulent flow of blood across the aortic valve during ventricular systole. Dyspnea, angina, and syncope are major symptoms that can be associated with it. In contrast, aortic regurgitation, pulmonic regurgitation, mitral stenosis, and tricuspid stenosis are all diastolic murmurs.

**267. The answer is b.** *(Ganong, pp 571-576. Widmaier, pp 379-382.)* Stroke volume is determined by preload, afterload, and contractility. Increasing heart rate decreases the time for filling during diastole and may decrease preload and therefore stroke volume. Increasing preload by increasing central venous pressure will increase stroke volume. Similarly, decreasing afterload by decreasing total peripheral resistance or systemic blood pressure will cause an increase in stroke volume. Increasing contractility will also increase stroke volume.

**268. The answer is b.** *(Ganong, pp 556-559.)* A premature ventricular beat originates from ventricular pacemaker cells. Most often, these pacemaker cells are reset with each heart beat and therefore do not produce ventricular activation. However, when the sinus rhythm is very slow (bradycardia), there is time for these pacemaker cells to reach threshold and produce a ventricular contraction. Because the patient is a well-trained athlete, his bradycardia is an index of his good aerobic conditioning and not a cause for alarm. An ECG that revealed a depressed ST segment would be significant, since it is a sign of ventricular ischemia. Although an inverted atrial wave can occur following a PVC (if the action potentials propagate into the atria) and a wide QRS complex, these are results, not causes of the premature contractions.

**269. The answer is e.** *(Fauci, pp 1393-1395. Ganong, pp 561-563.)* Abnormalities in coronary blood flow resulting in ischemia of the ventricular muscle will lead to a current of injury, which is reflected as an upward or downward shift in the ST segment of the ECG recording. The ECG presented shows marked ST-segment elevations in leads I, aVL, and $V_1$ to $V_6$ indicative of acute myocardial infarction. The electrical activity of the heart does not reflect changes in ventricular contractility, blood pressure, ejection fraction, or total peripheral resistance, although all of these can be altered by changes in coronary blood flow.

**270. The answer is c.** (*Ganong, pp 571-576. Widmaier, pp 379-382.*) Stroke volume is influenced by ventricular preload, afterload, and contractility. Decreasing total peripheral resistance may result in a decrease in afterload and therefore an increase in stroke volume. Decreasing ventricular compliance (making the heart stiffer) or increasing venous compliance will decrease ventricular filling and therefore preload and stroke volume. Similarly, increasing heart rate will decrease filling and stroke volume.

**271. The answer is b.** (*Ganong, pp 575-576, 586. Widmaier, pp 419-421.*) When the left ventricle fails, preload (left ventricular end-diastolic volume) is increased in an attempt to normalize stroke volume. The increase in radius of the dilated ventricle increases wall tension (stress) according to the Laplace relationship, $T = Pr/w$, where $T$ = tension, $P$ = systolic pressure, $r$ = ventricular radius, and $w$ = ventricular wall thickness. The increase in wall tension requires an increase in energy consumption. The increase in preload increases the left ventricular end-diastolic pressure. Because the pulmonary capillaries are supplying the blood to the left ventricle, an increase in left ventricular end-diastolic pressure must be accompanied by an increase in pulmonary capillary hydrostatic pressure. The decrease in left ventricular contractility associated with heart failure causes the ejection fraction to decrease. Heart rate will be increased by the increased sympathetic nerve activity that accompanies heart failure.

**272. The answer is b.** (*Ganong, pp 549-550, 565-569. Widmaier,pp 373-377.*) The PR interval starts at the beginning of the P wave and ends at the beginning of the QRS complex. The physiologic events that occur during this time period include atrial depolarization, which is responsible for the P wave, AV nodal depolarization, and depolarization of the bundle of His and the Purkinje fibers. SA nodal depolarization precedes the P wave. Since the mass of the SA node is so small, this event cannot be detected on the standard ECG recording. The mitral and aortic valves are closed during isovolemic contraction, which occurs after the QRS complex has begun. The second heart sound occurs at the end of systole.

**273. The answer is a.** (*Ganong, pp 569-570. Stead, pp 37-38.*) In aortic stenosis, the resistance of the aortic valve increases, making it more difficult for blood to be ejected from the heart. Because a pressure drop occurs across the stenotic aortic valve, the ventricular pressure is much larger than the aortic pressure. Although stroke volume typically decreases leading to a decrease in pulse pressure, a normal cardiac output and arterial pressure can still be maintained by increasing heart rate. However, the increased afterload will lead to a decreased ejection fraction and increased cardiac oxygen consumption.

**274. The answer is d.** (*Ganong, pp 78-81, 548-549.*) The plateau phase (phase 2) is the result of the influx of calcium. Although calcium channels begin to open during the upstroke (phase 0), the greatest number of calcium channels open during the plateau. The upstroke is primarily dependent on the opening of $Na^+$ channels. The initial repolarization (phase 1) is dependent on the inactivation of $Na^+$ channels and the opening of a transient $K^+$ channel. Repolarization (phase 3) is produced by the inactivation of $Ca^{2+}$ channels and the activation of the delayed rectifier $K^+$ channels.

**275. The answer is e.** (*Ganong, pp 550-551, 565-569. Widmaier, pp 373-377.*) The aortic valve closes when the pressure within the ventricle falls below the pressure within the aorta. This occurs when the ventricular muscle begins to relax. Relaxation begins at the end of the ventricular action potential, which is represented by the T wave (segment **E**) on the ECG recording.

**276. The answer is a.** (*Ganong, p 555. Stead, pp 6-8, 44-45.*) The PR interval represents the time it takes for the cardiac action potential to propagate from the SA node to the ventricular muscle. A delay in this interval, normally produced by a slowing in the conduction velocity through the AV node, is called a first-degree heart block. A second-degree heart block occurs when the action potential does not always propagate through the SA node. This produces an uneven heart beat. A third-degree block occurs when the action potential never reaches the ventricle. Under these conditions, pacemakers within the ventricle produce ventricular contraction but the rate is very slow. Inversion of the T wave and elevation of the ST segment of the ECG are indicators of membrane potential defects within the ventricular muscle.

**277. The answer is d.** (*Ganong, pp 565-568. Widmaier, pp 373-377.*) The graph illustrates the development of pressure in the aorta, the left atrium, and the left ventricle during a single cardiac cycle. At point **D**, the pressure within the left ventricle is less than the pressure in the left atrium, and therefore the mitral valve opens and ventricular filling begins. Although the volume in the left ventricle is increasing, the pressure is falling. During this time period, the recoil of the ventricle causes its pressure to decrease as it is filling. Later in diastole, the pressure of the blood returning from the lungs causes both volume and pressure in the ventricle to increase.

**278. The answer is c.** (*Fauci, pp 1407, 1469-1471. Ganong, pp 567, 569, 595-596.*) Regurgitation of the mitral valve results in backwards flow of blood from the left ventricle to the left atrium during systole, resulting in an increased v wave due to increased left atrial pressure. Blood pressure is typically normal in patients with mitral regurgitation. The greater left ventricular preload produces a greater-than-normal stroke volume. However, the forward stroke volume, the volume entering the aorta, does not increase, so there is no increase in pulse pressure or cardiac output.

**279. The answer is d.** (*Fauci, pp 1490-1492. Stead, pp 34-35.*) Cardiac tamponade is a disorder of the heart in which an increase in the volume of pericardial fluid compresses the heart and reduces ventricular filling during diastole. Pulsus paradoxus is a clinical sign in which there is an abnormally large decrease (> 10 mm Hg) in systolic pressure during inspiration. The drop in systolic pressure normally occurs during inspiration because the decreased intrathoracic pressure reduces the flow of blood from the lungs to the left ventricle. The decrease in intrathoracic pressure also increases venous return to the right ventricle. The decrease in ventricular filling during inspiration is exacerbated in cardiac tamponade because the increased volume of blood in the right ventricle cannot push out the right ventricular wall because of the increased fluid in the pericardial space. Instead, the blood pushes against the intraventricular septum, greatly reducing the volume of blood that can enter the left ventricle.

**280. The answer is b.** (*Ganong, pp 571-574.*) A normal Starling curve of the heart, showing stroke volume as a function of end-diastolic volume, is depicted by the curve on which an **X** is marked. The Starling curve below the normal one will result from a decrease in contractility (eg, with heart failure) or an increase in afterload. The Starling curve above the normal curve will result from an increase in contractility or a decrease in afterload. Digitalis is a positive inotropic agent that will cause a point on the lower curve to shift up and to the left, such that there is an increased stroke volume at a lower preload.

**281. The answer is e.** *(Ganong, pp 604-609, 637. Widmaier, pp 413-414.)* Loss of blood causes blood pressure to fall. The baroreceptor reflex response to the fall in blood pressure causes a reflex increase in sympathetic outflow, causing an $\alpha$-adrenergic receptor-mediated increase in arteriolar resistance, which further decreases capillary perfusing pressure. Because whole blood is lost, the concentration of circulating proteins remains normal and therefore the oncotic pressure remains the same. The decreased capillary pressure and normal oncotic pressure result in the transfer of fluid from the interstitium to the vascular bed, decreasing the hematocrit. The increased arteriolar constriction lowers blood flow to the kidney causing urine formation to decrease. Sympathetic stimulation causes peripheral constriction and produces sweating, resulting in the classic sign of hemorrhage: cold, pale skin. The baroreceptor reflex increases heart rate.

**282. The answer is a.** *(Ganong, pp 636-641.)* Anaphylactic shock is characterized by a decreased peripheral resistance and a high cardiac output. The decrease in peripheral resistance is so great that mean blood pressure falls below normal. Hypovolemic shock is caused by a decrease in circulating blood volume and pressure. In both types of shock, the baroreceptor reflex increases ventricular contractility and heart rate. Also, in both types of shock, blood is shunted away from the kidney, decreasing renal blood flow and glomerular filtration. As a result, plasma creatinine levels rise.

**283. The answer is c.** *(Fauci, pp 2269-2271. Ganong, pp 360, 642. Stead, pp 94-95.)* Pheochromocytoma is a tumor of the adrenal medulla characterized by an excessive release of catecholamines. Severe hypertension can result from the increase in heart rate and contractility ($\beta_1$-adrenergic activation by catecholamines) and vascular resistance ($\alpha$-adrenergic activation). Blocking the $\alpha$-adrenergic receptors will cause a decrease in TPR and a decrease in blood pressure. Glycoprotein IIb/IIIa antagonists inhibit platelet function and are used in patients with coronary heart disease, not in the treatment of hypertension.

**284. The answer is e.** *(Ganong, pp 574-575, 633-634.)* The diagram represents the cardiac (ventricular) function and venous function curves. Similar to the familiar Starling curves, cardiac output is graphed as a function of central venous pressure (preload). The cardiac function curves are shifted up and to the left by an increase in contractility and a decrease in afterload; they are shifted down and to the right by a decrease in contractility and an increase in afterload. The vascular function curves graph central venous pressure as a function of cardiac output. The independent variable, cardiac output, is represented on the y axis. An increase in cardiac output causes a fall in central venous pressure. A decrease in blood volume or venous tone shifts the vascular function curves to the left; an increase in blood volume or venous tone shifts the vascular function curves to the right. The point at which the two curves intersect represents the central venous pressure and cardiac output of the cardiovascular system. The shift from the resting state to point **E** represents an increase in vascular volume or venous tone without any change in TPR or ventricular contractility. This is consistent with an infusion of saline or a blood transfusion. The shift from the resting state to point **B** represents an increase in contractility with no change in TPR; this is consistent with the administration of a positive inotropic drug. With exercise, there is an increase in contractility and a decrease in TPR and venous compliance, consistent with a shift from control to point **C**.

**285. The answer is c.** *(Fauci, pp 1505-1507, 1509-1513. Ganong, pp 548-549, 565-568, 632-635.)* Sympathetic stimulation of the heart increases the activity of the sarcoplasmic reticulum (SR) $Ca^{2+}$ pump. Sympathetic stimulation also increases the rate of SA nodal firing, which increases heart rate, and decreases the duration of the total cardiac cycle. Norepinephrine secreted by the sympathetic nerve endings binds to $\beta_1$-adrenergic receptors, activating a G protein, which activates adenylyl cyclase and increases the intracellular concentration of cyclic AMP. Cyclic AMP activates protein kinase A, which leads to phosphorylation of the voltage-dependent $Ca^{2+}$ channels, causing them to spend more time in the open state. Cyclic AMP also increases the active transport of $Ca^{2+}$ to the sarcoplasmic reticulum (SR), thus accelerating relaxation and shortening systole, which is important when heart rate is increased to permit adequate diastolic filling in the face of a decrease in the duration of diastole.

**286. The answer is a.** *(Ganong, pp 80-81. Widmaier, pp 267-268.)* During exercise, sympathetic stimulation of the heart increases contractility, and thus stroke volume. A decrease in venous compliance, caused by sympathetic stimulation, increases venous return to the heart, which also increases stroke volume by a Frank-Starling mechanism. The increased stroke volume, coupled with an increase in heart rate, causes an increase in cardiac output. Systemic arterial pressure also increases in response to the increase in cardiac output. However, the fall in total peripheral resistance, which is caused by dilation of the blood vessels within the exercising muscles, results in a decrease in diastolic pressure. The pulmonary vessels undergo passive dilation as more blood flows into the pulmonary circulation. As a result, pulmonary vascular resistance decreases.

**287. The answer is b.** (*Ganong, pp 581-585.*) The ratio of the blood flow through vessels Y and Z is inversely proportional to their resistance. Because vessel Y has half the resistance of vessel Z, it has twice the blood flow. The blood flowing through vessel X is the sum of the blood flowing through vessels Y and Z ($2 + 1 = 3$). Therefore, the ratio of the blood flowing through vessels X and Y is 3:2.

$$Q_{Vessel\ Y} \propto 1/1;\ Q_{Vessel\ Z} \propto 1/2$$
$$Q_{Vessel\ Y}/Q_{Vessel\ Z} = \frac{1/1 \times 2/1}{1/2 \times 2/1}$$
$$= 2/1$$
$$Q_{Vessel\ X} = Q_{Vessel\ Y} + Q_{Vessel\ Z} = 2 + 1 = 3$$
$$Q_{Vessel\ X}/Q_{Vessel\ Y} = 3/2$$

**288. The answer is c.** (*Fauci, pp 1720-1723. Ganong, pp 604-608, 617.*) If intracranial pressure is rapidly elevated, cerebral blood flow is reduced. The increase in intracranial pressure stimulates the vasomotor center and produces an increase of systemic blood pressure that may lead to a restoration of cerebral blood flow. The increased blood pressure induces bradycardia mediated by the baroreceptor reflex.

**289. The answer is e.** (*Ganong, pp 576, 586. Widmaier, pp 371-373, 419.*) The factors that influence wall stress are given by the Laplace relationship— Tension (wall stress) = [$P \times r$/w]), where $P$ equals the transmural pressure across the wall of the ventricle, $r$, the radius of the ventricle (determined by end-diastolic volume), and w, the thickness of the ventricular wall. Tension (wall stress) is reduced if the wall thickness increases. Increasing the systolic pressure developed by the heart (ventricular transmural pressure) or increasing the end-diastolic volume will increase wall stress. Wall stress will also be increased if total peripheral resistance is increased or mean arterial blood pressure is increased because, under both conditions, the heart will have to develop more pressure. Losartan is an angiotensin II receptor (type $AT_1$) antagonist that helps to lower blood pressure as well as reduce left ventricular hypertrophy. The R wave of $\geq 11$ mm in aVL along with the findings of the S wave in $V_1$ + R wave in $V_5$ of $\geq 35$mm are suggestive of left ventricular hypertrophy.

**290. The answer is b.** *(Ganong, pp 547-554. Stead, p 7. Widmaier, pp 373-377.)* The bundle of His depolarizes during the PR segment (segment **B**), that is, during the interval between the end of atrial depolarization and the beginning of ventricular depolarization. Segment **A**, the **P** wave, represents atrial depolarization, segment **C**, the QRS complex, represents ventricular depolarization, segment **D**, the ST segment, represents the time interval during which all of the ventricular muscle is depolarized, and segment **E**, the T wave, represents ventricular repolarization.

**291. The answer is c.** *(Fauci, pp 1393-1394, 1532-1533. Ganong, pp 561-564.)* Within hours after an acute myocardial infarction of the anterior ventricle, ST-segment elevation appears in leads I, aVL, and the left precordial leads, $V_{3-6}$. Reciprocal ST depression occurs in leads II, III, and aVF. After some days or weeks, when the ST-segment abnormalities subside, the dead muscle and scar tissue become electrically silent. The infarcted area is therefore negative relative to the normal myocardium during systole, and it fails to contribute its share of positivity to the ECG complexes. Manifestations of this negativity include the appearance of Q waves and failure of progression of the R wave in the precordial leads.

**292. The answer is a.** *(Widmaier, p 415.)* Blood flow to the brain is kept relatively constant during both rest and exercise by local autoregulatory mechanisms. During aerobic exercise, vasodilation of blood vessels in the working muscles increases skeletal muscle blood flow. Coronary blood flow increases to meet the increased metabolic needs of the heart. Blood flow to the gut, the kidneys, and the nonexercising muscles is reduced by sympathetic constriction of the arterioles leading to these organs. Blood flow to the skin is increased to prevent overheating.

**293. The answer is b.** *(Ganong, pp 586-590. Widmaier, p 386.)* Pulse pressure is proportional to the amount of blood entering the aorta during systole and inversely proportional to aortic compliance. Pulse pressure increases with hypertension because hypertension causes aortic compliance to decrease. Whether the hypertension is a result of an increased cardiac output or an increased peripheral resistance, the higher arterial pressure is caused by an increase in arterial blood volume. The increased blood volume stretches the arterial wall, making it stiffer and decreasing its compliance. Stroke volume is decreased with tachycardia, hemorrhage, and heart failure, reducing pulse pressure in all three cases. In aortic stenosis, the ejection of blood from the ventricle is slowed and the increase in arterial blood volume during systole is less than normal.

**294. The answer is d.** (*Ganong, pp 605-607. Widmaier, pp 405-410.*) A reduction in carotid sinus pressure due to a decrease in mean blood pressure would elicit a baroreceptor reflex tending to restore blood pressure to normal. The reflex response includes an increase in sympathetic nervous system activity, which would cause an increase in heart rate and myocardial contractility, both of which would tend to increase cardiac output. Sympathetic stimulation would also cause constriction of both the arterioles and venous vessels. Arteriolar constriction would cause an increase in total peripheral resistance. Sympathetic stimulation of the venous vessels would cause a decrease in venous compliance.

**295. The answer is b.** (*Ganong, pp 612, 622, 632-634. Widmaier, p 393.*) The overall arteriovenous $O_2$ difference is determined by the oxygen consumption of a tissue and its blood flow. Because of the high rate of metabolism in the heart compared with its blood flow, it has the highest arteriovenous $O_2$ difference of any major organ of the body under normal conditions. The heart can extract a large amount of oxygen because of its high capillary density. Any substantial reduction in coronary blood flow (such as in the case of myocardial infarction) will curtail the delivery of oxygen to the myocardium since the extraction of oxygen from each unit volume of blood is nearly maximal even when blood flow is normal. Blood flow to the kidney and skin is far in excess of their metabolic needs, so little oxygen is removed from the blood as it passes through these organs. Therefore, their arteriovenous $O_2$ differences are rather small. Under normal conditions, the arteriovenous $O_2$ difference in skeletal muscle is quite low, but can increase substantially during vigorous exercise.

**296. The answer is e.** *(Widmaier, p 385.)* Compliance is defined as the change in volume divided by the change in pressure ($\Delta V/\Delta P$). The lower the compliance, the stiffer the vessel becomes. The venous system is much more compliant than the arterial system.

Arterial compliance = $\Delta V/\Delta P$ = 250 mL/160 mm Hg = 1.56 mL/mm Hg
Venous compliance = $\Delta V/\Delta P$ = 1500 mL/50 mm Hg = 30 mL/mm Hg
Arterial compliance/Venous compliance = 1.56 mL/mm Hg/30 mL/mm Hg = 1:19.2

**297. The answer is d.** *(Fauci, pp 1449-1450. Stead, p 26. Widmaier, pp 420, 508.)* Angiotensin converting enzyme (ACE) inhibitors such as captopril are a mainstay of treatment for congestive heart failure and their use has been shown to have a survival benefit. ACE inhibitors interfere with the renin-angiotensin system by blocking the conversion of angiotensin I to angiotensin II. Because angiotensin II is a potent vasoconstrictor, inhibiting this conversion leads to arteriolar vasodilation, thus reducing afterload. They also appear to stabilize ventricular remodeling. Bradykinin levels are increased with ACE inhibitor use and a nonproductive cough is a side effect as a result.

**298. The answer is a.** *(Ganong, pp 628-629.)* The fetus derives its oxygen from the maternal arterial blood supply by gas exchange across the placenta. The umbilical vein draining the placenta therefore has the highest oxygenation in the fetus, with a $PO_2$ of approximately 30 mm Hg and 80% oxygen saturation. The ductus venosus has only a slightly lower $PO_2$, and serves to direct much of the highly oxygenated blood from the umbilical vein to the inferior vena cava, bypassing the liver. From the right atrium, about two-thirds of the inferior venal caval flow (67% $O_2$ saturation) is diverted across the foramen ovale to the left atrium. The $PO_2$ in the left ventricular outflow tract going to the ascending aorta is approximately 25 mm Hg. The $PO_2$ in the ductus arteriosus is approximately 18 mm Hg, and blood in the descending aorta and umbilical arteries, is approximately 20 mm Hg with an oxygen saturation of approximately 60%.

**299. The answer is c.** *(Ganong, pp 628-629.)* The ductus arteriosus is a low-resistance arterial vessel of the fetus through which highly oxygenated blood flows from the pulmonary artery to the aorta, bypassing the lungs. The ductus arteriosus empties into the aorta just distal to the left subclavian artery. Because blood is oxygenated in the placenta, pulmonary blood flow in the fetus serves only a nutritive, not a gas exchange, function for the developing lungs, and thus only about 5% to 10% of the cardiac output flows through the lungs. Soon after birth with the onset of extrauterine respiration, the pulmonary vascular resistance falls, allowing blood to flow from the pulmonary artery to the lungs. The high oxygen tension in the blood of the baby causes the resistance of the ductus arteriosus to increase, with functional closure occurring within several hours after birth. When the ductus arteriosus does not close, it is called a patent ductus arteriosus. If there is normal oxygenation with a normal regression of the pulmonary vasculature after birth, blood flow will reverse across the ductus arteriosus after birth, flowing from the aorta to the pulmonary artery. The left-to-right shunt persists throughout the cardiac cycle yielding the characteristic thrill and continuous murmur with late systolic accentuation at the upper left sternal edge. Cyanosis does not occur with a left-to-right shunt; however, the chronic increase in blood flow through the lungs may induce structural changes in the pulmonary vasculature leading to obstruction and pulmonary hypertension (Eisenmenger syndrome). The resultant right-to-left flow across the ductus causes the toes, but not the fingers, to become cyanotic and clubbed, a finding termed differential cyanosis.

**300. The answer is a.** (*Ganong, pp 582-585. Widmaier, pp 362-364.*) Turbulence, and consequently the bruit, was produced by the high velocity of blood within the stenotic area of the carotid artery, as predicted by Reynolds number. The widening of a vessel associated with aneurysms can also produce bruits but these are not relieved by endarterectomy. An increase in hematocrit or blood viscosity would decrease Reynolds number and decrease the tendency for turbulent flow.

**301. The answer is b.** (*Ganong, pp 454-457, 601-602. Widmaier, pp 391-392.*) Angiotensin II is a powerful vasoconstrictor that is formed when renin is released from the kidney in response to a fall in blood pressure or vascular volume. Renin converts angiotensinogen to angiotensin I. Angiotensin II is formed from angiotensin I by angiotensin-converting enzyme localized within the vasculature of the lung. All the other listed substances cause vasodilation.

**302. The answer is c.** (*Ganong, pp 574-575, 633-634.*) This diagram depicts cardiac (ventricular) function and venous function curves. With the onset of exercise, there is an increase in contractility, which shifts the cardiac function curve up. Also accompanying the onset of exercise are decreases in total peripheral resistance and venous compliance, both of which shift the vascular function curve to the right and increase its slope. The point at which the cardiac function and venous function curves intersect (C) represents the central venous pressure and cardiac output of the cardiovascular system under these conditions.

**303. The answer is e.** (*Ganong, pp 565-566, 573.*) The left ventricular pressure-volume loop represents the changes in pressure and volume that occur during a cardiac cycle. Point **E** represents the end of the filling phase and the beginning of the isovolumic contraction phase. At this point, the pressure in the left ventricle increases above the pressure in the left atrium, causing the mitral valve to close. Systole is defined as the period between the first and second heart sounds and includes the isovolumic contraction and ejection phases. Aortic pressure continues to fall during the isovolumic contraction phase so that the rise in aortic blood pressure (which begins at point **D**) lags behind the beginning of systole. Point **B** represents the end of the ejection phase. At this point, the pressure in the left ventricle falls below the pressure in the aorta, and the aortic valve closes. Point **A** represents the end of the isovolumic relaxation phase and the beginning of the filling phase. At the point the pressure in the left ventricle falls below that in the left atrium, the mitral valve opens and blood begins to flow into the left ventricle.

**304. The answer is e.** (*Ganong, pp 628-629.*) At birth, with the onset of extrauterine respiration and elimination of the placental circulation, functional closure of the foramen ovale and the ductus venosus occur immediately, whereas functional closure of the ductus arteriosus generally begins within a few hours after birth, and is not complete until about 48 to 72 hours. Immediately after birth, flow through the ductus switches, with blood flowing from the aorta to the pulmonary artery. The ductus arteriosus is a systemic blood vessel, and thus it constricts in response to high oxygen tensions and dilates in response to hypoxemia (the opposite of the pulmonary vasculature). Ductal sensitivity to oxygen is age-dependent, however, and thus closure of the ductus arteriosus due to progressive constriction may be delayed in premature infants. Closure can be induced by infusion of cyclooxygenase inhibitors; drugs that inhibit both COX-1 and COX-2 have yielded the best results clinically.

**305. The answer is b.** *(Fauci, pp 1559-1561. Ganong, pp 78-84, 580-581.)* Smooth muscle contraction is regulated by a series of reactions that begins with the binding of calcium to calmodulin, in contrast to cardiac (and skeletal) muscle, where contraction is triggered by the binding of $Ca^{2+}$ to troponin C, which by altering the position of tropomyosin on the thin filament, allows cross-bridge cycling to begin. The calcium-calmodulin complex in smooth muscle binds to and activates a protein kinase called myosin light chain kinase (MLCK), which catalyzes the phosphorylation of the myosin light chains ($LC_{20}$). Once these light chains are phosphorylated, myosin and actin interaction can occur and vascular smooth muscle shortens and develops tension. Although β-adrenergic receptor agonists may lower blood pressure by relaxing vascular smooth muscle, they also increase the rate and strength of the heart beat.

**306. The answer is d.** *(Fauci, pp 1369-1370. Ganong, pp 65-67.)* Titin is a large protein that connects the Z lines to the M lines, thereby providing a scaffold for the sarcomere. Titin contains two types of folded domains that provide muscle with its elasticity. The resistance to stretch increases throughout a contraction, which protects the structure of the sarcomere and prevents excess stretch.

**307. The answer is d.** *(Fauci, pp 1522-1523. Widmaier, pp 423-424.)* Nitrates are commonly used for the treatment of angina. Myocardial oxygen demand is decreased primarily due to systemic venodilation and subsequent decrease in left ventricular wall stress due to decreased venous return. Nitrates also act on the arterial side, resulting in an increase in coronary blood flow and a decrease in blood pressure.

**308. The answer is e.** *(Ganong, pp 620-623. Widmaier, pp 373-378, 383.)* Blood flow through the coronary vessels of the left ventricle is determined by the ratio of perfusion pressure to vascular resistance. The perfusion pressure is directly related to the aortic pressure at the ostia of the coronaries. Myocardial vascular resistance is significantly influenced by the contractile activity of the ventricle. During systole, when the ventricle is contracting, coronary vascular resistance increases substantially and the first heart sound is auscultated due to closure of the mitral and tricuspid valves. Flow is highest just at the beginning of diastole because, during this phase of the cardiac cycle, aortic pressure is still relatively high and vascular resistance is low due to the fact that the coronary vessels are no longer being squeezed by the contracting myocardium. The second heart sound is due to closure of the aortic and pulmonic valves at the beginning of diastole.

**309. The answer is e.** *(Fauci, p 1371.)* Phospholamban is a protein contained within the sarcoplasmic reticulum (SR) that inhibits the activity of the SR calcium pump. Inactivation of phospholamban results in an increase in calcium sequestration by the SR. Increasing the concentration of calcium within the SR increases the force of the ventricular contraction.

**310. The answer is a.** *(Ganong, pp 565-569, 650, 660-662. Widmaier, pp 378-380, 400.)* Although the left and right preloads are not identical, they are very similar (right atrial pressure = 2 mm Hg; left atrial pressure = 5 mm Hg). The right and left ventricles are in series with one another such that the right and left ventricular outputs are essentially equal. Because the two ventricles beat at the same rate, their stroke volumes are the same. The resistance of the pulmonary vasculature is much lower than that of the systemic circulation, however, yielding much lower pressures in the pulmonary artery than the aorta (mean pulmonary artery pressure = 15 mm Hg; mean aortic pressure = 90 mm Hg). Thus, the afterload and stroke work are greater on the left side than on the right side. Because the same cardiac output is ejected into a higher resistance, peak systolic pressure is higher on the left side (120 mm Hg) than on the right side (25 mm Hg). Only about 10% of the blood volume is within the pulmonary circulation at any one time, whereas approximately two-thirds of the blood volume is stored within the systemic veins and venules.

# Gastrointestinal Physiology

## Questions

**311.** A 52-year-old man with diabetes mellitus type 1 has persistent nausea and vomiting due to gastroparesis with gastroesophageal reflux disease. Which of the following best describes the function of gastric emptying?

a. Solids empty more rapidly than liquids.
b. Meals containing fat empty faster than carbohydrate-rich food.
c. Hyperosmolality of duodenal contents initiates a decrease in gastric emptying.
d. Acidification of the antrum increases gastric emptying.
e. Vagal stimulation decreases receptive relaxation in the upper portion of the stomach.

**312.** A 27-year-old female medical student with irritable bowel syndrome (IBS) has an alteration in intestinal motility resulting in fluctuating constipation and diarrhea. Her condition has worsened in the past month as the date she has scheduled for her licensure examination approaches. Which of the following best describes small intestinal motility?

a. Contractile frequency is constant from duodenum to terminal ileum.
b. Peristalsis is the only contractile activity that occurs during feeding.
c. Migrating motor complexes occur during the digestive period.
d. Vagotomy abolishes contractile activity during the digestive period.
e. Contractile activity is initiated in response to bowel wall distention.

**313.** An 18-year-old man with pernicious anemia lacks intrinsic factor, which is necessary for the absorption of cyanocobalamin. Vitamin $B_{12}$ is absorbed primarily in which portion of the GI tract?

a. Stomach
b. Duodenum
c. Jejunum
d. Ileum
e. Colon

**314.** A 57-year-old man undergoes resection of the distal 100 cm of the terminal ileum as part of treatment for Crohn disease. The patient likely will develop malabsorption of which of the following?

a. Iron
b. Folate
c. Lactose
d. Bile salts
e. Protein

**315.** A 42-year-old salesman presents with the chief complaint of intermittent midepigastric pain that is relieved by antacids or eating. Gastric analysis reveals that basal and maximal acid outputs exceed normal values. The gastric acid hypersecretion can be explained by an increase in the plasma concentration of which of the following?

a. Somatostatin
b. Vasoactive intestinal peptide
c. Gastrin
d. Secretin
e. Cholecystokinin

**316.** A 27-year-old woman comes to the emergency room because of a 2-day bout of profuse watery diarrhea. Physical examination reveals dry lips and oropharynx. The patient is diagnosed with acute secretory diarrhea and dehydration, likely due to *Escherichia coli*. Which of the following sodium reabsorptive pathways is inhibited by the enterotoxin?

a. Sodium-glucose-coupled cotransport
b. Electroneutral NaCl transport
c. Sodium-phosphorous countertransport
d. Sodium-hydrogen countertransport
e. Sodium-bile salt cotransport

**317.** A 37-year-old man presents with dehydration and hypokalemic metabolic acidosis. This acid-base and electrolyte disorder can occur with excess fluid loss from which of the following organs?

a. Stomach
b. Ileum
c. Colon
d. Pancreas
e. Liver

**318.** Twenty years ago, a 65-year-old man underwent vagotomy for his refractory peptic ulcer disease. As a result, which of the following gastrointestinal motor activities will be affected most?

a. Secondary esophageal peristalsis
b. Distention-induced intestinal segmentation
c. Orad stomach accommodation
d. Migrating motor complexes

**319.** A 35-year-old male smoker presents with burning epigastric pain that is most pronounced on an empty stomach. A paroxysmal rise in serum gastrin in response to intravenous secretin further supports a diagnosis of Zollinger-Ellison syndrome. Normally, basal acid output is increased by which of the following?

a. Acidification of the antrum
b. Administration of an $H_2$-receptor antagonist
c. Vagotomy
d. Alkalinization of the antrum
e. Acidification of the duodenum

**320.** A 42-year-old man develops a gastric carcinoma affecting the proximal third of his stomach. He is scheduled for a partial gastrectomy of the affected region, which will primarily affect which of the following processes?

a. Accommodation
b. Peristalsis
c. Retropulsion
d. Segmentation
e. Trituration

**321.** A 68-year-old woman with rheumatoid arthritis, who has been taking nonsteroidal anti-inflammatory drugs (NSAIDS) for the past 10 years, complains of burning epigastric pain that is relieved by antacids, but worsened with food. Her doctor discontinues the NSAIDS and recommends cimetidine (Tagamet) because it is inexpensive and over-the-counter. Which of the following best describes the pharmacological blockade of histamine $H_2$ receptors in the gastric mucosa?

a. It inhibits both gastrin- and acetylcholine-mediated secretion of acid.
b. It inhibits gastrin-induced but not meal-stimulated secretion of acid.
c. It has no effect on either gastrin-induced or meal-stimulated secretion of acid.
d. It prevents activation of adenyl cyclase by gastrin.
e. It causes an increase in potassium transport by gastric parietal cells.

**322.** A 37-year-old man with AIDS presents with a fever, anorexia, weight loss, and GI bleeding. Physical examination reveals a palpable abdominal mass. Endoscopy and biopsy reveal a proximal small-bowel malignancy requiring surgical resection. Removal of proximal segments of the small intestine would most likely result in a decrease in which of the following?

a. Basal acid output
b. Maximal acid output
c. Gastric emptying of liquids
d. Gastric emptying of solids
e. Pancreatic enzyme secretion

**323.** A 63-year-old woman has an intractable duodenal ulcer failing all previous treatments. After consultation with a surgeon, a laparoscopic vagotomy is performed. Subsequently, the patient experiences nausea and vomiting after ingestion of a mixed meal. Which of the following best explains her symptoms?

a. Increased gastric emptying of solids
b. Decreased gastric emptying of solids
c. Increased gastric emptying of liquids
d. Decreased gastric emptying of liquids
e. Increased emptying of liquids and solids

**324.** A 17-year-old adolescent boy who is being treated with the macrolide antibiotic erythromycin complains of nausea, intestinal cramping, and diarrhea. The side effects are the result of the antibiotic binding to receptors in the GI tract that recognize which gastrointestinal hormone?
a. Gastrin
b. Secretin
c. Cholecystokinin
d. Motilin
e. Enterogastrone

**325.** A 23-year-old woman complains of abdominal cramps and bloating that are relieved by defecation. Subsequent clinical evaluation reveals an increased maximal acid output, decreased serum calcium and iron concentrations, and microcytic anemia. Inflammation in which area of the GI tract best explains these findings?
a. Stomach
b. Duodenum
c. Jejunum
d. Ileum
e. Colon

**326.** Gastric emptying studies performed on a 49-year-old woman who has vomiting shortly after a meal reveal a time to one-half emptying of liquids of 18 minutes (normal < 20 minutes) and a time to one-half emptying of solids to be 150 minutes (normal < 120 minutes). Which of the following best explains the data?
a. Increased amplitude of antral contractions
b. Colonic obstruction
c. Pyloric stenosis
d. Sectioning of the vagus nerves to the stomach
e. Inflammation of the proximal small intestine

**327.** A 57-year-old woman undergoes resection of the terminal ileum as part of treatment for her chronic inflammatory bowel disease. Removal of the terminal ileum will most likely result in which of the following?
a. Increased bile acid concentration in the enterohepatic circulation
b. Decreased glucose absorption
c. Increased water content of the feces
d. Increased iron absorption
e. Increased fat absorption

**328.** A 67-year-old man with a history of alcohol abuse presents to the emergency room with severe epigastric pain, hypotension, abdominal distension, and diarrhea with steatorrhea. Serum amylase and lipase are found to be greater than normal, leading to a diagnosis of pancreatitis. The steatorrhea can be accounted for by a decrease in the intraluminal concentration of which of the following pancreatic enzymes?

a. Amylase
b. Trypsin
c. Chymotrypsin
d. Lipase
e. Colipase

**329.** A 53-year-old man complains of a mild chronic cough and heartburn. Esophageal manometric and endoscopic evaluation reveal a hypotensive lower esophageal sphincter (LES) pressure and mild gastroesophageal reflux. Which of the following is the primary genesis of LES pressure in adults?

a. Tonic excitatory sympathetic nerve input to the smooth muscle
b. Tonic excitatory parasympathetic nerve input to the smooth muscle
c. Circulating gastrin
d. Myogenic properties of LES smooth muscle
e. Local production of nitric oxide by enteric nerves

**330.** A patient presents with a chronic cough. The history and physical findings rule out postnasal drip, asthma, and other pulmonary disease. Upon questioning, the patient also reports substernal burning pain that is most pronounced after ingestion of coffee, chocolate, french fries, and alcohol. Which of the following is the most likely cause of gastroesophageal reflux disease (GERD) in this patient?

a. Delayed gastric emptying
b. Decreased esophageal motility
c. Hiatal hernia
d. Decreased lower esophageal sphincter tone
e. Decreased upper esophageal sphincter tone

**331.** A 42-year-old man is referred to a gastroenterologist for evaluation of refractory peptic ulcer disease. Subsequent endoscopic and laboratory data are suggestive of Zollinger-Ellison syndrome. The increased basal acid output and maximal acid output of the patient is best explained by an increase in the plasma concentration of which of the following?

a. Gastrin-releasing peptide
b. Secretin
c. Somatostatin
d. Gastrin
e. Histamine

**332.** A 33-year-old woman who has been taking large doses of NSAIDs for her menstrual cramps presents with burning epigastric pain. The pain improves after eating a meal, suggesting a gastric versus duodenal ulcer. In the case of a duodenal ulcer, which of the following is the major factor that protects the duodenal mucosa from damage by gastric acid?

a. Pancreatic bicarbonate secretion
b. The endogenous mucosal barrier of the duodenum
c. Duodenal bicarbonate secretion
d. Hepatic bicarbonate secretion
e. Bicarbonate contained in bile

**333.** After a recent viral illness, a 20-year-old woman develops bilateral facial swelling consistent with parotitis. Which of the following best describes the salivary glands?

a. The parotid gland is the most mucinous of the salivary glands.
b. Starch digestion begins in the mouth via $\alpha$-amylase.
c. $\alpha$-Amylase works most efficiently in the stomach.
d. Approximately 4 L of saliva is secreted per day.
e. Cranial nerve VIII passes through the parotid gland.

**334.** A 70-year old woman presents with abdominal pain, microcytic anemia, and weight loss. Colonoscopy with biopsy confirms colon cancer. Which of the following best describes colonic function?

a. Absorption of $Na^+$ in the colon is under hormonal (aldosterone) control.
b. Bile acids enhance absorption of water from the colon.
c. Net absorption of $HCO_3^-$ occurs in the colon.
d. Net absorption of $K^+$ occurs in the colon.
e. The luminal potential in the colon is positive.

**335.** A 42-year-old woman presents to the ER with right upper quadrant pain that developed after eating dinner. She is diagnosed as having cholecystitis. Which of the following would be expected with contraction of the gallbladder following a meal?

a. It is inhibited by a fat-rich meal.
b. It is inhibited by the presence of amino acids in the duodenum.
c. It is stimulated by atropine.
d. It occurs in response to cholecystokinin.
e. It occurs simultaneously with the contraction of the sphincter of Oddi.

**336.** A 42-year-old airline pilot presents to his family physician with a chief complaint of midepigastric pain that is relieved by antacids or eating. Endoscopic evaluation reveals the presence of a duodenal ulcer. Based on the diagnosis, which of the following also would be expected?

a. Decreased basal acid output
b. Increased maximal acid output
c. Decreased gastric emptying of liquids
d. Decreased gastric emptying of solids
e. Increased gallbladder emptying

**337.** A 26-year-old man presents to the emergency room with a 48-hour bout of diarrhea with steatorrhea. Which of the following best accounts for the appearance of excess fat in the stool?

a. Decreased bile salt pool size
b. Delayed gastric emptying
c. Decreased gastric acid secretion
d. Decreased secretion of intrinsic factor
e. Decreased gastric accommodation

**338.** A 43-year-old woman presents with chief complaints of bulky and frequent diarrhea and weight loss. She experiences recurrent episodes of abdominal distension terminated by passage of stools. Laboratory data reveals a microcytic anemia, decreased serum calcium, and decreased serum albumin. After additional tests she is diagnosed with gluten-sensitive enteropathy. Her generalized decrease in intestinal absorption can be attributed to which of the following?

a. Decreased intestinal motility
b. Increased migrating motor complexes
c. Decreased intestinal surface area
d. Increased enterohepatic circulation of bile
e. Decreased gastric emptying

**339.** A 32-year-old woman presents to the emergency department with abdominal pain and diarrhea accompanied by steatorrhea. Gastric analysis reveals a basal acid output (12 mmol/h) greater than normal (< 5 mmol/h). The steatorrhea is most likely due to which of the following?

a. Inactivation of pancreatic lipase due to low duodenal pH
b. Delayed gastric emptying
c. Decreased gastric acid secretion
d. Decreased secretion of intrinsic factor
e. Decreased pyloric sphincter tone

**340.** A 37-year-old man is admitted to the hospital due to an exacerbation of his Crohn disease with severe inflammation of the ileum. Which of the following would be seen?

a. Increased vitamin $B_{12}$ absorption
b. Decreased bile acid pool size
c. Increased colon absorption of water
d. Decreased release of secretin
e. Increased absorption of dietary fats

**341.** A 30-year-old man with type 1 diabetes mellitus takes metoclopramide because of severe gastroparesis. Which of the following would be expected with the use of metoclopramide?

a. It is not associated with drug-induced parkinsonism.
b. It is a dopamine receptor agonist.
c. It decreases lower esophageal sphincter tone.
d. It increases peristalsis of the small intestine.
e. It may be used in patients with intestinal obstruction.

**342.** A 47-year-old man takes omeprazole for symptoms of his gastroesophageal reflux disease (GERD). Which of the following best describes the use of proton pump inhibitors (PPI)?

a. PPIs are not used in the treatment of Zollinger-Ellison syndrome.
b. PPIs inhibit H-K-ATPase in parietal cells.
c. PPIs are not effective as part of a treatment regimen for *Helicobacter pylori*.
d. PPIs must be dose-adjusted for renal insufficiency.
e. PPIs decrease gastrin levels.

**343.** A 62-year-old woman who takes an NSAID for her severe bilateral osteoarthritis of the knees is prescribed misoprostol. Which of the following would be expected with the use of misoprostol?

a. Diarrhea is not associated with its use.
b. It may be safely used in pregnancy.
c. It is used in the prevention of NSAID-induced gastric ulcers.
d. It is a histamine receptor antagonist.
e. It inhibits mucous bicarbonate secretion.

**344.** An 18-year-old college student reports that she experiences severe abdominal bloating and diarrhea within 1 hour of consuming dairy products. A subsequent hydrogen breath test is abnormal. The diarrhea and bloating can best be explained by which of the following?

a. A deficiency in the brush border enzyme lactase
b. Carbohydrate-induced secretory diarrhea
c. Decreased intestinal surface area
d. Decreased carbohydrate absorption
e. A decrease in exocrine pancreatic secretion

**345.** A 31-year-old man presents to the emergency department with the symptoms of heartburn and difficulty swallowing. Esophageal manometry reveals an inflamed esophageal mucosa and a hypotensive lower esophageal sphincter. A diagnosis of gastroesophageal reflux disease is made and the patient is subsequently treated with a proton pump inhibitor. Normally, which of the following is most likely regarding reflux of gastric acid into the esophagus?

a. It initiates primary esophageal peristalsis.
b. It inhibits gastric acid secretion.
c. It initiates secondary esophageal peristalsis.
d. It inhibits esophageal bicarbonate secretion.
e. It inhibits gastric motility.

**346.** A 42-year-old obese woman presents to the emergency department with right upper quadrant pain, nausea, and vomiting. The pain is not related to food intake and lasts for several hours before resolving slowly. Ultrasound images are suggestive of gallstones with cystic duct obstruction. Which of the following is the primary physiological stimulus of gallbladder contraction in the digestive period?

a. Acid-induced release of secretin from the small intestine
b. Fat-induced release of cholecystokinin from the small intestine
c. Acid-induced release of motilin from the small intestine
d. Distension-induced release of glucagon from the small intestine
e. Amino acid-induced release of motilin from the small intestine

**347.** A 20-year-old woman presents with symptomatic hyperglycemia, and a diagnostic workup confirms type 1 diabetes mellitus. The patient is started on insulin glargine. The metabolic effects of insulin include which of the following?

a. Decreased glucose utilization
b. Decreased lipolysis
c. Increased proteolysis
d. Increased gluconeogenesis
e. Increased ketogenesis

**348.** A 56-year-old man presents with postprandial diarrhea persisting since an ileal resection. The gastric surgeon suspects bile acid malabsorption. Which of the following best describes bile acid function?

a. They are essentially water insoluble.
b. The majority of bile acids are absorbed by passive diffusion.
c. Glycine conjugates are more soluble than taurine conjugates.
d. The amount lost in the stool each day represents the daily loss of cholesterol.
e. The bile acid-dependent fraction of bile is stimulated by the hormone secretin.

**349.** A 14-year-old ballerina reports that she has chronic diarrhea. A detailed history reveals that she frequently drinks skim milk, that she does not use laxatives, and that she has noticed that her condition improves during times that she fasts for religious observances. In contrast to secretory diarrhea, which of the following is most likely seen with osmotic diarrhea?

a. It is characterized by an increase in the stool osmotic gap.
b. It is the result of increased crypt cell secretion.
c. It is the result of decreased electroneutral sodium absorption.
d. It is caused by bacterial toxins.
e. It occurs only in the colon.

**350.** A newborn with severe diarrhea is found to have an inherited defect in a glucose transporter resulting in glucose/galactose malabsorption, necessitating a glucose- and galactose-free diet. Which of the following is the transport protein responsible for entry of glucose into the intestinal enterocyte?

a. Glut-2
b. Glut-5
c. SGLT 1
d. SGLT 2
e. SGLT 5

**351.** An 83-year-old woman with constipation is prescribed a high-fiber diet, which leads to an increased production of short-chain fatty acids (SCFAs). SCFA absorption occurs almost exclusively from which of the following segments of the GI tract?

a. Stomach
b. Duodenum
c. Jejunum
d. Ileum
e. Colon

**352.** A 42-year old man with alcoholism presents to the ER with epigastric abdominal pain associated with nausea and vomiting. He is diagnosed with acute pancreatitis. Which of the following best describes pancreatic function?

a. Secretin inhibits $HCO_3$ secretion from the pancreas.
b. Pancreatic lipase converts triglycerides to monoglycerides and free fatty acids.
c. Serum amylase would be decreased in this patient.
d. Serum lipase would be decreased in this patient.
e. Hypertriglyceridemia is not associated with pancreatitis.

**353.** A 47-year-old woman with hypermenorrhea develops an iron-deficiency anemia requiring iron supplements. Which of the following best describes iron digestion and absorption?

a. About 100 mg of iron is absorbed per day.
b. Iron is absorbed rapidly from the small intestine.
c. Iron is transported in the blood bound to transferrin.
d. In general, iron must be oxidized from the ferrous to the ferric state for efficient absorption.
e. Iron is transported into enterocytes by a ferroportin transporter on the apical membrane.

**354.** A patient with alcoholic cirrhosis presents to the emergency room with hematemesis. After stabilizing him with IV fluids, the gastroenterologist administers an agonist/analog of which of the following agents to inhibit gastric acid secretion and visceral blood flow?

a. Gastrin
b. Somatostatin
c. Histamine
d. Pepsin
e. Acetylcholine

**355.** A 56-year-old man presents with weight loss, cough, and diffuse chest pain. A chest x-ray reveals normal heart and lungs, but the radiologist detects a "bird's beak" narrowing of the terminal esophagus, which is also seen with a barium swallow. Follow-up history indicates that the patient also has dysphagia and regurgitation. Manometry shows increased lower esophageal sphincter pressure with no relaxation upon swallowing, indicating a diagnosis of achalasia. Which of the following is the putative inhibitory neurotransmitter responsible for relaxation of gastrointestinal smooth muscle?

a. Dopamine
b. Vasoactive intestinal peptide
c. Somatostatin
d. Substance P
e. Acetylcholine

**356.** A patient has vomiting and severe watery diarrhea after eating spoiled shellfish. Intravenous fluid and electrolyte replacement was started, and a stool specimen was taken, which came back positive for *Vibrio cholerae*. Which of the following statements best describes water and electrolyte absorption in the GI tract?

a. Osmotic equilibration of chime occurs in the ileum.
b. The small intestine and colon have similar absorptive capacities.
c. Osmotic equilibration of chyme occurs in the stomach.
d. The majority of absorption occurs in the jejunum.
e. The incubation period for *V cholerae* is 1 week.

**357.** A 38-year-old man has dinner one evening at his favorite steakhouse. Several hours later, the chyme reaches the duodenum. After secretion of trypsinogen into the duodenum, the enzyme is converted into its active form, trypsin, by which of the following?

a. Enteropeptidase
b. Procarboxypeptidase
c. Pancreatic lipase
d. Chymotrypsin
e. An alkaline pH

**358.** A 52-year-old patient with past medical history significant for cirrhosis and recent total colectomy presents to the ER with hepatic encephalopathy. Removal of the entire colon would be expected to cause which of the following?

a. Decreased urinary urobilinogen
b. An increase in blood ammonia
c. Megaloblastic anemia
d. Severe malnutrition
e. Death

**359.** An 18-year-old woman decides to get a tattoo for her birthday. Two months later she presents with a fever, right upper quadrant pain, nausea, vomiting, and jaundice. Which of the following laboratory values would most likely be found in a patient with infectious hepatitis?

a. An increase in plasma alkaline phosphatase
b. An increase in plasma bile acids
c. An increase in both direct and indirect plasma bilirubin
d. A decrease in plasma alkaline phosphatase
e. A decrease in both direct and indirect plasma bilirubin

**360.** A 27-year-old female patient with a history of irritable bowel syndrome presents with a chief complaint of flatulence. Gas within the colon is primarily derived from which of the following sources?

a. $CO_2$ liberated by the interaction of $HCO_3^-$ and $H^+$
b. Diffusion from the blood
c. Fermentation of undigested oligosaccharides by bacteria
d. Swallowed atmospheric air
e. Air pockets within foodstuffs

**361.** A 60-year-old woman presents to her family physician with complaints of paresthesias in her lower legs bilaterally. On physical examination she is found to have a shiny tongue. During the workup, a complete blood count reveals a macrocytic anemia with hypersegmented neutrophils on peripheral smear. She is subsequently diagnosed with pernicious anemia. With respect to cobalamin-intrinsic factor binding in a normal individual, nearly all binding of cobalamin to intrinsic factor occurs in which of the following organs?

a. Stomach
b. Duodenum
c. Jejunum
d. Ileum
e. Colon

**362.** A 29-year-old internal medicine resident has a breakfast buffet after a long night of call. The rate of gastric emptying increases with an increase in which of the following?

a. Intragastric volume
b. Intraduodenal volume
c. Fat content of duodenum
d. Osmolality of duodenum
e. Acidity of duodenum

**363.** Following an anastomosis of the jejunum to the stomach, a patient presents with discomfort after meals, including weakness, dizziness, and sweating. The symptoms of dumping syndrome are caused in part by which of the following?

a. Increased blood pressure
b. Increased secretion of glucagon
c. Increased secretion of cholecystokinin
d. Hypoglycemia
e. Hyperglycemia

**364.** A 52-year-old woman who has been dieting for several weeks breaks down and eats half a pan of frosted brownies. Insulin secretion following a carbohydrate-rich meal is stimulated by which of the following?

a. Gastrin
b. Cholecystokinin (CCK)
c. Serotonin
d. VIP
e. GLP-1 (7-36) amide

**365.** A new mother calls the pediatrician because she is concerned that her infant defecates after every meal. Which of the following is the cause of these normal bowel movements in newborns?

a. The gastroileal reflex
b. The gastrocolic reflex
c. The intestino-intestinal reflex
d. The defecation reflex
e. Peristaltic rushes

**366.** A 10-year-old boy presents with below-average body weight and height, signs of vitamin K deficiency, steatorrhea, and bloating. He is found to have the MHC class II antigen HLA-DQ2. Which of the following is the most appropriate dietary treatment for malabsorption in this condition?

a. Fat-free diet
b. Lactose-free diet
c. Gluten-free diet
d. High-fiber diet
e. Low-salt diet

**367.** A 47-year-old woman presents to her primary care physician with jaundice. She is found to have elevated levels of direct (conjugated) plasma bilirubin. Which of the following is the most likely diagnosis?

a. Gilbert syndrome
b. Crigler-Najjar syndrome type I
c. Crigler-Najjar syndrome type II
d. Obstruction of the common bile duct
e. Hemolytic anemia

**368.** After a long workout, a third-year medical student drinks a bottle of an electrolyte containing sports drink. Which of the following is the major mechanism for absorption of sodium from the small intestine?

a. $Na^+-H^+$ exchange
b. Cotransport with potassium
c. Electrogenic transport
d. Neutral NaCl absorption
e. Solvent drag

**369.** A morbidly obese man presents with hypertension, hyperlipidemia, and type 2 diabetes mellitus. Dietary fat, after being processed, is extruded from the mucosal cells of the gastrointestinal tract into the lymphatic ducts in the form of which of the following?

a. Monoglycerides
b. Diglycerides
c. Triglycerides
d. Chylomicrons
e. Free fatty acids

**370.** A 42-year-old healthy man takes a daily multivitamin to complement his diet. Which of the following is required for absorption of the fat soluble vitamins contained in his supplement?

a. Intrinsic factor
b. Chymotrypsin
c. Pancreatic lipase
d. Pancreatic amylase
e. Secretin

**371.** A 63-year-old woman presents with diarrhea, abdominal pain, and flushing. The urinary excretion of the serotonin metabolite, 5-hydroxyindoleacetic acid (5-HIAA) is elevated. Abdominal CT reveals a tumor in the terminal ileum. Surgical resection of the terminal ileum will most likely result in which of the following?

a. A decrease in absorption of amino acids
b. An increase in the water content of the feces
c. An increase in the concentration of bile acid in the enterohepatic circulation
d. A decrease in the fat content of the feces
e. An increase in the absorption of iron

# Gastrointestinal Physiology

## Answers

**311. The answer is c.** *(Fauci, pp 240-241, 2289-2290. Ganong, pp 480-482, 494-496. Stead, pp 109-110. Widmaier, pp 548-551.)* Gastroparesis is delayed emptying of food from the stomach, and is a common cause of gastroesophageal reflux disease (GERD). The rate of gastric emptying depends upon neural (enterogastric reflex) and hormonal inhibitory feedback from the proximal small bowel. Gastroparesis is common in diabetes mellitus because hyperosmolality of the duodenum initiates a decrease in gastric emptying, which is probably neural in origin and is sensed by duodenal osmoreceptors. Because solids must be liquefied prior to emptying from the stomach, the gastric emptying of liquids begins before the emptying of solids. Emptying is fastest with a carbohydrate meal, and slowest after a fatty meal. Acid in the antrum inhibits gastrin secretion, which may inhibit gastric motility. The vagus mediates receptive relaxation, the process in which the fundus and upper portion of the body of the stomach relax in response to movement in the pharynx and esophagus in order to accommodate food that enters the stomach.

**312. The answer is e.** *(Fauci, pp 1899-1903. Ganong, pp 480-482, 506-507.)* Contractile activity in the small intestine is initiated in response to distention of the bowel wall. Three types of smooth muscle contractions contribute to small intestinal motility—peristalsis, segmental contractions, and tonic contractions. A fourth type of contraction, peristaltic rushes, are very intense peristaltic waves that may occur in intestinal obstruction. The basal electrical rhythm (BER) are the spontaneous rhythmic fluctuations in membrane potential in the smooth muscle along the GI tract. The BER itself rarely causes muscle contraction, but contractions only occur during the depolarizing phase of BERs, which function to coordinate the various types of contractile activity. The BER is initiated by the interstitial cells of Cajal, which, in the small intestine, are located in the outer circular muscle layer near the myenteric plexus. There are an average of approximately 12 BER cycles/min in the duodenum and proximal jejunum and 8/min in the distal ileum. During fasting between periods of digestion, cycles of motor activity, called migrating motor complexes (MMC), migrate from the stomach to the distal ileum. The MMCs immediately stop with ingestion of food. After vagotomy, contractile activity becomes irregular and chaotic.

**313. The answer is d.** *(Fauci, pp 643-649, 1877-1878. Ganong, pp 313, 315, 477, 496. Stead, pp 150-151.)* Most vitamins are absorbed in the upper small intestine, but vitamin $B_{12}$ (cobalamin) is absorbed primarily in the terminal ileum. Vitamin $B_{12}$ binds with intrinsic factor, a glycoprotein secreted by the parietal cells of the gastric mucosa. The vitamin $B_{12}$-intrinsic factor complex is propelled along the small intestine to the terminal ileum, where specific active transporters located on the enterocyte microvilli bind the vitamin $B_{12}$-intrinsic factor complex and the complex is absorbed across the ileal mucosa. Pernicious anemia is a disease in which there is autoimmune destruction of the parietal cells. Vitamin $B_{12}$ can also be produced by gastrectomy with removal of the intrinsic factor-secreting tissue or by diseases of the terminal ileum. Binding of the Vitamin $B_{12}$-intrinsic factor complex requires $Ca^{2+}$. Whereas vitamin $B_{12}$ and folate absorption are $Na^+$ independent, all seven of the other water-soluble vitamins are absorbed by carriers that are $Na^+$ cotransporters.

**314. The answer is d.** *(Fauci, p 1874. Ganong, pp 470, 472, 474-477. Widmaier, pp 536-537.)* The terminal ileum contains specialized cells responsible for the absorption of primary and secondary bile salts by active transport. Bile salts are necessary for adequate digestion and absorption of fat. Resection of the ileum prevents the absorption of bile acids, which leads to steatorhea. In addition, diarrhea results because the unabsorbed bile acids enter the colon where they increase adenylate cyclase activity, thus promoting the secretion of water into the lumen of the colon causing an increase in the water content of the feces. Iron, folate, carbohydrate, and protein absorption occur primarily in the upper portions of the small intestine.

**315. The answer is c.** *(Ganong, pp 484-488, 492-496. Widmaier, pp 540-543, 545-548.)* Increases in basal and maximal acid output are suggestive of inflammation or removal of the proximal small intestine. Intestinal receptors monitor the composition of chyme and elicit feedback mechanisms that regulate gastric acid secretion and gastric emptying. Absence of feedback leads to an increased presence of excitatory mediators of gastric function. Gastrin is the primary stimulus of meal-induced acid secretion by the parietal cells. Somatostatin, vasoactive intestinal peptide, secretin, and cholecystokinin inhibit gastric acid secretion.

**316. The answer is b.** *(Ganong, pp 476, 512. Stead, pp 139-141. Fauci, p 814.)* Diarrhea is the abnormal passage of fluid or semisolid stool with increased frequency. The general approach to the primary evaluation of patients with diarrhea is differentiating between an infectious versus non-infectious etiology. Although sodium is absorbed from the small intestine by several mechanisms, bacterial toxins specifically inhibit neutral NaCl absorption. In addition, the toxins augment diarrhea by increasing salt and water secretion by intestinal crypt cells. Oral rehydration involves utilizing the sodium-glucose-coupled cotransport pathway.

**317. The answer is c.** *(Ganong, pp 475-477, 491-492. Widmaier, pp 556-557.)* Loss of gastric juice results in hypokalemic, metabolic alkalosis. Excessive loss of fluid from the gastrointestinal tract can lead to dehydration and, depending on the origin of the fluid loss, electrolyte and acid-base disturbances. The hydrogen ion and potassium ion concentration of gastric juice exceeds that of the plasma. As a result, excess fluid loss leads to metabolic alkalosis accompanied by hypokalemia. Because the pancreas, liver, ileum, and colon secrete bicarbonate, excessive loss leads to metabolic acidosis. In addition, the colon secretes potassium. Thus, the acidosis is accompanied by hypokalemia.

**318. The answer is c.** *(Ganong, pp 479-482, 494-495. Widmaier, pp 540-541, 548-550.)* Orad stomach accommodation depends exclusively on an intact vago-vagal reflex. Vagal innervation of the gastrointestinal tract extends from the esophagus to the level of the transverse colon. Preganglionic fibers from cell bodies in the medulla synapse with ganglion cells located in the enteric nervous system. Distention-induced contraction of gastrointestinal smooth muscle develops as the result of long (vago-vagal) and local (enteric nerves) reflexes. The importance of long versus local reflex pathways varies along the gut. Secondary esophageal peristalsis, intestinal segmentation, and migrating motor complexes are unaffected by vagotomy.

**319. The answer is d.** *(Fauci, pp 1868-1869. Ganong, pp 484-488, 494-496. Le, pp 302, 307. Stead, p 111.)* Alkalinization of the antrum releases the gastrin-containing cells from the inhibitory influences of somatostatin and increases acid secretion. Acidification of the antrum promotes the release of somatostatin from cells in the gastrointestinal mucosa, which inhibits gastrin release and gastric acid secretion. Acidification of the duodenum elicits inhibitory neural and hormonal reflexes that also inhibit acid output. Administration of a histamine antagonist, proton pump inhibitor, and vagotomy all reduce acid secretion.

**320. The answer is a.** *(Ganong, pp 480, 494, 506. Widmaier, pp 548-550.)* Increases in intragastric volume normally are not associated with large increases in intragastric pressure because of receptive relaxation or the accommodation reflex, which is vagally mediated. The reflex, which is abolished by vagotomy, is a property of the orad stomach only and counterbalances the stretch-induced myogenic contraction of the gastric smooth muscle. Peristalsis, trituration (grinding), and retropulsion (mixing) are terms referring to the contractile activity and functions of the caudad stomach. Segmental contractions are the primary contractile pattern of the small intestine during the digestive period.

**321. The answer is a.** *(Fauci, pp 244-245. Ganong, pp 493-496.)* Histamine ($H_2$) receptor antagonists inhibit both gastrin-induced and vagal-mediated secretion of acid. Secretion of acid by gastric parietal cells involves stimulation of adenyl cyclase and cyclic AMP-mediated stimulation of the active transport of chloride and potassium-hydrogen ion exchange. Neither gastrin nor vagal stimulation activates adenyl cyclase directly; both depend on concomitant release of histamine and histamine-induced activation of adenyl cyclase.

**322. The answer is e.** *(Ganong, pp 495, 497-498. Widmaier, p 552.)* Inflammation or removal of the upper small intestine leads to a decrease in pancreatic and hepatobiliary function. The proximal small intestine contains a number of receptors that monitor the physical (volume) and chemical (pH, fat content, caloric density, osmolality) composition of the chyme emptied from the stomach. Stimulation of these receptors releases secretin, which acts on pancreatic ductal cells to increase $HCO_3^-$ secretion, as well as cholecystokinin, which acts on pancreatic acinar cells to increase pancreatic enzyme secretion (lipases, amylases, and proteases). Stimulation of proximal small intestine receptors also activates neural reflexes, which initiate pancreatic enzyme and bicarbonate secretion, stimulate gallbladder emptying, and provide feedback for inhibitory regulation of gastric function. Removal of these reflexes decreases pancreatic secretion and gallbladder emptying and increases gastric emptying and acid output.

**323. The answer is b.** *(Fauci, pp 1866-1867. Ganong, p 494.)* The vagus nerve is the primary neural mediator of gastric function. Activation of distension-mediated vago-vagal reflexes in response to the presence of food in the stomach will (1) increase gastric compliance (receptive relaxation or accommodation reflex) and promote gastric retention of food, (2) increase the strength of antral peristaltic contractions necessary for trituration of solids, and (3) increase gastric acid secretion. Sectioning of the vagus nerve fibers to the antral region of the stomach will decrease the strength of contractions thereby prolonging the emptying of solids. The emptying of liquids will be unaffected.

**324. The answer is d.** *(Ganong, pp 482-487. Widmaier, p 556.)* Motilin is the gastrointestinal peptide hormone associated with the initiation of migrating motor complexes during the interdigestive period. The hormone stimulates increased contractions by a direct action on smooth muscle and by activation of excitatory enteric nerves. Erythromycin belongs to the group of macrolide antibiotics and also shows an ability to excite motilin-like receptors on enteric nerves and smooth muscle. As a result, a common side effect of the antibiotic is abdominal cramping and diarrhea.

**325. The answer is b.** *(Fauci, p 2368. Ganong, pp 477, 504-505.)* Inflammation of the duodenum may lead to increased acid output, hypocalcemia, and microcytic anemia. Increased basal and maximal acid outputs may result from excessive stimulation of the parietal cell (eg, hypergastrinemia) or reduced inhibitory feedback (ie, reduced effect of enterogastrone and the enterogastric reflex). The latter may occur when the proximal small intestine is inflamed. Although calcium is absorbed along the entire length of the small intestine, it is absorbed primarily in the duodenum. Similarly, iron is absorbed primarily in the duodenum and the microcytic anemia is the result of reduced stores of iron.

**326. The answer is c.** *(Fauci, pp 241-242 Ganong, pp 494-495.)* The emptying of solids from the stomach is determined by the strength of antral peristaltic contractions and the resistance offered by the pyloric sphincter.

Either a decrease in the amplitude of the antral contractions or an increase in sphincter resistance will delay the emptying of solids from the stomach. Liquid emptying is regulated by the proximal stomach and is primarily a function of the difference between the intragastric pressure and the intraduodenal pressure.

**327. The answer is c.** *(Ganong, pp 474-475, 507.)* Removal of the terminal ileum can lead to diarrhea and steatorrhea. The terminal ileum contains specialized cells responsible for the absorption of primary and secondary bile salts by active transport. Bile salts are necessary for adequate digestion and absorption of fat. In the absence of the terminal ileum there will be an increase in the amounts of bile acids and fatty acids delivered to the colon. Fats and bile salts in the colon increase the water content of the feces by promoting the influx (secretion) of water into the lumen of the colon.

**328. The answer is d.** *(Ganong, pp 473-475. Widmaier, pp 537-538.)* The process of fat digestion begins in the stomach and is completed in the proximal small intestine, predominately by enzymes synthesized and secreted by the pancreatic acinar cells. The major lipolytic pancreatic enzyme is the carboxylic esterase, known as lipase. Full activity requires the protein cofactor colipase, as well as an alkaline pH, bile salts, and fatty acids.

**329. The answer is d.** *(Ganong, p 490. Stead, pp 109-110.)* The lower esophageal sphincter is a high-pressure zone that exists between the esophageal body and the gastric fundus. The high pressure limits reflux of gastric contents into the esophageal body. Although excitatory vagal input contributes to the high-pressure zone, the principal determinant is intrinsic (myogenic) properties of the circular smooth muscle of the sphincter. Excess acid in the esophagus creates the pain sensation referred to as heartburn.

**330. The answer is d.** *(Fauci, pp 1851-1852. Ganong, pp 232, 489-490. Stead, pp 109-110. Widmaier, p 545.)* Delayed gastric emptying, hiatal hernia, and decreased esophageal motility are all causes of GERD, but the most likely cause of GERD in this patient is a relaxed or incompetent lower espophageal sphincter (LES), which allows the gastric contents to reflux into the esophagus. The hydrochloric acid from the stomach irritates the esophageal walls, producing the substernal pain of indigestion, called heartburn. Causes of decreased LES tone include alcohol, cigarettes, coffee (caffeine), and chocolate, as well as certain drugs (nitrates and calcium channel blockers) and hormones (estrogen and progesterone). The LES is comprised of smooth muscle at the junction of the esophagus and the stomach. The upper esophageal sphincter is located between the pharynx and the esophagus and is comprised of skeletal muscle.

**331. The answer is d.** *(Fauci, pp 1867-1869. Ganong, p 496. Stead, pp 111-113, 233.)* Zollinger-Ellison (ZE) has a triad of peptic ulcer disease, gastric acid hypersecretion, and an elevated gastrin level. In ZE, a pancreatic acinar cell adenoma (gastrinoma) is the site for the synthesis and secretion of large amounts of gastrin. Unlike gastrin released from the antrum in response to normal physiological stimuli, the pancreatic release of gastrin from the pancreas is not under physiological control, that is, intestinal feedback and gastric pH. ZE can be part of a multiple endocrine tumor (MEN I). Proton pump inhibitors (omeprazole, lansoprazole) are the treatment of choice for peptic ulcer disease in ZE, and have decreased the need for total gastrectomy.

**332. The answer is a.** *(Le, p 307. Stead, pp 111-113. Widmaier, p 557.)* Pancreatic bicarbonate secretion into the small intestine is essential for neutralization of gastric acid emptied into the small intestine. Unlike the gastric mucosal lining, the mucosal surface of the small intestine does not provide a significant endogenous defense mechanism against the insult of HCl. Upon delivery into the proximal small intestine, hydrogen ions stimulate the release of the hormone secretin from the intestinal wall, which in turn stimulates pancreatic bicarbonate secretion. In fact, the acid output of the stomach during a meal is matched equally by the pancreatic output of bicarbonate. Although the liver secretes bicarbonate and bile contains bicarbonate, the amounts are not sufficient for acid neutralization.

**333. The answer is b.** *(Fauci, p 220. Ganong, pp 467-469, 488-489. Widmaier, pp 530-531)* Starch digestion begins in the mouth via α-amylase, which is inactivated by the acidity of the stomach. The parotid gland is the most serous of the salivary glands and cranial nerve VII, not VIII, runs through the parotid (though it does not innervate the gland). Approximately 1.5 L of saliva is secreted per day.

**334. The answer is a.** *(Fauci, p 246. Ganong, pp 475-477, 508-509.)* Both the absorption of Na⁺ and secretion of K⁺ from the colon are affected by changes in circulating levels of aldosterone. The major route of absorption of sodium in the colon is electrogenic transport. Because of the "tight" nature of the tight junctions that connect cells in the colon, a relatively large potential difference exists between the mucosal (negative) and serosal (positive) surfaces of the absorptive cells. This electrical difference favors the net secretion of $K^+$ into the lumen. Secretion of $HCO_3^-$ occurs in exchange for absorption of $Cl^-$. No counterbalancing cation exchange pumps are present in the colon.

**335. The answer is d.** *(Fauci, pp 1991-1992. Ganong, pp 485-487, 500-503. Widmaier, pp 541-542, 552.)* Cholecystokinin is released from the upper small intestine in response to partially hydrolyzed dietary lipids and proteins and promotes gallbladder emptying. Gallbladder contraction and sphincter of Oddi relaxation are necessary for delivery of bile into the duodenum. These muscular actions are under both hormonal and neural control. Cholecystokinin contracts gallbladder smooth muscle by a direct action on the muscle and through activation of vagal afferent fibers leading to a vago-vagal reflex. Relaxation of sphincter of Oddi smooth muscle occurs via activation of inhibitory enteric nerves. Gallbladder contraction is also promoted by vagal stimulation, which is cholinergically mediated and blocked by the muscarinic receptor antagonist, atropine.

**336. The answer is b.** *(Fauci, pp 1855-1862. Ganong, pp 504-508.)* Inflammation of the proximal small intestine results in a decrease in the feedback regulation of gastric function by reducing the input of the enterogastric reflex and enterogastrones to gastric emptying and gastric acid secretion. Absent inhibitory input, basal and maximal acid outputs are increased, and the gastric emptying of liquids and solids is increased.

**337. The answer is a.** *(Fauci, pp 250-251. Ganong, pp 474-475, 507. Widmaier, p 559.)* Steatorrhea is defined as excess loss of fat in the stool. Numerous pathophysiological situations can cause the loss of excess fat in the stool including a decrease in bile acid pool size, inactivation or decreased intraluminal concentration of pancreatic lipase in the small intestine, and decreased intestinal absorptive surface area. A decrease in bile acid pool size results in an increased delivery of fats into the colon, which in turn inhibits fat absorption and promotes water secretion.

**338. The answer is c.** *(Fauci, pp 250-251, 1872, 1877-1878, 1880-1881. Ganong, p 507. Stead, pp 142-143.)* Gluten-sensitivity enteropathy, also known as celiac sprue, is characterized by an autoimmune-induced decrease in the absorptive surface area of the small intestine in response to gluten and other proteins in grain foods. In addition to a decrease in the area available for absorption of nutrients, minerals, electrolytes, and water, the membrane transporters of the remaining villous tip cells are impaired or absent.

**339. The answer is a.** (*Ganong, pp 473-475.*) The process of fat digestion begins in the stomach and is completed in the proximal small intestine, predominately by enzymes synthesized and secreted by the pancreatic acinar cells. The major lipolytic pancreatic enzyme is the carboxylic esterase, known as lipase. Full activity requires the protein cofactor colipase, bile salts, fatty acids, as well as an alkaline pH. Excess delivery of acid into the proximal small intestine leads to reduced lipolytic activity.

**340. The answer is b.** (*Fauci, pp 1890-1892. Le, p 308. Stead, pp 132-134.*) Individuals with inflammatory disease of the ileum have decreased bile acid pool size due to decreased bile acid reabsorption. This results in reduced absorption of dietary triglycerides and fat-soluble vitamins, including vitamin K. The efficient absorption of dietary fats requires the presence of critical concentrations of primary and secondary bile salts (1-5 mmol/L). Because the absolute amount of bile acids available for fat digestion during a meal (the bile acid pool size) is generally less than the amounts required for complete digestion and absorption, bile acids must be recirculated via the enterohepatic circulation. Conservation of bile acids during a meal is highly efficient and occurs primarily from the distal ileum via sodium-dependent, secondary active transport. The increased delivery of dietary fat and bile acids into the colon decreases colonic absorption of water. The loss of bile salts in the stool cannot be fully compensated for by increased hepatic synthesis, and, thus, there is a resultant decrease in bile acid pool size.

**341. The answer is d.** (*Fauci, pp 2553, 2559. Le, p 318.*) Metoclopramide is used as a motility agent in patients with diabetic gastroparesis. It increases peristalsis of the small intestine and increases lower esophageal sphincter tone. It is contraindicated in patients with intestinal obstruction. Metoclopramide is a dopamine receptor antagonist and Parkinsonian-like symptoms are a known side effect of its use.

**342. The answer is b.** (*Fauci, pp 1851-1852. Stead, pp 109-110.*) Proton pump inhibitors are used for the treatment of acid-related conditions such as Zollinger-Ellison syndrome. They work by inhibiting the H-K-ATPase of the gastric parietal cells and cause an increase in gastrin levels. They are used in conjunction with various antibiotics as treatment for the eradication of *H pylori*. They do not need to be dose-adjusted for renal insufficiency.

**343. The answer is c.** *(Fauci, pp 257-258, 1862-1864. Le, pp 303, 317.)* Misoprostol is used in the prevention of NSAID-induced gastric ulcers. It is a prostaglandin $E_1$ analog that helps maintain the gastric mucosal barrier, which can become compromised with prostaglandin inhibitors such as NSAIDs. Misoprostol enhances mucous bicarbonate secretion in the stomach. Diarrhea is the most common side effect and its use is contraindicated in pregnancy.

**344. The answer is a.** *(Fauci, p 1876. Ganong, pp 469-470. Widmaier, p 560.)* Lactase is a brush border enzyme that hydrolyzes milk sugar (lactose) into glucose and galactose. Patients with a lactase deficiency may experience diarrhea, cramps, and intestinal gas. The diarrhea and cramping reflect the osmotic effect of the sugar on water flux across the intestine. Colonic bacteria metabolize lactose to fatty acids, $CO_2$, and $H_2$.

**345. The answer is c.** *(Fauci, pp 1851-1852. Ganong, pp 489-491. Stead, pp 109-110.)* Reflux of gastric contents into the smooth-muscle region of the esophagus leads to the development of secondary esophageal peristalsis, characterized by enteric nerve-initiated peristalsis, beginning at the site of irritation and LES relaxation. Primary peristalsis is initiated by the medullary swallowing center and is preceded by an oral-pharyngeal phase.

**346. The answer is b.** *(Ganong, pp 482-488, 503. Widmaier, pp 541-542.)* The delivery of food into the small intestine is characterized by prompt emptying of the gallbladder, resulting from fat-induced release of cholecystokinin. Secretin stimulates pancreatic bicarbonate secretion. Glucagon is involved in nutrient metabolism and motilin is an interdigestive hormone responsible for migrating motor complex activity.

**347. The answer is b.** *(Ganong, pp 333-337, 354-355. Stead, pp 63-65.)* Insulin, a pancreatic hormone, decreases tissue lipolysis. The main function of insulin is to stimulate anabolic reactions involving carbohydrates, fats, proteins, and nucleic acids. Therefore, insulin increases glucose utilization while also stimulating lipogenesis and proteogenesis. By promoting glucose utilization by cells, insulin decreases the need for gluconeogenesis and ketogenesis.

**348. The answer is d.** (*Ganong, pp 501-502. Widmaier, pp 553-554.*) Although only small amounts of bile acids are lost in the stool each day, the loss represents the only route of elimination of cholesterol from the body. The predominant organic component of bile is the bile salts, which make up about 67% of the total solutes. Bile salts are amphiphilic molecules, that is, they exhibit both water and lipid solubility. Primary bile acids, cholic acid, and chenodeoxycholic acid are synthesized from cholesterol. Secondary bile acids, deoxycholic acid, and lithocholic acid are produced by biotransformation of primary bile acids by intestinal bacteria. Prior to secretion, the bile acids are conjugated with either glycine or taurine, which greatly enhances their water solubility. In general, taurine conjugates are more water-soluble than glycine conjugates. The majority of bile acid is absorbed via a Na-K ATPase in the terminal ileum.

**349. The answer is a.** (*Fauci, pp 249-253. Ganong, p 512. Stead, pp 139-141.*) Osmotic diarrhea occurs when ingested, poorly absorbable, osmotically active solutes draw fluid into the lumen of the small intestine or colon leading to osmotic water loss in the stool. In osmotic diarrhea, the stool osmotic gap $(290 − 2[Na^+ + K^+])$ exceeds 50 mOsm, consistent with an unmeasured solute contributing to the fecal electrolyte content. Osmotic diarrhea generally ceases with fasting or discontinued ingestion of the solute. The most common causes of osmotic diarrhea are (1) lactase (and other disaccharide) deficiency with resultant lactose intolerance and carbohydrate malabsorption, (2) ingestion of magnesium-containing antacids or laxatives, and (3) ingestion of nonabsorbable sugars, such as sorbitol. Secretory diarrhea, on the other hand, is caused by the overproduction of water by the small and large bowel. In contrast to osmotic diarrhea, secretory diarrhea has a normal stool osmotic gap and is not remedied with fasting. The other major pathophysiologic mechanisms of chronic diarrhea include steatorrheal, inflammatory, infectious, dysmotile, radiation injury, and factitial causes.

**350. The answer is c.** (*Ganong, pp 336-338, 470-472.*) The transport protein responsible for the sodium-dependent glucose transport in the small intestine is termed the SGLT1 (Na⁺-glucose transporter). The absorption of glucose occurs through the coordinated action of transport proteins located in the brush border and basolateral membranes of the enterocyte. Glucose uptake into the enterocyte from the lumen of the GI tract occurs primarily via the sodium-dependent SGLT1 secondary active transport mechanism. Glucose exit from the enterocyte into the extracellular fluid occurs by facilitated diffusion and is mediated by the membrane transporter, Glut-2. The Na⁺-glucose cotransporter also transports galactose. Thus, when the cotransporter is congenitally defective, the resulting glucose and galactose malabsorption causes severe diarrhea that can be fatal if glucose and galactose are not removed from the diet. A similar secondary active transport process (Na⁺-glucose cotransport) occurs in the renal tubules via SGLT1 and SGLT2. Glut-5 is the membrane transporter located on the apical portion of the enterocyte responsible for the facilitated entry of fructose into the cell.

**351. The answer is e.** *(Fauci, pp 253-255. Ganong, pp 474-475.)* The colon is the major site for the generation and absorption of short-chain fatty acids. They are products of bacterial metabolism of undigested complex carbohydrates derived from fruits and vegetables. In addition to exhibiting trophic effects on the colonic mucosa, they are believed to promote sodium absorption from the colon. The mechanism of action remains controversial.

**352. The answer is b.** *(Fauci, pp 2005-2009. Ganong, pp 497-498. Widmaier, pp 541-542, 552.)* Pancreatic lipase converts triglycerides to monoglycerides and free fatty acids. Secretin stimulates bicarbonate secretion from the pancreas. Serum amylase and lipase would be expected to be increased in a patient presenting with acute pancreatitis. Gallstones are the most common cause of pancreatitis. Alcohol, hypertriglyceridemia, drugs, and endoscopic retrograde cholangiopancreatography (ERCP) are other common causes.

**353. The answer is c.** *(Ganong, pp 477-478. Widmaier, p 540.)* Iron is transported in the blood bound to the β globulin, transferrin. Excess iron is stored in all cells, but especially in hepatocytes where it combines with apoferritin. The stored form is called ferritin. The rate of iron absorption is extremely slow, with a maximum of only a few milligrams per day. Iron is absorbed primarily in the ferrous form. Therefore, ferrous iron compounds, rather than ferric compounds, are effective in treating iron deficiency.

**354. The answer is b.** (*Fauci, pp 1976-1977. Ganong, p 487. Stead, pp 121-123.*) Somatostatin, located within the gastric antral mucosa, is the principal paracrine secretion involved in the inhibitory feedback of gastric acid secretion by parietal cells. Somatostatin has a short half-life of several minutes, which limits its clinical use. The analog octreotide (Sandostatin), however, can be administered subcutaneously to inhibit the secretion of gastrin and gastric acid and visceral blood flow in patients with bleeding esophageal varices secondary to portal hypertension, after stabilizing with IV fluids, as acute variceal bleeds have a 50% mortality. Acid secretion is stimulated by acetylcholine (via $M_3$ muscarinic receptors), histamine (via $H_2$ receptors), and gastrin (directly via gastrin receptors and principally via stimulation of histamine secretion by enterochromaffin-like [ECL] cells). Gastrin secretion is stimulated by the amino acids and peptides produced by pepsin's action in protein digestion.

**355. The answer is b.** (*Fauci, pp 1847-1850. Ganong, pp 486, 490. Stead, pp 106-107.*) Important inhibitory neurotransmitters in the gastrointestinal tract include vasoactive intestinal peptide and nitric oxide. Relaxation of gastrointestinal smooth muscle occurs following activation of nonadrenergic, noncholinergic (NANC) enteric nerve fibers. Acetylcholine, substance P, and dopamine are excitatory neurotransmitters. Somatostatin is a paracrine secretory product with multiple effects on gastrointestinal function.

**356. The answer is d.** (*Ganong, pp 475-477. Stead, pp 139-140.*) Most water and electrolyte absorption occurs in the jejunum, with the duodenum serving primarily as the site of osmotic equilibration of chyme. Water absorption is passive and occurs as the direct result of active sodium absorption. The small intestine and colon absorb approximately 9 to 12 L of fluid per 24-hour period, most of which comes from gastrointestinal secretions. In contrast to the small intestine, the colon has a limited capacity to absorb water (approximately 3 to 6 L/d); most water absorption in the colon occurs in the proximal colon. The incubation period for *V. cholerae* is 24 to 48 hours.

**357. The answer is a.** (*Ganong, pp 468, 497-498. Widmaier, p 552.*) Liberation of the enzyme enteropeptidase (enterokinase) from the duodenal mucosal cells causes the inactive trypsinogen to be converted to the active form, trypsin. Enteropeptidase contains 41% polysaccharide. It is this high level of polysaccharide that protects enteropeptidase from digestion. Trypsin is responsible for the conversion of chymotrypsinogens and other proenzymes into their active forms.

**358. The answer is b.** *(Fauci, pp 1971-1972. Ganong, pp 293-296, 470-478, 501-502, 509-511. Stead, pp 121, 123.)* One of the actions of colonic bacteria is to convert $NH_3$ to $NH_4^+$. Thus, a total colectomy would increase blood ammonia levels, which would be exacerbated in a person with cirrhosis. $NH_3$ is in equilibrium with $NH_4^+$. Most of the $NH_4^+$ formed by oxidative deamination of amino acids in the liver is converted to urea, and the urea is excreted in the urine. The $NH_4^+$ forms carbamoyl phosphate, and in the mitochondria it is transferred to ornithine by ornithine carbamoyltransferase forming citrulline. Citrulline is converted to arginine, after which urea is split off and ornithine is regenerated (urea cycle). Most of the urea is formed in the liver, and in severe liver disease the blood urea nitrogen falls and blood $NH_3$ rises. Normally, about 5% to 10% of bile salts enter the colon. In the colon, bacteria convert the two primary bile acids, cholic acid and chenodeoxycholic acid, to the secondary bile acids, deoxycholic acid and lithocholic acid, respectively. Lithocholate is relatively insoluble and is mostly excreted in the stool, but deoxycholate is reabsorbed from the colon, where it is transported back to the liver in the portal vein and reexcreted in the bile (enterohepatic circulation). Humans can survive after total removal of the colon if fluid and electrolyte balance is maintained. When total colectomy is performed, the ileum is brought out through the abdominal wall (ileostomy). Advances in surgical techniques make ileostomies relatively trouble-free and patients with them can lead essentially normal lives.

**359. The answer is c.** *(Fauci, pp 1932-1946. Ganong, pp 500-503. Stead, pp 124-127.)* Infectious hepatitis is a systemic infection predominantly affecting the liver. When jaundice appears, serum bilirubin rises, and, in most instances, total bilirubin is equally divided between the conjugated (direct) and unconjugated (indirect) fractions. The bilirubin in serum represents a balance between input from production of bilirubin and hepatic/biliary removal of the pigment. Hyperbilirubinemia may result from (1) overproduction of bilirubin; (2) impaired uptake, conjugation, or removal of bilirubin; or (3) regurgitation of unconjugated or conjugated bilirubin from damaged hepatocytes or bile ducts. Alkaline phosphatase, which is excreted in bile, increases in patients with jaundice due to bile duct obstruction, but generally not when the jaundice is due to hepatocellular disease. Bile acids are synthesized in the liver by a series of enzymatic steps that also involve cholesterol catabolism. Liver disease decreases bile acid synthesis.

**360. The answer is c.** *(Fauci, p 1900. Ganong, p 491. Widmaier, p 557.)* Gas within the colon is derived primarily from fermentation of undigested material by intestinal bacteria to produce $CO_2$, $H_2$, and methane. The digestive tract normally contains about 150 to 200 mL of gas, most of which is in the colon (100-150 mL). Most of the gas in the stomach is derived from air swallowed during eating or in periods of anxiety. Gas is produced in the small intestine by interaction of gastric acid and bicarbonate in the intestinal and pancreatic secretions but does not accumulate because it is either reabsorbed or quickly passed into the colon. The amount of gas varies markedly from one person to another and is influenced by diet; for example, ingestion of large amounts of beans, which contain indigestible carbohydrates in their hulls, will increase gas formation by intestinal bacteria. Diffusion of gas from the blood to the intestinal lumen is responsible for the $N_2$ present in intestinal gas and is influenced by the atmospheric pressure. While many patients with irritable bowel syndrome complain of increased flatus, most produce no more than that seen in normal individuals.

**361. The answer is b.** *(Fauci, p 1878. Ganong, pp 313, 315, 496. Stead, pp 150-151.)* Although intrinsic factor is secreted by the parietal cells of the gastric mucosa, binding to cobalamin occurs in the duodenum. Cobalamin, also known as vitamin $B_{12}$, is provided almost entirely from animal products in the human diet. Gastric digestion of food liberates cobalamin where, at low pH, it binds primarily to R-binder protein, derived primarily from salivary secretions. In the duodenum, pancreatic proteases release cobalamin from the R-binder protein where cobalamin then rapidly complexes with intrinsic factor and is transported along the gut to the terminal ileum, where specific receptors located on the villus tip cells bind the cobalamin-intrinsic factor complex. In this patient, the neurologic symptoms, glossitis, and findings on the peripheral smear are characteristic of cobalamin deficiency.

**362. The answer is a.** *(Ganong, pp 494-496. Widmaier, pp 548-551.)* The initial rate of emptying varies directly with the volume of the meal ingested. Increasing the volume, fat content, acidity, or osmolarity of the lumen of the small intestine inhibits gastric emptying via neural, hormonal, and paracrine feedback mechanisms.

**363. The answer is d.** *(Fauci, p 1867. Ganong, pp 496-497. Widmaier, pp 550-551.)* Weakness, dizziness, and sweating, due in part to hypoglycemia, underlie the presentation of "dumping syndrome," which may develop in patients in whom part of the stomach has been removed or the jejunum has been anastomosed to the stomach. Another cause of the symptoms is rapid entry of a hypertonic meal into the intestine, which promotes the movement of an abundance of water into the gut, producing significant hypovolemia and hypotension.

**364. The answer is e.** *(Fauci, p 2278. Ganong, pp 347-348, 486-487.)* Glucagon-like polypeptide 1 (GLP-1) is a product of glucagon metabolism in the L cells of the lower intestinal tract. GLP-1 has no definite biological activity by itself but is processed further by removal of its amino-terminal amino acid residues, and the product, GLP-1 (7-36), is a potent stimulator of insulin secretion that also increases glucose utilization.

**365. The answer is b.** *(Ganong, pp 506-511. Widmaier, pp 555-557.)* Distention of the stomach by food initiates contraction of the rectum and often, a desire to defecate. This response is called the gastrocolic reflex, but it may be mediated by the action of gastrin on the colon rather than being neurally mediated. This response leads to defecation after meals in infants and children. The gastroileal reflex refers to the relaxation of the cecum and passage of chyme through the ileocecal valve when food leaves the stomach. Peristaltic rushes are very intense peristaltic waves that may occur with intestinal obstruction. The intestino-intestinal reflex refers to a complete cessation of intestinal motility that may be caused by large distensions of the intestine, injury to the intestinal wall, or various intestinal bacterial infections. The defecation reflex refers to the sudden distention of the walls of the rectum produced by mass movement of fecal material into the rectum.

**366. The answer is c.** *(Fauci, pp 1880-1881. Ganong, p 507. Stead, p 142.)* Malabsorption syndrome refers to the inability to adequately absorb nutrients and vitamins from the intestinal tract. One example of a malabsorption syndrome is the autoimmune disease, celiac sprue, which is also called gluten enteropathy. The disease is characterized by a deficiency in MHC class II antigen HLA-DQ2, which causes an allergic response to ingestion of gluten and related proteins. Elimination of these proteins, which are found in wheat, rye, barley, and oats, can restore normal bowel function in these patients.

**367. The answer is d.** *(Ganong, pp 502-503. Le, p 304.)* When plasma bilirubin is increased due to bile duct obstruction, it is generally the conjugated form of bilirubin that increases due to reabsorption of bilirubin glucuronide into the blood. All other choices are found in conditions with an increase in the indirect (unconjugated) form of bilirubin.

**368. The answer is d.** *(Ganong, pp 475-477. Widmaier, p 540.)* Although multiple pathways exist for the absorption of $Na^+$, neutral absorption is the major mechanism. Absorption of sodium is the primary absorptive event in the small intestine. Absorption of $Na^+$ is necessary for absorption of water and other electrolytes. Neutral absorption may occur in two ways: $Na^+$ cotransported with $Cl^-$ or in exchange for $H^+$ ions.

**369. The answer is d.** *(Ganong, pp 473-475. Widmaier, pp 538-539.)* Long-chain fatty acids are extruded from enterocytes in the form of chylomicrons into the lymphatic system. Triglycerides are hydrolyzed to monoglycerides and taken into mucosal cells. If the fatty acids are short chains (less than 10-12 carbon atoms), they are extruded in the form of free fatty acids into the portal blood. Chylomicrons represent triglycerides and esters of cholesterol that have been invested in the intestinal mucosa with a coating of phospholipid, protein, and cholesterol.

**370. The answer is c.** *(Ganong, p 477. Widmaier, pp 537-539.)* Absorption of the fat-soluble vitamins (A, D, E, K) is diminished if there is a lack of pancreatic lipase. Lipase is required to produce monoglycerides that, in combination with bile salts, make it possible to bring the fat-soluble vitamins close to the mucosal cell surface for absorption. With the exception of vitamin $B_{12}$, which is absorbed bound to intrinsic factor in the ileum, vitamins are absorbed chiefly in the upper small intestine.

**371. The answer is b.** *(Fauci, pp 2350-2353. Ganong, pp 505-506.)* Removal of the terminal ileum can lead to diarrhea and steatorrhea. The terminal ileum contains specialized cells responsible for the absorption of primary and secondary bile salts by active transport. Bile salts are necessary for adequate digestion and absorption of fat. In the absence of the terminal ileum there will be an increase in the amounts of bile acids and fatty acids delivered to the colon. Fats and bile salts in the colon increase the water content of the feces by promoting the influx (secretion) of water into the lumen of the colon. Amino acids are absorbed in the jejunum. Iron is primarily absorbed in the duodenum. Gastrointestinal neuroendocrine tumors are derived from the diffuse neuroendocrine system of the GI tract, which is composed of amine- and acid-producing cells with different hormonal profiles, depending on the site of origin. The tumors they produce are generally divided into carcinoid tumors (ectodermal stem cells) and pancreatic endocrine tumors. One third of all primary gut tumors are carcinoid. Carcinoid tumors are frequently classified according to their anatomic area of origin (foregut, midgut, hindgut). Small intestinal (midgut) carcinoid tumors arise from the argentaffin cells of the crypts of Lieberkühn in the terminal ileum, and have a high serotonin content. Small intestinal carcinoids are the most common cause of the carcinoid syndrome (cutaneous flushing, diarrhea, bronchospasm, right heart valvular lesions), which is manifest when they metastasize, but only occurs in 5% to 10% of carcinoid tumors.

# Renal and Urinary Physiology

## Questions

**372.** A 65-year-old man with uncontrolled type 2 diabetes and sustained hyperglycemia (serum glucose = 550 mg/dL) and polyuria (5 L/d) is evaluated in the hospital's clinical laboratory because his urine glucose concentration (<100 mM) was much lower than expected. The graph below illustrates the relationship between plasma glucose concentration and renal glucose reabsorption for this patient. The glomerular filtration rate (GFR) is 100 mL/min. Which of the following is the $T_{max}$ for glucose?

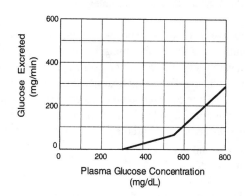

a. 100 mg/min
b. 200 mg/min
c. 300 mg/min
d. 400 mg/min
e. 500 mg/min

**373.** A 16-year-old girl presents for her annual high school athletic physical. She states that she seems more tired than usual, that she has been having muscle cramps in her calves, and that her legs get very weak and sore after running and playing soccer. Her blood pressure is 160/100 mm Hg, and her EKG shows a prolonged QT interval and the presence of a U wave. Blood analysis shows hypokalemia and metabolic alkalosis. Plasma renin activity and aldosterone concentration are lower than normal. Her clinical condition is reversed after she is placed on the diuretic amiloride, which blocks tubular epithelial sodium channels. Based on this finding, which of the following renal transport processes is the major defect causing her metabolic disorder?

a. Greater than normal sodium reabsorption by the proximal tubules
b. Greater than normal sodium reabsorption by the distal tubules
c. Inability of the distal nephron to secrete potassium ion
d. Inability of the distal nephron to secrete hydrogen
e. Inability of the distal nephron to concentrate urine

**374.** A previously well 12-year-old boy is brought to the emergency department with vomiting and severe abdominal cramps after a prolonged period of exercise. Elevated levels of serum creatinine and blood urea nitrogen suggest acute renal failure. Following treatment and recovery, his serum uric acid concentration (0.6 mg/dL) remains consistently below normal. To determine if his low serum uric acid level is related to renal dysfunction, uric acid clearance studies are conducted and the following data are obtained:

Urine flow rate = 1 mL/min
Urine (uric acid) = 36 mg/dL

Which of the following is the patient's uric acid clearance?

a. 6 mL/min
b. 12 mL/min
c. 24 mL/min
d. 48 mL/min
e. 60 mL/min

**375.** A 69-year-old man presents with symptoms of thirst and dizziness, and physical evidence of orthostatic hypotension and tachycardia, decreased skin turgor, dry mucous membranes, reduced axillary sweating, and reduced jugular venous pressure. He was recently placed on an angiotensin-converting enzyme inhibitor for his hypertension. Urinalysis reveals a reduction in the fractional excretion of sodium and the presence of acellular hyaline casts. The internist suspects acute renal failure of prerenal origin, which has increased renin secretion by the kidney. A stimulus for increasing renal renin secretion is an increase in which of the following?

a. Angiotensin II
b. Atrial natriuretic peptide
c. Glomerular filtration rate
d. Mean blood pressure
e. Sympathetic nerve activity

**376.** A patient with uncontrolled hypertension is placed on a new diuretic targeted to the $Na^+$ reabsorption site from the basolateral surface of the renal epithelial cells. Which of the following transport processes is the new drug affecting?

a. $Na^+/H^+$ exchange
b. $Na^+$-glucose cotransport
c. $Na^+$-$K^+$ pump
d. Facilitated diffusion
e. Solvent drag

**377.** A 28-year-old woman presents to her physician's office with fatigue, malaise, and orthostatic dizziness. When asked what medications she is taking, she stated that she has a prescription for oral contraceptives for her endometriosis and that she had been taking 800 mg ibuprofen 4 to 6 times a day for her painful menstrual cramps. Which of the following is most likely to produce an increase in GFR in patients with acute renal failure?

a. Administration of angiotensin II
b. Increased renin release from the juxtaglomerular apparatus
c. Contraction of glomerular mesangial cells
d. Dilation of afferent arterioles
e. Volume depletion

**378.** A 32-year-old man complaining of fatigue and muscle weakness is seen by his physician. Blood tests reveal a serum glucose level of 325 mg/dL and serum creatinine of 0.8 mg/dL. Results of a 24-hour urine analysis are as follows:

Total volume = 5 L
Total glucose = 375 g
Total creatinine = 2.4 g

The patient's GFR is approximately which of the following?

a. 75 mL/min
b. 100 mL/min
c. 125 mL/min
d. 200 mL/min
e. 275 mL/min

**379.** A 38-year-old woman is admitted to the hospital by her physician because of decreased urine output. Prior to admission, she was rehearsing for a dance performance and had been taking ibuprofen (Motrin) for pain. Laboratory data reveal: blood urea nitrogen, 49 mg/dL; serum sodium, 135 mmol/L; serum creatinine, 7.5 mg/dL; urine sodium, 33 mmol/L, and urine creatinine, 90 mg/dL. Her fractional sodium excretion is approximately which of the following?

a. 0.5%
b. 1.0%
c. 1.5%
d. 2.0%
e. 3.0%

**380.** An 85-year-old woman presents with a fever and hypovolemic hypotension. To assess her renal function, the filtration fraction is determined using a freely filterable substance that is neither reabsorbed nor secreted. The infusate yields a renal artery concentration of 12 mg/mL and a renal vein concentration of 9 mg/mL. Which of the following is her filtration fraction?

a. 0.05
b. 0.15
c. 0.25
d. 0.35
e. 0.45

**381.** A 17-year-old girl went on a starvation diet for 3 days before prom so that she would look thin in her new dress. Her mother found her lethargic and hyperventilating, and took her to the emergency department for evaluation. Based on the following laboratory values, which of the following is her net acid excretion?

Plasma pH = 7.26
Urine flow = 1.2 L/d
Urine bicarbonate = 2 mEq/L
Urine titratable acids = 24 mEq/L
Urine ammonium = 38 mEq/L
Urine pH = 5.4

a.  60 mEq/L
b.  64 mEq/L
c.  68 mEq/L
d.  72 mEq/L
e.  76 mEq/L

**382.** A 68-year-old woman presents with hypertension and oliguria. A CT of the abdomen reveals a hypoplastic left kidney. Based on the following laboratory data, which of the following is her estimated renal plasma flow (RPF)?

Renal artery PAH = 6 mg/dL
Renal vein PAH = 0.6 mg/dL
Urinary PAH = 25 mg/mL
Urine flow = 1.5 mL/min
Hematocrit = 40%

a.  475 mL/min
b.  550 mL/min
c.  625 mL/min
d.  700 mL/min
e.  775 mL/min

**383.** An 83-year-old woman with a history of hypertension presents to her family physician's office with oliguria. Serum creatinine and BUN are elevated and a CT reveals that the patient's left kidney is hypoplastic. Renal function studies are performed to assess the renal handling of various substances. Substance X is injected into an arterial line. All of substance X appears in the urine and none is detected in the renal vein. What do these findings indicate about the renal handling of substance X?

a. It must be filtered by the kidney.
b. It must be reabsorbed by the kidney.
c. Its clearance is equal to the glomerular filtration rate.
d. Its clearance is equal to the renal plasma flow.
e. Its urinary concentration must be higher than its plasma concentration.

**384.** A 46-year-old man presents to his physician with a 12-week history of frontal headaches. A computed tomography (CT) of the brain shows a mass in the posterior pituitary, and the posterior pituitary "bright spot" is absent on MRI. The patient also complains of increased thirst and waking up frequently during the night. Which of the following best describes his urine?

a. A higher-than-normal flow of hypotonic urine
b. A higher-than-normal flow of hypertonic urine
c. A normal flow of hypertonic urine
d. A lower-than-normal flow of hypotonic urine
e. A lower-than-normal flow of hypertonic urine

**385.** A 63-year-old woman is brought to the emergency department complaining of fatigue and headaches. She appears confused and apathetic. She has been taking diuretics to treat her hypertension and paroxetine for her depression. Laboratory results are as follows:

Urine flow = 1 L/d
Plasma sodium = 125 mmol/L
Plasma potassium = 4 mmol/L
Urine osmolality = 385 mOsm/L
Urine sodium = 125 mmol/L
Urine potassium = 25 mmol/L

Which of the following is this patient's approximate free water clearance?

a. −0.20 L/d
b. −0.50 L/d
c. −0.75 L/d
d. +0.2 L/d
e. +0.50 L/d

**386.** A 28-year-old woman with systemic lupus erythematosus (SLE) is brought to the emergency department after developing hypokalemic paralysis. Arterial blood-gas analysis shows a $PaO_2$ of 102 mm Hg and a pH of 7.1. She is diagnosed with type I RTA caused by an autoimmune response that damages the $H^+$-ATPase on the distal nephron. Which of the following laboratory measurements will most likely be normal in this patient?

a. Anion gap
b. Aldosterone secretion
c. Net acid excretion
d. Serum bicarbonate
e. Urine ammonium

**387.** A 24-year-old man with a history of renal insufficiency is admitted to the hospital after taking a large amount of ibuprofen. His BUN is 150 mg/dL. This patient's high serum urea nitrogen was most likely caused by which of the following?

a. Decreased secretion of urea by the distal tubules
b. Decreased glomerular filtration rate
c. Increased synthesis of urea by the liver
b. Increased reabsorption of urea by the proximal tubules
e. Increased renal blood flow

**388.** A 60-year-old woman presents to her gynecologist with progressive fatigue, weakness, and diffuse bony pain. She has been postmenopausal for 5 years and her medical history is notable for hypertension and recurrent kidney stones. Physical examination is insignificant except for a slight dorsal kyphosis. A bone scan confirms osteoporosis. Serum calcium and parathyroid hormone (PTH) are increased and serum phosphate is decreased. PTH increases $Ca^{2+}$ reabsorption at which of the points along the nephron pictured below?

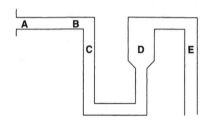

a. A
b. B
c. C
d. D
e. E

**389.** A 52-year-old man presents to his internist for a 6-month check-up following diuretic therapy and recommended diet changes for his essential hypertension. His blood pressure is 145/95 mm Hg and serum aldosterone levels are increased. Aldosterone secretion is increased when there is a decrease in the plasma concentration of which of the following?

a. ACTH
b. Angiotensin II
c. Potassium
d. Renin
e. Sodium

**390.** A 92-year-old man presents with dehydration following four days of persistent diarrhea. Under these circumstances, hypotonic fluid would be expected in which of the following?

a. Glomerular filtrate
b. Proximal tubule
c. Loop of Henle
d. Cortical collecting tubule
e. Distal collecting duct

**391.** A 76-year-old man presents at the emergency department with headache, vomiting, shortness of breath, insomnia, and confusion. He is found to be oliguric with an increased BUN and creatinine. Urine specific gravity is low and there is proteinuria. Which of the following statements concerning the normal renal handling of proteins is correct?

a. Proteins are more likely to be filtered if they are negatively charged than if they are uncharged.
b. Proteins can be filtered and secreted but not reabsorbed by the kidney.
c. Most of the protein excreted each day is derived from tubular secretion.
d. Protein excretion is directly related to plasma protein concentration.
e. Protein excretion is increased by sympathetic stimulation of the kidney.

**392.** A 19-year-old man presents for his annual football physical examination. He is asymptomatic but urinalysis reveals macroscopic hematuria. Microscopic examination is positive for deformed erythrocytes and RBC casts. Where in the renal-urinary system is the most likely origin of the blood in his urine?

a. Bowman capsule
b. Glomerulus
c. Peritubular capillaries
d. Renal artery
e. Urinary bladder

**393.** An 18-year-old man presents with muscle weakness, cramps, and tetany. Blood pressure is normal and no edema is present. Laboratory analysis reveals hypokalemic alkalosis, hyperaldosteronism, and high plasma renin activity, diagnostic of Bartter syndrome. Which of the following statements best describes the secretion or action of renin?

a. It is secreted by cells of the proximal tubule.
b. Its secretion leads to loss of sodium and water from plasma.
c. Its secretion is stimulated by increased mean renal arterial pressure.
d. It converts angiotensinogen to angiotensin I.
e. It converts angiotensin I to angiotensin II.

**394.** A 56-year-old man with hypertension presents with complaints of flushing and orthostatic hypertension. Blood analysis reveals an increased plasma renin activity and hyperlipidemia. Urinalysis reveals a decreased GFR and an increase in urinary albumin excretion. Gadolinium-enhanced three-dimensional magnetic resonance angiography is suggestive of renal artery stenosis. Measurement of renal blood flow (RBF) and a renal arteriogram are ordered to evaluate the patient for atherosclerotic renal vascular disease (ARVD = renal artery stenosis and ischemic nephropathy). The effective renal plasma flow (RPF), determined, from the clearance of $p$-aminohippuric acid (PAH), is less than the true RPF because of which of the following?

a. The fraction of PAH filtered is less than the filtration fraction.
b. The plasma entering the renal vein contains a small amount of PAH.
c. The cortical and medullary collecting ducts are able to reabsorb some PAH.
d. The calculated clearance of PAH depends on the urinary flow rate.
e. The measured value of the plasma PAH concentration is less than the actual PAH concentration.

**395.** A 63-year-old hospitalized woman becomes oliguric and confused. Her blood glucose is found to be only 35 mg/dL. An IV access is obtained and an ampule of 50% dextrose is given followed by a continuous infusion of 10% dextrose. Most of the glucose that is filtered through the glomerulus undergoes reabsorption in which of the following?

a. Proximal tubule
b. Descending limb of the loop of Henle
c. Ascending limb of the loop of Henle
d. Distal tubule
e. Collecting duct

**396.** A patient with multiple myeloma develops a defect in renal bicarbonate reabsorption, which involves the proximal tubule, that is, type II RTA. Which of the following structural features distinguishes the epithelial cells of the proximal tubule from those of the distal tubule?

a. The distal tubule has a thicker basement membrane.
b. The proximal tubule has a thicker basement membrane.
c. The proximal tubule has a more extensive brush border.
d. The proximal tubule forms the juxtaglomerular apparatus.
e. The distal tubule has fewer tight intercellular junctions.

**397.** A 35-year-old man with polycystic kidney disease has a decrease in both GFR and RBF. The nephrologists wants to administer a drug that will increase both GFR and RBF. GFR and RBF would both increase if which of the following occurred?

a. The efferent and afferent arterioles are both dilated.
b. The efferent and afferent arterioles are both constricted.
c. Only the afferent arteriole is constricted.
d. Only the efferent arteriole is constricted.
e. The afferent arteriole is constricted and the efferent arteriole is dilated.

**398.** A 39-year-old woman with diabetes mellitus presents with a chief complaint of weakness and chest discomfort. Her blood pressure is 150/98 mm Hg and an EKG reveals tall, peaked T-waves. Blood results show hyperkalemia, and decreased aldosterone and plasma renin activity, suggestive of type IV RTA. In type IV RTA, there is a defect in aldosterone secretion, as well as ammonium ($NH_4^+$) excretion. What characteristics best describe the ammonia ($NH_3$) present in the kidney?

a. It is impermeable to the epithelial cells of the proximal tubule.
b. It is classified as a titratable acid.
c. It is produced by epithelial cells in the distal nephron.
d. It reduces the concentration of bicarbonate in the plasma.
e. Its synthesis is increased in respiratory acidosis.

**399.** A 47-year-old woman presents for her annual physical examination. A year ago, the patient was started on a diet and exercise regimen when her blood pressure was 130/85 mm Hg. She has lost 10 lb and reduced her BMI to 25 kg/m$^2$, but her blood pressure on this visit is found to be 145/98 mm Hg. The patient is started on a combination of a low dose of hydrochlorothiazide with the K$^+$-sparing diuretic, triamterene. The amount of potassium excreted by the kidney will decrease if which of the following occurs?

a. Distal tubular flow increases.
b. Circulating aldosterone levels increase.
c. Dietary intake of potassium increases.
d. Na$^+$ reabsorption by the distal nephron decreases.
e. The excretion of organic ions decreases.

**400.** A 23-year-old woman presents with burning epigastric pain. A careful history reveals that the burning is exacerbated by fasting and improved with meals. The woman is prescribed the H$_2$ receptor antagonist, cimetidine, for suspected peptic ulcer disease (PUD). Cimetidine may also have an adverse effect on proximal tubular function. Which of the following substances will be more concentrated at the end of the proximal tubule than at the beginning of the proximal tubule?

a. Bicarbonate
b. Creatinine
c. Glucose
d. Phosphate
e. Sodium

**401.** A 69-year-old man with chronic hypertension presents to his physician's office. His blood pressure is 165/105 mm Hg despite treatment with a diuretic, β-blocker, and an angiotensin receptor antagonist. It is decided that a fourth drug is needed for the patient's resistant hypertension, and he is prescribed the vasodilator diltiazem, a calcium channel antagonist. The effect of decreasing the resistance of the afferent arteriole in the glomerulus of the kidney is to decrease which of the following aspects of renal function?

a. Filtration fraction
b. Glomerular filtration rate
c. Oncotic pressure of the peritubular capillary blood
d. Renal plasma flow
e. Renin release from juxtaglomerular cells

**402.** A 38-year-old man presents in the emergency department with severe back pain. He is writhing around, unable to find a comfortable position, and nauseated. A CT scan reveals nephrocalcinosis and urinalysis reveals decreased urinary chloride and calcium. Blood analysis reveals hypokalemia and hypochloremic metabolic alkalosis. The clinical findings suggest a defect in electrically neutral renal NaCl transport. Electrically neutral active transport of sodium and chloride occurs in which of the following areas of the kidney?

a. Distal tubule
b. Descending limb of the loop of Henle
c. Thin ascending limb of the loop of Henle
d. Cortical collecting duct
e. Medullary collecting duct

**403.** A 73-year-old woman develops a thready pulse, tachycardia, and hypotension 60 minutes following a hysterectomy. Laboratory analysis shows an increase in plasma renin activity and angiotensin II accompanied by a decrease in creatinine clearance. Under euvolemic conditions, a decrease in GFR would decrease proximal tubular reabsorption of salt and water by a process called glomerulotubular balance. One of the mechanisms for glomerulotubular balance is related to the Starling forces. According to this mechanism, how would a decrease in GFR promote a decrease in proximal tubular reabsorption of salt and water?

a. Via a decrease in peritubular capillary hydrostatic pressure
b. Via a decrease in peritubular oncotic pressure
c. Via a decrease in proximal tubular flow
d. Via a decrease in peritubular capillary flow
e. Via an increase in peritubular sodium concentration

**404.** A 27-year-old man with bipolar disorder presents to his psychiatrist complaining that since he started his lithium treatment six months ago, he is frequently thirsty and with gets up three or four times each night to urinate. Head-neck examination reveals slightly dry mucous membranes. Urinalysis reveals polyuria with a dilute urine. Serum ADH is normal. A diagnosis of lithium-induced nephrogenic diabetes insipidus is suspected. In the absence of ADH or when the kidney lacks responsiveness to ADH, the luminal Na⁺ concentration will be lowest at which of the points along the nephron shown schematically in the diagram below?

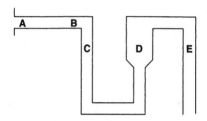

a. A
b. B
c. C
d. D
e. E

**405.** A 36-year-old African American man presents with low renin essential hypertension. Renin release from the juxtaglomerular apparatus is normally inhibited by which of the following?

a. Aldosterone
b. β-Adrenergic agonists
c. Increased pressure within the afferent arterioles
d. Prostaglandins
e. Stimulation of the macula densa

**406.** A patient undergoing surgery develops an increase in the secretion and plasma levels of ACTH, cortisol, and aldosterone. What best characterizes the production and actions of aldosterone in the body?

a. It produces its effect by activating cAMP.
b. It produces its effect by increasing distal tubular permeability to sodium.
c. It causes an increased reabsorption of hydrogen ion.
d. It has its main effect on the proximal tubule.
e. It is secreted in response to an increase in blood pressure.

**407.** A trauma patient with multiple rib fractures requires intubation and mechanical ventilation. Mechanical ventilation causes an increase in the patient's vasopressin secretion and plasma levels. Which of the following is the effect of vasopressin on the kidney?

a. Increased diameter of the renal artery
b. Increased glomerular filtration rate
c. Increased excretion of Na⁺
d. Increased excretion of water
e. Increased permeability of the distal nephron to water

**408.** A 44-year-old woman presents with abdominal pain, fever, and chills. Physical examination reveals costovertebral angle tenderness, previously undiagnosed hypertension, and a mid-systolic click. Urine culture shows bacteriuria and free water clearance is positive, indicating excretion of dilute urine. The ability of the kidney to excrete concentrated urine will increase if which of the following occurs?

a. The reabsorption of Na⁺ by the proximal tubule decreases.
b. The glomerular capillary pressure increases.
c. The flow of filtrate through the loop of Henle increases.
d. The activity of the Na⁺-K⁺ pump in the loop of Henle increases.
e. The permeability of the collecting duct to water decreases.

**409.** A 16-year-old pregnant girl is admitted to the hospital in labor. Her blood pressure is 130/85 mm Hg and her plasma creatinine is 2.7 mg/dL (normal 0.6-1.2 mg/dL). Renal ultrasonography demonstrates severe bilateral hydronephrosis (enlarged kidney). Which of the following is the most likely cause of this patient's high creatinine levels?

a. Increased sympathetic nerve activity
b. Coarctation of the renal artery
c. Hyperproteinemia
d. Ureteral obstruction
e. Hypovolemia

**410.** A 54-year-old man with small cell lung cancer presents with lethargy, confusion, and muscle cramps. Blood work shows an increase in plasma levels of antidiuretic hormone (ADH), possibly from the ectopic production of ADH. In patients with the syndrome of inappropriate antidiuretic hormone (SIADH), which of the following will increase?

a. The concentration of plasma sodium
b. Intracellular volume
c. Urinary flow
d. Plasma oncotic pressure
e. Plasma osmolarity

**411.** A patient with congestive heart failure is given the loop diuretic, furosemide, along with the potassium sparing diuretic, spironolactone. How does the distal nephron differ functionally from the proximal tubule?

a. The distal nephron is more permeable to hydrogen ion than the proximal tubule.
b. The distal nephron is less responsive to aldosterone than the proximal tubule.
c. The distal nephron has a more negative intraluminal potential than the proximal tubule.
d. The distal nephron secretes less potassium than the proximal tubule does.
e. The distal nephron secretes more hydrogen ion than the proximal tubule does.

**412.** An 82-year-old man presents with polyuria and polydipsia. Blood analysis reveals hypernatremia and urinalysis shows hypotonicity and an increased free water clearance. In which of the following conditions is an increased free water clearance a hallmark of the disease?

a. Diabetes insipidus
b. Diabetes mellitus
c. Diuretic therapy
d. Heart failure
e. Renal failure

**413.** A 42-year-old man presents with fatigue, loss of stamina, and frequent urination. He is not taking any medications currently. Physical examination is normal except for a blood pressure of 165/95 mm Hg. Serum electrolytes show: sodium, 152 mEq/L; potassium, 3.1 mEq/L; chloride, 112 mEq/L; and bicarbonate, 32 mEq/L. Aldosterone concentration is elevated and plasma renin activity is low, consistent with primary hyperaldosteronism. Aldosterone increases $Na^+$ reabsorption at which of the points depicted in this schematic diagram of the nephron?

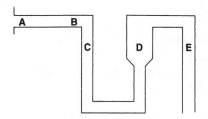

a. A
b. B
c. C
d. D
e. E

**414.** A 58-year-old man is hospitalized following an acute myocardial infarction. Several days later, the patient's 24-hour urine output is lower-than-normal. An increase in which of the following contributes to a reduced urine flow in a patient with congestive heart failure and reduced effective circulating volume?

a. Atrial natriuretic peptide
b. Renal natriuretic peptide (urodilantin)
c. Renal perfusion pressure
d. Renal sympathetic nerve activity
e. Sodium delivery to the macula densa

**415.** A 55-year-old hypertensive patient is placed on a potassium-sparing diuretic. Potassium-sparing diuretics inhibit $Na^+$ reabsorption in which of the following?

a. Proximal tubule
b. Distal tubule
c. Thin descending limb of loop of Henle
d. Thick descending limb of loop of Henle
e. Thick ascending limb of loop of Henle

**416.** A patient has suffered from persistent diarrhea lasting for the past seven days. Which of the following would be decreased in this patient?

a. The filtered load of $HCO_3^-$
b. The production of ammonia by the proximal tubule
c. $H^+$ secretion by the distal nephron
d. The anion gap
e. The production of new bicarbonate by the distal nephron

**417.** A 27-year-old graduate student from China presents at the Student Medical Center for mandatory tuberculosis screening. Quantiferon testing is positive and physical examination reveals cough, cachexia, and mild respiratory distress. Chest x-ray reveals a cavitary lesion in the right upper lobe. Blood analysis reveals a serum sodium of 118 mg/dL and increased ADH concentration. In addition to increasing the permeability of the collecting duct to water, ADH increases the permeability of the collecting duct to which of the following?

a. Hydrogen
b. Ammonium
c. Potassium
d. Sodium
e. Urea

**418.** A 54-year-old woman presents with a chief complaint of edema. Physical examination is otherwise normal. The only medication she reports taking is ibuprofen *prn* for headaches, backaches, and muscle soreness. Filtration fraction can be increased by an increase in which of the following?

a. Afferent arteriolar resistance
b. Efferent arteriolar resistance
c. Hydrostatic pressure within Bowman capsule
d. Plasma oncotic pressure
e. Renal blood flow

**419.** A 23-year-old man expresses concern about his upcoming skiing trip to Breckenridge, Colorado (elevation = 10,000 ft). He states that every time he goes there, he gets high altitude sickness that is relieved when he is given oxygen. The family physician gives the patient a prescription for oxygen to use when he arrives in Colorado, as well as a prescription for acetazolamide to take for 2 days prior and throughout his four-day trip. Carbonic anhydrase inhibitors exert their diuretic effect by inhibiting the reabsorption of $Na^+$ in which of the following parts of the nephron?

a. The proximal tubule
b. The thick ascending limb of loop of Henle
c. The distal convoluted tubule
d. The cortical collecting duct
e. The outer medullary collecting duct

**420.** A patient with atherosclerosis shows signs of chronic renal failure attributed to poor renal perfusion and ischemic necrosis of the nephrons. Which of the following endogenous substances causes RBF to decrease?

a. Nitric oxide
b. Atrial natriuretic peptide
c. Acetylcholine
d. Angiotensin II
e. Dopamine

**421.** A 67-year-old woman presents for her annual gynecological examination. Her major complaint is leaking urine, which she has had for 20 years. She has started wearing pads because it seems to be getting worse. It used to happen with coughing, sneezing, or jogging, but now she has the urge to urinate throughout the day and night with some leakage during sleep, as well. She takes insulin for her diabetes, a diuretic for her hypertension, and a baby aspirin daily. Urinalysis is positive for bacteria. Administration of which of the following drugs may mitigate her incontinence?

a. Acetylcholine
b. Anticholinergics
c. Antiestrogens
d. α-Adrenergic blockers
e. β-Blockers

**422.** A patient develops acute renal failure due to an autoimmune disorder affecting the proximal tubules. What percentage of the filtered load of sodium is reabsorbed by the proximal tubule?

a. 15%
b. 25%
c. 45%
d. 65%
e. 95%

**423.** A patient with congestive heart failure presents with jugular venous distention, ascites, and peripheral edema. Blood work shows elevated levels of plasma atrial natriuretic peptide (ANP). ANP decreases $Na^+$ reabsorption within which of the following?

a. The proximal tubule
b. The thick ascending limb of loop of Henle
c. The distal convoluted tubule
d. The cortical collecting duct
e. The inner medullary collecting duct

**424.** An elderly woman presents with spiking fever, shaking chills, nausea, and costovertebral angle tenderness. Urine cultures are positive and she is hospitalized for pyelonephritis. Her GFR decreases with a resultant increase in the concentration of NaCl delivered in the intraluminal fluid to the thick ascending limb of the loop of Henle. Under these conditions, the macula densa will increase the formation and release of which of the following substances?

a. Adenosine
b. Aldosterone
c. Antidiuretic hormone
d. Angiotensinogen
e. Renin

**425.** A 39-year-old man presents with severe writhing back pain, hematuria, and nausea. An intravenous pyelogram (IVP) confirms a diagnosis of renal calculi. The presence of strongly opaque stones on the plain film is suggestive of calcium oxalate stones, which have an increased incidence with hypophosphatemia. The renal clearance of phosphate is increased by which of the following hormones?

a. Aldosterone
b. Parathyroid hormone
c. Norepinephrine
d. Vasopressin
e. Angiotensin

**426.** A 41-year-old woman presents with hemoptysis and hematuria. Laboratory findings include markedly elevated BUN, creatinine, and erythrocyte sedimentation rate. Serum is positive for antiproteinase-3 ANCA and negative for anti-glomerular basement membrane antibody, suggesting Wegener granulomatosis rather than Goodpasture disease. Urinalysis reveals proteinuria and RBC casts, in addition to the hematuria. Progressive renal failure makes it difficult for the patient to excrete a normal dietary potassium load. Which of the following will produce the greatest increase in potassium secretion?

a. A decrease in circulating blood volume
b. A decrease in renal blood flow
c. A decrease in urine flow rate
d. An increase in distal nephron sodium concentration
e. An increase in sympathetic nerve activity

**427.** A 36-year-old man suffers third-degree burns over 70% of his body while responding to a three-alarm fire. His effective circulating volume and renal perfusion pressure drop precipitously and the concentration of NaCl in the intraluminal fluid in the kidney decreases. These conditions cause the juxtaglomerular apparatus to release which of the following hormones?

a. Adenosine
b. Aldosterone
c. Angiotensinogen
d. Antidiuretic hormone
e. Renin

**428.** A hypertensive patient develops chronic renal failure from progressive nephrosclerosis. Which of the following should you expect to occur as a result?

a. A decrease in the fractional excretion of sodium
b. An increase in the free water clearance
c. A decrease in net acid excretion
d. A decrease in the excretion of creatinine
e. No change in the anion gap

**429.** A patient with renal failure develops symptoms caused by the loss of a hormone produced by the kidney. Which of the following is the most likely diagnosis?

a. Edema
b. Hypertension
c. Anemia
d. Uremia
e. Acidosis

**430.** Renal and pulmonary biopsies in a 35-year-old woman with Wegener granulomatosis demonstrate a granulomatous vasculities in the lungs and glomerulonephritis. In adults, which of the following is greater in the pulmonary circulation compared to the renal circulation?

a. Arterial pressure
b. Blood flow
c. Capillary hydrostatic pressure
d. Capillary oncotic pressure
e. Vascular resistance

**431.** A 25-year-old man qualifies to run in the Boston Marathon. He presents at his physician's office with a request to have his oxygen consumption measured. Which of the following is correct regarding the consumption of oxygen by the kidney?

a. It decreases as blood flow increases.
b. It is regulated by erythropoietin.
c. It remains constant as blood flow increases.
d. It directly reflects the level of sodium transport.
e. It is greatest in the medulla.

**432.** A 57-year-old woman with chronic cardiac failure presented at the University Medical Center to participate in a clinical research study on the genetics of heart failure. Genetic analysis showed an increase in vasopressin gene expression and associated hypothalamic biosynthesis of the hormone, in addition to increased release of the hormone from the posterior pituitary. In the presence of antidiuretic hormone (ADH), the filtrate will be isotonic to plasma in which of the following parts of the kidney?

a. Ascending limb of the loop of Henle
b. Descending limb of the loop of Henle
c. Cortical collecting tubule
d. Medullary collecting tubule
e. Renal pelvis

**433.** A 65-year-old man presents in the emergency department with a fracture of his right arm after slipping and falling on the ice. He reports that he has had back pain for the past 6 months. Blood results show Hb = 9 gm/dL; Hct = 30%; BUN = 35 mg/dL; Creatinine = 3 mg/dL. Urinalysis shows pH > 5.3 and is positive for Bence Jones proteins. The patient is diagnosed with type II (proximal) RTA secondary to multiple myeloma. The transport of $H^+$ into the proximal tubule is primarily associated with which of the following?

a. Excretion of potassium ion
b. Excretion of hydrogen ion
c. Reabsorption of calcium ion
d. Reabsorption of bicarbonate ion
e. Reabsorption of phosphate ion

**434.** A 58-year-old man presents with hematuria, abdominal pain, and fatigue. Physical examination reveals a flank mass and an abdominal CT reveals a large solid mass on the left kidney. Laboratory studies show anemia and increased creatinine and BUN suggestive of advanced disease. A decrease in GFR would result from which of the following?

a. Constriction of the efferent arteriole
b. An increase in afferent arteriolar pressure
c. Compression of the renal capsule
d. A decrease in the concentration of plasma protein
e. An increase in renal blood flow

# Renal and Urinary Physiology

## *Answers*

**372. The answer is e.** *(Ganong, pp 709-712. Widmaier, pp 496.)* The renal threshold for glucose is the plasma concentration at which glucose first appears in the urine. The graph shows that glucose is excreted at a plasma concentration of 300 mg/dL. (This is higher than the typical value of 200 mg/dL.) Glucose appears in the urine at a filtered load less than the $T_{max}$ for glucose because of the differences in the reabsorptive capacity of the nephrons. Some nephrons can only reabsorb a small amount of glucose. When their reabsorptive capacity is exceeded, glucose is excreted. Other nephrons can absorb much more glucose. The $T_{max}$ represents the average reabsorptive capacity of all the renal nephrons. The $T_{max}$ for glucose is the maximum rate of glucose reabsorption from the kidney. Typically, the $T_{max}$ is 375 mg/min. However, the $T_{max}$ in this patient is 500 mg/min. The higher-than-normal reabsorptive capacity accounts for the lower-than-expected urinary concentration. The $T_{max}$ is calculated by subtracting the amount of glucose excreted from the filtered load at any plasma concentration at which the amount of glucose excreted increases linearly as plasma glucose concentration increases. For example, when the plasma glucose concentration is 600 mg/dL, the filtered load of glucose is 600 mg/min, the amount of glucose excreted is 100 mg/min, and the amount of glucose reabsorbed (the $T_{max}$) is 500 mg/min.

**373. The answer is b.** *(Ganong, pp 642-643, 723.)* Sodium reabsorption in the distal nephron is normally under the control of aldosterone. In patients with Liddle syndrome, the distal nephron reabsorbs excess $Na^+$ despite low levels of aldosterone and renin in the plasma, because a mutation in the genes for the renal epithelial sodium channels (ENaC) increases ENaC activity and sodium retention. Metabolic alkalosis, hypokalemia, and hypertension are also present secondary to the increased sodium (and water) reabsorption.

**374. The answer is e.** (*Fauci, pp 268-271, 1744, 2447, 2475. Ganong, pp 706-708.*) Clearance is a measure of how much plasma is totally cleared of a substance. It is calculated using the formula

$$\text{Clearance} = U_{\text{uric acid}} \times V/P_{\text{uric acid}} = 36 \text{ mg/dL} \times 1 \text{ mL/min} / 0.6 \text{ mg/dL}$$
$$= 60 \text{ mL/min}$$

The boy's hypouricemia is an inherited defect in the ability to reabsorb uric acid by the anion/urate exchangers on proximal tubule cells rather than an increased secretion of uric acid. Patients with hypouricemia sometimes develop exercise-induced acute renal failure. Although the mechanism is not known, some investigators suggest that uric acid has an important antioxidant role in the kidney and that the oxygen radicals produced during prolonged exercise are responsible for the acute renal failure in patients with low uric acid levels.

**375. The answer is e.** (*Fauci, pp 1748, 2250-2251. Ganong, pp 454-459.*) Renin secretion is stimulated by the sympathetic nerves innervating the juxtaglomerular apparatus. Increasing mean blood pressure decreases sympathetic activity. Changes in GFR are detected by the macula densa. Decreases in GFR lead to an increase in renin release, whereas increases in GFR lead to the secretion of a mediator, perhaps adenosine or ATP, which contracts the afferent arteriole (tubuloglomerular feedback). ANP and angiotensin II decrease renin release.

**376. The answer is c.** (*Ganong, pp 709-710, 715, 724-725.*) The intracellular $Na^+$ concentration of renal epithelial cells is pumped out of renal epithelial cells by $Na^+$-$K^+$ pump located on the basolateral surface of the epithelial cells. The $Na^+/H^+$ exchanger and the $Na^+$-glucose cotransporter are located on the apical surface of the epithelial cells. $Na^+$ is transported from the peritubular spaces to the capillaries by solvent drag.

**377. The answer is d.** (*Ganong, pp 705-708. McPhee and Ganong, pp 459-469.*) The GFR is proportional to the glomerular capillary hydrostatic pressure, the renal plasma flow (RPF), and the surface area and hydraulic conductivity of the diffusion barrier between the glomerular capillary and Bowman space. Dilating the afferent arteriole causes an increase in glomerular capillary pressure and, therefore, an increase in GFR. Contraction of the mesangial cells causes a decrease in the surface area of the diffusion barrier between the glomerular capillary and Bowman space. Volume depletion causes a release of renin from the juxtaglomerular cells, leading to an increase in angiotensin II (AII) that causes constriction of the glomerular capillaries and contraction of the mesangial cells. Nonsteroidal anti-inflammatory drugs can induce acute renal failure in patients dependent on prostaglandin-mediated vasodilation to maintain renal perfusion.

**378. The answer is d.** (*Ganong, pp 705-708. Widmaier, pp 497-498.*) Glomerular filtration rate (GFR) is approximately equal to the clearance of creatinine, which in this case is

Creatinine clearance = creatine excreted/plasma creatinine concentration
Creatinine clearance = 2.4 g/d/0.8 mg/dL = 300 L/d = 300,000 mL/d
= 300,000 mL/24 h = 300,000 mL/1440 min = 208 mL/min

**379. The answer is d.** (*Stead, pp 237-238.*) The fractional excretion (FE) is the fraction of the filtered load that is excreted. It is calculated using the formula

$$FE = \text{amount excreted/amount filtered} = (U_{Na} \times \dot{V})/(P_{Na} \times GFR)$$
$$\text{Because GFR} = (U_{creatinine} \times \dot{V}/P_{creatinine})$$
$$FE = (U_{Na} \times \dot{V})/[P_{Na} \times (U_{creatinine} \times \dot{V}/P_{creatinine})]$$
$$= (U_{Na} \times P_{creatinine})/(P_{Na} \times U_{creatinine})$$
$$= 33 \text{ mM} \times 7.5 \text{ mg/dL}/135 \text{ mM} \times 90 \text{ mg/dL} = 0.02$$

Fractional excretion is used to distinguish between a prerenal state, such as volume depletion, and intrinsic renal failure, such as acute tubular necrosis. A fractional excretion of less than 1% is consistent with volume depletion, whereas a fractional excretion of 2% or greater is consistent with acute renal failure. This patient, with a fraction excretion of 2%, was diagnosed with acute renal failure caused by excessive intake of ibuprofen (Motrin).

**380. The answer is c.** (*Ganong, pp 705-708.*) Because the amount of fluid excreted by the kidney is only a small fraction of the RPF, the volume of fluid in the vein is essentially equal to that in the artery. Thus, the difference between the arterial and venous concentrations is due to the loss of solute. Because the material is neither reabsorbed nor secreted, its removal from the plasma must have been by glomerular filtration. Therefore the filtered solute equals (12 mg/mL − 9 mg/mL), and the percent of the arterial concentration that is filtered (and therefore, the fraction of plasma filtered) is

$$3 \text{ mg/mL}/2 \text{ mg/mL} = 0.25$$

**381. The answer is d.** (*Ganong, pp 720-722. Widmaier, pp 518-520.*) Net acid excretion is the amount of acid excreted each day. It is calculated using the formula

$$\text{Net acid excretion (NAE)} = (TA + NH_4^+ - HCO_3^-) \times V$$
$$NAE = (24 \text{ mEq/L} + 38 \text{ mEq/L} - 2 \text{ mEq/L}) \times 1.2 \text{ L/d} = 72 \text{ mEq/L/d}$$

Almost all of the acid excreted is buffered by either phosphate, called titratable acid, and ammonia. The titratable acid is equal to the mM of NaOH that must be added to the urine to raise its pH back to that of plasma. Bicarbonate must be subtracted from the sum of acid excreted because each milliequivalent of excreted bicarbonate represents the addition of 1 mEq of acid to the plasma.

**382. The answer is c.** (*Ganong, pp 702-704.*) The clearance of PAH is a good estimate of RPF because, under normal circumstances, almost all (more than 90%) of the PAH passing through the kidney is excreted.

$$C_{PAH} = U_{PAH} \times \dot{V}/P_{PAH} = (25 \text{ mg/mL} \times 1.5 \text{ mL/min})/6 \text{ mg/100 mL}$$
$$= 625 \text{ mL/min}$$

If the clearance of PAH is 90% of the actual renal blood flow, then the true renal blood flow (RBF) is approximately 695 mL/min.

**383. The answer is d.** (*Ganong, p 309. Widmaier, pp 497-498.*) If a substance disappears from the circulation during its passage through the kidney, it usually indicates that it has been totally secreted into the nephron. In this case, its clearance will be equal to the RPF. If the substance is bound to plasma proteins, it can be secreted without being filtered. Even if it is entirely secreted by the kidney, its urinary concentration may be less than its plasma concentration if the urinary flow rate is very high.

**384. The answer is a.** *(Fauci, pp 2218-2220. McPhee and Ganong, pp 561-563. Stead, pp 76-77.)* The presence of a mass in the posterior pituitary, coupled with the presentation of thirst and nocturia, suggest that the patient has a central diabetes insipidus with inadequate pituitary secretion of antidiuretic hormone (ADH). As a result of decreased ADH, the urine will have a low tonicity. On MRI, the absence of the normal bright spot in the region of the posterior pituitary further supports the diagnosis.

**385. The answer is a.** *(Ganong, pp 719-720.)* Free water clearance is the amount of water excreted in excess of that required to excrete urine that is isoosmotic to plasma. When the urine is concentrated, the value of $C_{H_2O}$ is negative, indicating that solute-free water is retained in the body. In other words, the amount of water excreted is less than that required to excrete urine that is isoosmotic to plasma. When the urine is dilute, the value of $C_{H_2O}$ is positive, indicating that solute-free water is excreted. Free water clearance is calculated using the formula:

Free water clearance $(C_{H_2O})$ = urine flow − osmolar clearance $(C_{osm})$
where $C_{osm} = U_{osm} \times$ urine flow$/P_{osm}$,
$U_{osm} = 2(U_{Na}^+ + U_K^+)$,
and $P_{osm} = 2 \times [Na^+]$

The urine osmolarity is estimated from the concentration of effective osmoles, that is, sodium and potassium, because these electrolytes determine the shift of water between intracellular and extracellular compartments. The total measured osmolarity is not used because it includes urea, which has no effect on body fluid distribution. Similarly, effective plasma osmolarity is used in calculating free water clearance, rather than total plasma osmolarity.

$$C_{H_2O} = \text{urine flow} -[2(U_{Na}^+ + U_K^+) \times \text{urine flow}/P_{osm}]$$
$$= 1 \text{ L/d} - [2(125 + 25 \text{ mOsm/kg H}_2\text{O}) \times 1 \text{ L/d}/2 \times 125 \text{ mOsm/kg H}_2\text{O}]$$
$$= 1 \text{ L/d} - 1.2 \text{ L/d} = -0.2 \text{ L/d}$$

This patient has a negative free water clearance, and thus she is producing concentrated urine. This means that she is diluting her plasma despite her low serum sodium. The negative free water clearance is probably caused by the combination of diuretics and antidepressants, which stimulate the release of ADH. The serum hypotonicity (250 mOsm/L) causes brain swelling, accounting for her signs and symptoms.

**386. The answer is a.** *(Stead, p 246.)* The rise in $H^+$ and fall in $HCO_3^-$ that occurs in type I (distal) renal tubular acidosis (RTA) does not increase the anion gap because the decrease in $HCO_3^-$ is accompanied by an increase in $Cl^-$. The failure of the distal nephron $H^+$ ATPase causes a reduction in net acid excretion and a reduced $H^+$ secretion, which causes less ammonium to be excreted in the urine. The low $HCO_3^-$ in the glomerular filtrate reduces $Na^+$ reabsorption by the Na-H exchanger and therefore more $Na^+$ is delivered to the distal nephron. The increased $Na^+$ delivery results in salt wasting and a secondary hyperaldosteronism which, in turn, causes $K^+$ concentration to fall.

**387. The answer is b.** *(Fauci, pp 268-271. Ganong, pp 294-296, 710, 718.)* Urea is synthesized primarily in the liver. Its excretion is dependent on its concentration in plasma and the GFR. Approximately 50% to 60% of filtered plasma urea is passively reabsorbed in the proximal tubule at normal GFR. In renal insufficiency, in which GFR is decreased, less urea is filtered and therefore less urea is excreted. The decreased excretion of urea results in an increase in its plasma concentration.

**388. The answer is d.** *(Ganong, pp 391, 709-710, 716-718. McPhee and Ganong, pp 460, 485-487, 493-498, 504-508, 509-510, 715.)* Parathyroid hormone (PTH) acts in the kidney to stimulate $Ca^{2+}$ reabsorption and to inhibit phosphate reabsorption. Although most of the filtered $Ca^{2+}$ is reabsorbed in the proximal tubule, the regulation of $Ca^{2+}$ excretion by PTH occurs in the medullary thick ascending limb and the distal convoluted tubule, where the action of PTH increases $Ca^{2+}$ reabsorption. The major effect of PTH inhibits on phosphate handling is to promote its excretion by inhibition of sodium-dependent phosphate transport in the proximal and distal tubules. PTH also increases urinary excretion of bicarbonate through its action on the proximal tubule, which may produce proximal renal tubular acidosis. These physiological responses to PTH are the basis for hyphosphatemia and hyperchloremic acidosis commonly observed in patients with hyperparathyroidism. Primary hyperparathyroidism, in which there is excessive secretion of PTH in relation to serum calcium, accounts for most cases of hypercalcemia in the outpatient setting. The *PRAD1* gene, which produces the cell cycle regulatory protein D1 cyclin, has been implicated in the pathogenesis of primary hyperparathyroidism.

**389. The answer is e.** *(Ganong, pp 362-365, 377-381.)* A decrease in plasma sodium increases aldosterone secretion. Aldosterone secretion increases in response to an increase in all of the other answer choices. The effects of sodium on aldosterone secretion are mediated via the renin angiotensin system. Hyponatremia, as may occur with a low-sodium diet, is associated with a decrease in extracellular volume, which increases renin secretion, probably due to a reflex increase in renal sympathetic nerve activity. Increased renin leads to increased production of angiotensin II, which binds to $AT_1$ receptors in the zona glomerulosa, which act via a G protein to activate phospholipase C. The resultant increase in protein kinase C fosters the conversion of cholesterol to pregnenolone and facilitates the action of aldosterone synthase, resulting in the conversion of deoxycorticosterone to aldosterone. Increased potassium concentration directly stimulates aldosterone secretion. Like angiotensin II, $K^+$ stimulates the conversion of cholesterol to pregnenolone and the conversion of deoxycorticosterone to aldosterone by aldosterone synthase. Potassium exerts effect on aldosterone secretion by depolarizing the the zona glomerulosa cells, which opens voltage-gated $Ca^{2+}$ channels, increasing intracellular $Ca^{2+}$. Adrenocorticotropic hormone (ACTH) stimulates aldosterone synthesis and secretion via increases in cyclic AMP and protein kinase A. The stimulatory effect of ACTH on aldosterone secretion is usually transient, declining in 1 to 2 days, but persists in patients with glucocorticoid-remediable aldosteronism, an autosomal dominant disorder in which the 5′ regulatory region of the 11β-hydroxylase gene is fused to the coding region of aldosterone synthase gene, producing an ACTH sensitive aldosterone synthase.

**390. The answer is c.** *(Ganong, pp 716-719, 240-246.)* When a person is dehydrated, ADH secretion increases. In the presence of ADH, the cortical and medullary collecting tubules become permeable to water, and the filtrate within these portions of the nephron reaches osmotic equilibrium with the interstitial fluid surrounding them. The ascending limb of the loop of Henle is not affected by ADH and so remains impermeable to water. As sodium and other electrolytes are reabsorbed from the ascending limb, its filtrate becomes hypotonic. The glomerular filtrate and proximal tubular fluid remain isotonic to plasma, which in the case of dehydration is higher than normal.

**391. The answer is e.** (*McPhee and Ganong, p 463. Stead, pp 248-249.*) Protein excretion is increased by sympathetic stimulation, such as that occurring during exercise. In this situation, renal vasoconstriction reduces the GFR, which, by increasing the transit time of glomerular filtrate, favors diffusion of proteins across the basement membrane. Approximately two-thirds of the 40 to 150 mg of protein excreted per day by the kidney is derived from plasma proteins; the remainder is derived from the tubular secretion of Tamm-Horsfall protein, a mucoprotein present in tubular casts appearing in urinary sediment. Not all plasma proteins are filtered equally because glomerular permeability is related to molecular size and charge. The larger and negatively charged proteins are poorly filtered. Most of the filtered protein is reabsorbed in the proximal tubule unless the filtered load exceeds the tubular capacity. Such overload would occur following damage to the glomerular basement membrane and breakdown of normal barriers, or following an increase in the plasma concentration of a small protein, such as myoglobin. The presence of protein in the urine indicates glomerular dysfunction. Progressive elevation of BUN serum creatinine results in uremia, a clinical syndrome manifest by headache, vomiting, dyspnea, insomnia, and delirium progressing to convulsions and coma.

**392. The answer is b.** (*Ganong, pp 714-715. Stead, pp 241-242.*) Abrupt onset hematuria with RBC casts are pathognomonic of any glomerulonephritis, also known as nephritic syndrome. IgA nephropathy is the most common glomerulonephritis. It generally presents in young men during or after a viral infection or after trauma or exercise. Pathologically, IgA nephropathy has immune complex deposition of IgA and C3 in the mesangial matrix, hence the alternative name, mesangial proliferative glomerulonephritis. There is no effective treatment.

**393. The answer is d.** (*Ganong, pp 454-459, 715. Stead, p 230.*) Renin is secreted by the juxtaglomerular cells (near the afferent arterioles) in response to decreased renal arterial pressure. It acts on angiotensinogen to form angiotensin I. Angiotensin I is then converted to angiotensin II, a highly potent pressor agent that, despite a short half-life in humans, has numerous regulatory functions, including the control of aldosterone secretion and sodium and water conservation.

**394. The answer is b.** (*Fauci, pp 1811-1812. Ganong, pp 702-704.*) The clearance of PAH would equal the true RPF only if the kidney reabsorbs all of the filtered PAH, that is, if no PAH appears in the renal vein. Because the kidney is only able to reabsorb approximately 85% to 90% of the filtered PAH, some PAH appears in the renal vein, and the PAH clearance is less than the true RPF. A number of clinical trials have focused on the rate of urinary albumin excretion as an early and powerful predictor of atherosclerotic vascular disease. Renal artery stenosis accounts for approximately 5% of cases of hypertension. The most common cause of renal artery stenosis in the middle-aged and elderly is an atheromatous plaque at the origin of the renal artery. Atherosclerotic renal vascular disease (ARVD) with renal artery stenosis and ischemic nephropathy stimulate renin release and increase sympathetic activity, resulting in the frequently described flushing, rapid blood pressure swings, and autonomic instability. The low GFR in these patients is a strong independent predictor of cardiovascular risk; in other words, patients with ARVD are more likely to suffer from stroke, myocardial infarction, or heart failure than to progress to end-stage renal disease. Gadolinium-enhanced 3D-MRA has replaced previous imaging modalities as the most sensitive and specific test for RAS. The most definitive diagnostic procedure is contrast-enhanced arteriography.

**395. The answer is a.** *(Stead, pp 69-70.)* Glucose reabsorption employs an active transport mechanism located in the proximal tubule. The same mechanism also transports fructose, galactose, and xylose. Essentially all filtered glucose is reabsorbed, inasmuch as the transport maximum $(T_{max})$ for glucose (320 mg/min) is not exceeded in normal persons. In diabetes mellitus, hyperglycemia results in a tubular filtration load that exceeds the $T_{max}$, and glycosuria ensues.

**396. The answer is c.** *(Ganong, pp 714-715. Stead, p 246.)* The major structural differences between epithelial cells of the proximal and distal tubules account for the fact that 65% of glomerular filtrate is reabsorbed in the proximal tubule and that the proximal tubule is more permeable to water. The proximal tubule has an extensive brush border composed of numerous microvilli, which markedly increase the surface area for reabsorption, and the tubule also has an extensive network of intracellular channels. The distal tubule has many more tight junctions between cells, which makes it less permeable to water. No significant difference in basement membrane thickness is observed between the proximal and distal tubules. Cells of the distal tubule lying adjacent to the afferent arteriole form the juxtaglomerular apparatus.

**397. The answer is a.** (*Ganong, pp 702-705. Stead, p 245.*) The renal artery pressure and the resistance of the renal vascular bed determine renal blood flow. Decreasing the resistance of either the afferent or efferent arterioles could increase RBF. Alternatively, if the resistance of one of these vessels decreased more than the resistance of the other one increased, RBF would also increase. GFR will increase if glomerular capillary pressure increases. This can occur if the afferent arteriolar resistance decreases or if the efferent arteriolar resistance increases.

**398. The answer is e.** (*Fauci, pp 283-285, 1751, 1764. Ganong, pp 293-294, 721-722. Stead, p 246. Widmaier, pp 520-521.*) Ammonia ($NH_3$) is produced from amino acids in the cells of the renal tubules (mainly the proximal tubules), and its rate of production increases during acidosis. This is important in acidosis because it increases the total amount of $H^+$ ion that can be excreted in a given volume of urine. The $NH_3$ freely diffuses into the tubular lumen, and because of the high $pK_a$ (9.2) of the reaction, essentially all of it combines with $H^+$ to form $NH_4^+$. This maintains the driving force for more $NH_3$ to passively diffuse into the lumen. The $NH_4^+$ that is formed gets "trapped" in the tubules and excreted because the tubules are impermeable to this cation. The combination of hyperkalemia and hyperchloremic metabolic acidosis, known as type IV RTA or hyporeninemic hypoaldosteronism, is often seen in patients with diabetic nephropathy.

**399. The answer is d.** (*Fauci, pp 1559-1561. Ganong, pp 710-712, 724.*) The amount of potassium excreted is controlled by the amount of potassium secreted by the distal tubule. Potassium secretion is a passive process that depends on the electrochemical gradient between the distal tubular cells and the tubular lumen and the permeability of the luminal cells to potassium. By inhibiting $Na^+$ reabsorption, the intraluminal potential becomes less negative and $K^+$ secretion is reduced. $K^+$-sparing diuretics such as amiloride act in this fashion. Aldosterone increases the intracellular potassium concentration by augmenting the activity of the Na-K pump and increasing the potassium permeability of the luminal membrane. Increasing dietary intake increases the plasma potassium concentration, which in turn stimulates aldosterone production. Increasing the rate of distal tubular flow increases the rate of $K^+$ secretion. The high flow maintains a low tubular $K^+$ concentration and therefore increases the electrochemical gradient for $K^+$ secretion. Low-dose thiazide diuretics, such as hydrochlorothiazide, are often used as first-line antihypertensive agents, and are often combined with a potassium-sparing diuretic to prevent hypokalemia. Health-promoting lifestyle modifications are recommended for individuals with pre-hypertension and as an adjunct to therapy in hypertensive individuals.

**400. The answer is b.** *(Fauci, pp 1744-1745, 1855, 1862-1863. Ganong, pp 705-714.)* Because creatinine cannot be reabsorbed from the tubule, its concentration rises as water is reabsorbed. The $H_2$ receptor antagonist, cimetidine, competes with creatinine for proximal tubule transport by the organic cation pathways. This may elevate serum creatinine levels, but this change does not reflect changes in GFR. Phosphate is almost completely reabsorbed in the proximal tubule, so its concentration decreases along the length of the tubule. The concentrations of glucose and bicarbonate are also less at the end of the proximal tubule than at the beginning. Sodium is isosmotically reabsorbed from the proximal tubule; that is, when sodium is reabsorbed, water flows out of the proximal tubule to maintain a constant osmolarity; thus, the concentration of sodium does not normally change as the filtrate flows through the proximal tubule.

**401. The answer is e.** *(Fauci, pp 1550-1551, 1559-1561. Ganong, pp 702-728.)* Decreased pressure or stretch in the afferent arteriole is one of three primary stimuli for increasing renin secretion. RPF, filtration fraction, the oncotic pressure, and the filtration rate all increase when the afferent arteriolar resistance is decreased. The RBF increases because total renal resistance is less. Decreasing renal resistance also increases the glomerular capillary pressure, which results in an increase in filtration fraction. Because more fluid is filtered out of the glomerular capillaries and no plasma protein is removed, the oncotic pressure rises. The GFR is proportional to the glomerular capillary pressure and the RPF. Because both of these increase, so does the GFR. Vasodilators are used in the treatment of hypertension to improve both cardiovascular and renal outcomes. The concomitant use of an ACE inhibitor or angiotensin receptor antagonist, protects against the effects of renin on angiotensin generation or action, respectively.

**402. The answer is a.** *(Fauci, pp 1743-1747, 1801-1803. Ganong, pp 710-711, 715.)* The distal convoluted tubule reabsorbs approximately 5% of the filtered NaCl via an electrically neutral thiazide-sensitive $Na^+/Cl^+$ cotransporter on the apical membrane. Loss-of-function mutations of SLC12A3 encoding the apical Na$^+$/Cl$^+$ co-transporter causes Gitelman syndrome, a salt-wasting disorder associated with hypokalemic alkalosis, hypomagnesemia, hypocalciuria, and decreased urine chloride. The thick ascending limb of loop of Henle employs a carrier that binds one sodium, one potassium, and two chloride ions. It is also electrically neutral. Diffusion of Na$^+$ through channels on the apical surface of principal cells of the cortical and medullary collecting ducts is electrogenic.

**403. The answer is b.** *(Fauci, pp 275-277. Ganong, pp 706-708.)* Under euvolemic conditions, when water is filtered across the glomerulus, the protein concentration (and thus the oncotic pressure) within the capillaries increases, which in turn increases the efficiency by which sodium and water is reabsorbed from the proximal tubule and returned to the circulatory system. If GFR decreases, it results in a decreased oncotic pressure, which in turn decreases the amount of water reabsorbed from the proximal tubule. Postoperative hemorrhage causes hypovolemic hypotension, which overrides glomerulotubular balance via baroreceptor-mediated activation of the sympathetic nervous system and the renin-angiotensin system. Increased sympathetic tone increases proximal tubular sodium reabsorption despite a decreased GFR caused by preferential afferent arteriolar vasoconstriction.

**404. The answer is e.** *(Ganong, pp 391, 709-710, 716-718. McPhee and Ganong, pp 561-563, 565-566, 719.)* The ascending limb of the loop of Henle dilutes the fluid within the nephron by reabsorbing Na$^+$ without water. In the absence of antidiuretic hormone (ADH), or when the nephron is resistant to ADH, the reabsorption of Na$^+$ without water continues along the collecting duct, making the Na$^+$ concentration lower and lower. In the presence of ADH, water is reabsorbed from the collecting duct making the luminal fluid isotonic in the cortical collecting duct and hypertonic in the medullary collecting duct. Diabetes insipidus is a syndrome of polyuria resulting from the inability to concentrate urine and thus to conserve water due to a lack of action of ADH. Diabetes insipidus is classified as central (affecting the synthesis or secretion of ADH) or nephrogenic (due to loss of the kidney's ability to respond to circulating ADH). Both types of diabetes insipidus have hereditary and acquired causes.

**405. The answer is c.** *(Fauci, pp 1551-1552, 1555-1556, 2250-2251. Ganong, pp 378-380, 454-459.)* Juxtaglomerular (JG) cells are sensitive to changes in afferent arterial intraluminal pressure. Increased pressure within the afferent arteriole leads to a decrease in renin release, whereas decreased pressure tends to increase renin release. Angiotensin appears to inhibit renin release by initiating the flow of calcium into the JG cells. Renin release is increased in response to increased activity in the sympathetic neurons innervating the kidney. Prostaglandins, particularly $PGI_2$ and $PGE_2$, stimulate renin release. Stimulation of the macula densa leads to an increase in renin release, and although the mechanism is not fully understood, it appears that increased delivery of NaCl to the distal nephron is responsible for stimulating the macula densa. Aldosterone does not appear to have any direct effect on renin release.

**406. The answer is b.** (*Ganong, pp 367, 375-381. Widmaier, pp 318, 507-509, 513-514.*) Aldosterone binds to an intracellular receptor that causes an increased synthesis of a variety of proteins, including $K^+$ and $Na^+$ ion channels and $Na^+$-$K^+$-ATPase, which together act to increase $Na^+$ reabsorption and $K^+$ secretion by the tubular cells of the distal nephron. The secretion of $H^+$ is also enhanced by aldosterone. Aldosterone secretion is stimulated by a decrease in blood volume (through the renin-angiotensin system) and by increased plasma $K^+$ concentrations.

**407. The answer is e.** (*Ganong, pp 95, 113, 242-247, 456, 604, 713-716, 729-730. Widmaier, pp 319, 502-503.*) The principal physiologic action of antidiuretic hormone (ADH) is to increase water retention by the kidney. Antidiuretic hormone acts on the distal nephron to increase its permeability so that water more readily enters the hypertonic interstitium of the renal pyramids. Thus, the concentration of solutes in the urine is increased. Antidiuretic hormone increases $Na^+$ reabsorption so that the actual amount of $Na^+$ excreted is decreased. It also acts as a vasoconstrictor; hence, it is called arginine vasopressin (AVP). ADH has no effect on GFR, and because it increases water reabsorption, it would decrease urine formation.

**408. The answer is d.** (*Fauci, pp 418-420, 1472, 1557, 1769-1771, 1797-1799, 1806-1807. Ganong, pp 719-720. Stead, pp 181-183, 245. Widmaier, pp 503-506.*) Concentrated urine is produced by the reabsorption of water from the medullary collecting ducts down an osmotic gradient that is created by the reabsorption of sodium from the loop of Henle. If the $Na^+$-$K^+$ pump activity in the loop of Henle is increased, the osmotic gradient, and the ability to excrete concentrated urine, is increased. Water reabsorption will be reduced if the permeability of the collecting duct principal cells is reduced. Also, concentrated urine will be more difficult to produce if an increase in glomerular capillary increases the filtered load of $Na^+$ or if the reabsorption of $Na^+$ is decreased in the proximal tubule. Patients with autosomal dominant polycystic kidney disease typically present in their 30s or 40s with flank pain. Complications include recurrent urinary tract infections and pyelonephritis, and cardiovascular complications, including hypertension, valvular disorders (especially mitral valve prolapse and aortic regurgitation), and berry aneurysms (subarachnoid hemorrhage). Approximately 50% of patients will develop end-stage renal disease, requiring dialysis or renal transplantation.

**409. The answer is d.** (*Fauci, 1755-1761. McPhee and Ganong, pp 462-466.*) The most likely cause of acute renal failure in this patient is ureteral obstruction, as evidenced by the swelling of the kidneys. The ureteral obstruction raises the hydrostatic pressure within Bowman space, which reduces glomerular filtration. The decrease in GFR (postrenal renal failure) increases creatinine. The normal blood pressure rules out sympathetic discharge, coarctation of the renal artery, and hypovolemia as causes of her renal failure. Hyperproteinemia, although possibly a cause of renal failure, would not produce an enlarged kidney.

**410. The answer is b.** (*Stead, pp 77-78, 227, 277.*) The increased secretion of antidiuretic hormone (ADH) increases the permeability of the distal nephron to water and therefore increases the reabsorption of water from the kidney. The excessive reabsorption of water dilutes the extracellular fluid, producing a decrease in plasma sodium, osmolarity, and oncotic pressure. The decreased extracellular osmolarity causes water to flow from the extracellular fluid compartment into the intracellular fluid compartment, increasing intracellular volume. Because more water is being reabsorbed, less is excreted and urinary flow is decreased.

**411. The answer is c.** (*Fauci, pp 1448-1451. Ganong, pp 724-725, Widmaier, pp 486-517, 523.*) The distal nephron has a negative luminal potential because it is poorly permeable to negatively charged ions. Therefore, when $Na^+$ is reabsorbed, negatively charged ions, primarily $Cl^-$, lag behind, producing a negative intraluminal potential. Although a similar situation occurs in the proximal tubule, the proximal tubule has a higher permeability to $Cl^-$ and, therefore, does not develop as large a negative intraluminal potential. The distal nephron is less permeable to hydrogen than the proximal tubule. Aldosterone increases $Na^+$ reabsorption from the distal nephron but has no effect on the proximal tubule. $K^+$ is reabsorbed from the proximal tubule and secreted by the distal nephron. Although the amount of $H^+$ excreted each day is determined by the amount of $H^+$ secreted into the distal nephron, the proximal tubule secretes much more $H^+$ than the distal nephron. However, almost all of the $H^+$ secreted in the proximal tubule is reabsorbed in association with the reabsorption of $HCO_3^-$.

**412. The answer is a.** (*Ganong, pp 719-720. McPhee and Ganong, pp 559-566, 719.*) Free water clearance is the amount of water excreted in excess of that required to make the urine isotonic to plasma. It is calculated using the formula: $C_{H_2O} = urine\ flow - C_{osm}$. Free water clearance is positive when the urine is dilute (more than a sufficient amount of water is excreted), and free water clearance is negative when the urine is concentrated (not enough water is excreted to make the urine isotonic to plasma). An increase in free water clearance can lead to hypernatremia; a decrease in free water clearance can lead to hyponatremia. In diabetes insipidus, very little water is reabsorbed in the distal nephron, and, therefore, the free water clearance is very high. In heart failure or renal failure, very little free water can be generated even if the urine is dilute because the GFR is decreased. With diuretic therapy, $Na^+$ excretion is increased. Therefore, the increased water excretion is accompanied by an increased $Na^+$ excretion and the amount of free water generated is limited. Although the water loss is proportionally greater than the solute loss in diabetes mellitus, the amount of water excreted is much less and the solute concentration significantly higher than in diabetes insipidus, so the free water clearance is much less in diabetes mellitus than in diabetes insipidus.

**413. The answer is e.** (*Ganong, pp 391, 709-710, 716-718. McPhee and Ganong, pp 615-618, 621, 722-723.*) Aldosterone increases the reabsorption of $Na^+$ from the principal cells within the cortical and medullary collecting ducts. Aldosterone increases $Na^+$ reabsorption by increasing the luminal permeability to $Na^+$ on the apical surface and the activity of the Na-K pump on the basal lateral surface of the principal cells. Aldosterone also increases the secretion of $K^+$ and $H^+$ from the collecting ducts. Up to 15% of patients diagnosed as having essential hypertension have primary hyperaldosteronism. The ratio of plasma aldosterone concentration to plasma renin activity is high in primary aldosteronism and low in secondary hyperaldosteronism, in which plasma renin activity is high.

**414. The answer is d.** (*Fauci, pp 232-234, 1443-1453, 1742-1748. Ganong, pp 340, 707-708, 718-719. Stead, pp 63-64, 76-77. Widmaier, pp 500-511*) Patients with congestive heart failure frequently have a paradoxical increase in NaCl and water retention despite an increase in extracellular fluid volume. An increase in renal sympathetic nerve activity promotes a decrease in NaCl and water excretion by decreasing GFR, increasing renin secretion, and increasing tubular NaCl reabsorption. All of the other factors an increase in NaCl and water excretion.

**415. The answer is b.** (*Ganong, pp 724-725.*) Diuretics produce an increase in water excretion primarily by blocking $Na^+$ reabsorption. If $Na^+$ reabsorption is blocked in the proximal portions of the nephron, then the amount of $Na^+$ in the filtrate flowing through the distal nephron increases. The increased $Na^+$ load in the distal nephron results in an increased $Na^+$ reabsorption and, as a result, an increased $K^+$ secretion. If $Na^+$ reabsorption in the distal nephron is blocked, then a diuresis can be produced without an excess loss of $K^+$. These diuretics, some of which block the aldosterone receptor, others of which block the Na channels on the apical surface of the distal nephron tubular cells, are called potassium-sparing diuretics.

**416. The answer is a.** (*Ganong, pp 734-735.*) Persistent diarrhea will result in a metabolic acidosis, due to the loss of the bicarbonate-rich secretions from the pancreas and gallbladder. The ensuing metabolic acidosis will decrease the plasma concentration of $HCO_3^-$, decreasing the amount of bicarbonate that is filtered into the proximal tubule. At the same time, the metabolic acidosis will increase ammonia production by the proximal tubule as well as $H^+$ secretion and production of new bicarbonate by the distal nephron. Because the metabolic acidosis is produced by the loss of bicarbonate, the anion gap will remain within normal limits.

**417. The answer is e.** (*Fauci, pp 277-279. Ganong, pp 713-718. McPhee and Ganong, pp 563-566, 719.*) ADH increases the permeability of the distal nephron to urea as well as to water. The increased urea permeability increases the urea concentration and osmolarity of the interstitial fluid surrounding the loop of Henle and the distal nephron. The high interstitial urea concentration helps to increase the osmolarity of the fluid within the descending limb of the loop of Henle, the reabsorption of Na⁺ from the ascending limb of the loop of Henle, and the reabsorption of water from the distal nephron. The cardinal clinical presentation in patients with the syndrome of inappropriate ADH secretion (SIADH) is hyponatremia without edemas. SIADH is due to the secretion of ADH in excess of what is appropriate for plasma osmolality or intravascular volume depletion. Tuberculosis is one of many causes of SIADH.

**418. The answer is b.** *(Fauci, pp 231-236. Ganong, pp 702-708. Widmaier, pp 489-494.)* The filtration fraction (FF) is defined as the ratio of GFR to RBF. FF will therefore increase with increases in GFR, such as occurs with an increase in glomerular capillary (hydrostatic) pressure. Increasing the resistance of the efferent arteriole increases the glomerular capillary pressure and, therefore, the filtration fraction. An increase in afferent arteriolar resistance, such as occurs with inhibition of vasodilatory prostaglandins by NSAIDS, will decrease glomerular capillary pressure and, therefore, the filtration fraction. Increasing the plasma oncotic pressure or the hydrostatic pressure within Bowman capsule will decrease the filtration fraction because both of these Starling forces oppose filtration. Increasing RBF at a constant GFR causes a decrease in the filtration fraction.

**419. The answer is a.** *(Ganong, pp 720-725. Levitzky, p 238.)* Carbonic anhydrase is the enzyme that catalyzes the formation of $CO_2$ and $H_2O$ from $HCO_3^-$ and $H^+$. In the proximal tubule, the efficient reabsorption of bicarbonate requires the presence of carbonic anhydrase. Carbonic anhydrase inhibitors like acetazolamide prevent the formation of $CO_2$ and therefore block the reabsorption of bicarbonate (and $Na^+$), resulting in a diuresis. Because almost all of the filtered bicarbonate is reabsorbed in the proximal tubule, inhibiting carbonic anhydrase has little effect on bicarbonate reabsorption from other segments of the nephron. Acetazolamide taken for a few days before ascending to high altitude can prevent the symptoms of acute mountain sickness. The mechanisms are unclear, but likely relate to (1) prevention of fluid retention via diuresis, (2) production of metabolic acidosis from decreased bicarbonate reabsorption, which may offset the respiratory alkalosis at high altitude, and (3) inhibition of hypoxic pulmonary vasoconstriction.

**420. The answer is d.** (*Ganong, pp 703-705. Stead, pp 242-243. Widmaier, pp 486-517.*) Blood flow through the kidney is controlled by numerous humoral agents. Angiotensin II decreases renal blood flow. It vasoconstricts efferent arterioles more than afferent arterioles, which helps to maintain GFR in the face of decreases in renal perfusion pressure. This may account for the renal failure that sometimes develops in patients with decreased renal perfusion who are taking angiotensin-converting enzyme inhibitors. Nitric oxide dilates the afferent arteriole and constricts the efferent arteriole, producing a rise in glomerular capillary pressure (and glomerular filtration) without having much of an effect on renal blood flow. Dopamine synthesized in the kidney increases RBF and sodium excretion. Acetylcholine and atrial natriuretic peptide (ANP) also produce renal vasodilation and an increase in renal blood flow.

**421. The answer is b.** (*Fauci, pp 58-59. Widmaier, pp 498-499.*) Contraction of the detrusor muscle in the bladder causes micturition. The detrusor muscle is innervated by parasympathetic neurons, which cause contraction. The internal urethral sphincter at the base or neck of the bladder is innervated by sympathetic neurons, which constrict the sphincter to prevent urination. Incontinence is the involuntary release of urine, and is generally classified as stress incontinence (due to sneezing, coughing, exercise), urge incontinence (associated with the desire to urinate), or mixed. This patient has mixed incontinence. Anticholinergics, such as tolterodine or oxybutin, would be useful for the treatment of her urge incontinence. Any irritation to the bladder or urethra, for example, a bacterial infection, can cause urge incontinence. Urge incontinence acetylcholine and adrenergic blockers would promote micturition. In women, stress incontinence is usually due to a loss of urethral support provided by the anterior vagina. Estrogen replacement therapy can often improve vaginal tone and thus relieve stress incompetence.

**422. The answer is d.** (*Ganong, pp 709-713.*) About two-thirds of the filtered load of sodium is reabsorbed by the proximal tubule. This percentage is maintained when there are spontaneous changes in the filtered load by a process called glomerular tubular balance. However, the percentage of reabsorption can be changed when necessary to maintain homeostasis. For example, the production of angiotensin II during volume depletion can result in the reabsorption of as much as 75% of the filtered load of $Na^+$.

**423. The answer is e.** (*Ganong, pp 460-462, 706-707, 723-724.*) ANP increases Na⁺ excretion by decreasing the amount of Na⁺ reabsorbed from the inner medullary collecting duct via a decrease in the permeability of the apical membrane of the collecting duct epithelial cells. Less Na⁺ is able to enter the epithelial cells and therefore, less Na⁺ is reabsorbed. ANP also increases Na⁺ excretion by increasing the filtered load of Na⁺.

**424. The answer is a.** (*Ganong, pp 712-713. Stead, pp 181-183.*) The macula densa senses the chloride concentration of the fluid flowing from the ascending limb of loop of Henle into the distal convoluted tubule. An increase in NaCl concentration occurs when the amount of fluid flowing through the ascending limb increases because there is less time available for the reabsorption of NaCl. The resulting increase in Cl⁻ concentration results in the release of adenosine (and/or ATP) from the macula densa. Adenosine constricts the afferent arteriole, resulting in a decrease in filtration and a return of the flow rate within the nephron toward normal. This response is referred to as tubuloglomerular feedback. If the NaCl concentration decreases (eg, when circulating blood volume decreases), the decreased Cl⁻ concentration results in the release of renin from granular cells of the juxtaglomerular apparatus. Spironolactone acts by competitive inhibition of aldosterone, thereby blocking Na⁺ reabsorption in the distal tubules and collecting ducts. Potassium-sparing diuretics are relatively weak and therefore are most effective when administered in combination with loop and/or thiazide diuretics.

**425. The answer is b.** (*Ganong, pp 391-393, 710. Stead, pp 246-249.*) Between 85% and 90% of the filtered phosphate is reabsorbed in the proximal tubule by a sodium-dependent secondary active transport system. The transporter is electrically neutral, requiring two Na⁺ molecules for every $HPO_4^{2-}$ molecule that it transports. The transporter is inhibited by parathyroid hormone (PTH). The decreased reabsorption of phosphate results in an increased clearance from the plasma. PTH is released from the parathyroid gland in response to lowered plasma $Ca^{2+}$ concentrations. In addition to inhibiting the reabsorption of phosphate from the proximal tubule, PTH increases the reabsorption of $Ca^{2+}$ from the loop of Henle.

**426. The answer is d.** (*Fauci, pp 1744-1752, 2121-2124. Ganong, pp 710, 724. Stead, pp 241-243.*) Potassium is secreted from the principal cells lining the cortical and medullary collecting ducts. Secretion is passive and is increased by increasing the electrochemical gradient driving the diffusion through the potassium channels on the apical surface of the principal cells. Increasing $Na^+$ concentration within the distal nephron increases $Na^+$ reabsorption, which, in turn, increases the negativity of the luminal electrical potential. The increased negativity drives $K^+$ into the lumen at a greater rate. Decreasing the distal flow rate, which occurs when circulating blood volume or RBF decreases or when sympathetic nerve activity to the renal vessels increases, will allow the $K^+$ concentration within the distal nephron to increase. The increase in $K^+$ concentration decreases the driving force for $K^+$ diffusion and, therefore, decreases $K^+$ secretion.

**427. The answer is e.** (*Fauci, pp 270-271. Ganong, pp 454-459. Widmaier, pp 508-509.*) The juxtaglomerular apparatus (JGA) is responsible for releasing renin when the effective circulating blood volume is decreased. The JGA releases renin when the $Cl^-$ concentration in the luminal fluid bathing the macula densa is decreased or when renal perfusion pressure is decreased. The decrease in $Cl^-$ (and $Na^+$) concentration occurs when the flow rate within the nephron decreases and ample time is available for the loop of Henle to remove NaCl from the lumen. Adenosine is released from the macula densa cells when the luminal $Cl^+$ concentration increases in response to an increase in luminal flow rate. Adenosine decreases RBF by constricting the afferent arteriole and, therefore, the blood flow through the glomerular capillary. Decreased renal perfusion accounts for 40% to 80% of acute renal failure. The etiologies of prerenal failure include any cause of decreased circulating blood volume (burns, diarrhea, diuretics, GI hemorrhage), volume sequestration (pancreatitis, rhabdomyoloysis, peritonitis), or decreased effective arterial volume (cardiogenic shock, sepsis).

**428. The answer is d.** (*Ganong, pp 705-708, 725-726. Stead, pp 242-243.*) The excretion of creatinine, which is neither reabsorbed nor secreted in any significant amount, is dependent on filtration, which is in turn dependent on RPF. The decrease in RPF that accompanies chronic renal failure results in a decrease in creatinine excretion and an increase in plasma creatinine concentration. The increase in plasma creatinine concentration is used to assess the percentage of non functioning nephrons in renal failure. Interestingly, the remaining nephrons adapt to renal failure. To maintain $Na^+$

balance, less $Na^+$ is reabsorbed, so the fractional excretion (the fraction of filtered $Na^+$ that is excreted) goes up. Although the remaining nephrons are able to excrete a larger than normal amount of $H^+$, secretion cannot fully compensate for the reduced number of nephrons because there is a limit to the amount of $NH_4^+$ that can be synthesized by the proximal tubules. Therefore, despite the overall increase in net acid excretion, $H^+$ accumulation leads to a metabolic acidosis. Even creatinine secretion can be increased so the plasma creatinine concentration does not increase proportionally to the amount of renal damage. The anion gap increases because of the reduced excretion of phosphate and other anions that are included in the anion gap. Free water clearance decreases because there is decreased filtration. Therefore, to prevent overhydration in patients with renal failure, water intake must be limited.

**429. The answer is c.** *(Ganong, pp 459-460.)* The kidney produces a number of important hormones, including erythropoietin. Erythropoietin is necessary for the normal production of red blood cells. The anemia associated with renal failure results from the decrease in the synthesis of erythropoietin. Often, the first clinical sign of renal failure is the fatigue produced by anemia.

**430. The answer is b.** *(Fauci, pp 2120-2123. Ganong, pp 650, 661-662, 702-705. Levitzky, pp 86-92.)* Because the lungs are in series with the heart, pulmonary blood flow constitutes 100% of the cardiac output, whereas the kidneys receive approximately 25% of the cardiac output. As part of the systemic circulation, the renal circulation has higher vascular pressures, including both arterial pressure and capillary hydrostatic pressure. The capillary oncotic pressures in the renal and pulmonary circulations are essentially equal.

**431. The answer is d.** *(Ganong, pp 612, 705.)* Oxygen consumption by the kidney is directly proportional to the amount of sodium reabsorbed and is greatest in the cortex, where most tubular reabsorption of sodium occurs. An increase in RBF will raise the GFR and increase the quantity of solute to be transported, so that oxygen consumption increases as blood flow increases and the arteriovenous oxygen difference remains constant. This is in contrast to the situation in other organs where increases in blood flow are accompanied by a decrease in arteriovenous oxygen difference.

Erythropoietin is released in response to renal hypoxia and acts to increase erythrocyte production.

**432. The answer is c.** (*Ganong, pp 240-246, 716-719.*) In the absence of antidiuretic hormone (ADH, vasopressin), the cortical and medullary collecting tubules and ducts are impermeable to water. ADH increases the water permeability of these nephron segments and allows the filtrate to reach osmotic equilibrium with the interstitial fluid surrounding the nephron. The interstitial fluid in the cortex of the kidney is isotonic to plasma, and, therefore, the filtrate can become isotonic to plasma in the cortical collecting tubule. The interstitial fluid is hypertonic to plasma in the medullary collecting tubule, and so the filtrate becomes hypertonic to plasma in this region of the nephron and remains hypertonic as it passes through the renal pelvis. ADH has no effect on the water permeability of the loop of Henle. The filtrate is hypertonic to plasma in the descending limb and becomes hypotonic to plasma by the time it reaches the end of the ascending limb of the loop of Henle.

**433. The answer is d.** (*Fauci, pp 1742-1745, 1802-1805. Ganong, pp 709-710, 722. Stead, p 246.*) In the proximal tubule, a large amount of $H^+$ ion is secreted into the tubule lumen via an $Na^+$-$H^+$ antiporter (exchanger). Most of this $H^+$ combines with bicarbonate ion in the tubular fluid to form $CO_2$ and water. The $CO_2$ diffuses into the proximal tubular cells, where the opposite reaction takes place to form $H^+$ and $HCO_3^-$. The $HCO_3^-$ exits the cells on the basolateral side and enters the blood as reabsorbed bicarbonate. Carbonic anhydrase is located on the luminal surface of the cells as well as inside the cells to facilitate the above reactions. In type II RTA, a defect in proximal tubular bicarbonate reabsorption causes normal anion gap metabolic acidosis and bicarbonate wasting in the urine (increased pH). Multiple myeloma, heavy metals, and carbonic anhydrase inhibitors are causes of type II RTA. The most common presenting symptom of multiple myeloma is bone pain and compression fractures. Bence-Jones proteins in the urine are pathognomonic.

**434. The answer is c.** (*Fauci, pp 592-593. Ganong, pp 706-708.*) GFR will decrease if there is a decrease in the net glomerular capillary pressure or the flow of fluid through the glomerulus. The net glomerular capillary pressure (for Starling forces) is equal to the glomerular capillary pressure minus the sum of the plasma oncotic pressure and intrarenal pressure. Compression of the renal capsule increases the intrarenal pressure and therefore decreases the net capillary filtration pressure. Constriction of the efferent arteriole increases glomerular capillary pressure. Decreasing the concentration of plasma protein will decrease the plasma oncotic pressure and lead to an increase in GFR. In clinical practice, any solid renal masses should be considered malignant until proven otherwise. Renal cell carcinomas account for 90% to 95% of malignant neoplasms arising from the kidney.

# Reproductive Physiology

## Questions

**435.** A 15-year-old boy presents for his annual athletic physical. A thorough examination reveals unilateral cryptorchidism. The physician schedules a follow-up visit with the boy and his parents to discuss his recommendation for surgery to correct the defect because of his concerns of possible infertility in the future. Which of the following best describes spermatogenesis?

a. Mature spermatozoa are present at birth, but cannot be released until puberty is reached.
b. Spermatogenesis requires a temperature lower than internal body temperature.
c. Spermatogenesis requires continuous release of gonadotropin-releasing hormone (GnRH).
d. Leydig cell secretion of testosterone requires follicle-stimulating hormone (FSH).
e. Luteinizing hormone (LH) acts directly on Sertoli cells to promote cell division.

**436.** A 32-year-old man taking chlorpromazine for his schizophrenia presents with diminished libido and decreased beard growth. His blood prolactin level of 75 µg/L confirms the presence of hyperprolactinemia. Which of the following is most likely regarding prolactin?

a. Normal adult serum levels of prolactin are much higher in women than men.
b. Prolactin causes milk ejection during suckling.
c. Prolactin inhibits the growth of breast tissue.
d. Prolactin inhibits gonadotropin releasing hormone secretion by the hypothalamus.
e. Prolactin inhibits gonadotropin secretion by the pituitary gland.

### Questions 437 and 438

**437.** A 32-year-old woman medical student develops nausea and breast tenderness after missing her menstrual period. She discovers that she is 4 weeks pregnant. With respect to hormonal changes during pregnancy, which of the following is the source of estrogen and progesterone during the first 2 months of pregnancy?

a. Ovary
b. Placenta
c. Corpus luteum
d. Anterior pituitary
e. Posterior pituitary

**438.** Other than lower back pain, occasional headaches, and frequent urination, the pregnancy progresses to the second trimester without complications. Which of the following is the source of estrogen and progesterone during the last 7 months of pregnancy?

a. Ovary
b. Placenta
c. Corpus luteum
d. Anterior pituitary
e. Posterior pituitary

**439.** In the graph below showing plasma hormone levels as a function of time, ovulation takes place at which of the lettered points on the time axis?

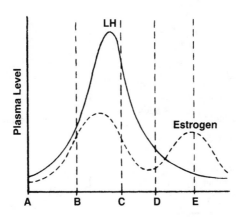

a. A
b. B
c. C
d. D
e. E

**440.** The normal pattern of progesterone secretion during the menstrual cycle is exhibited by which of the following curves?

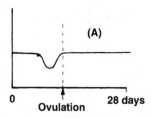

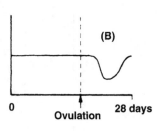

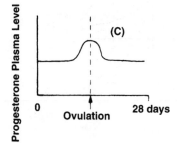

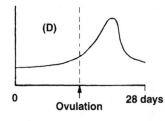

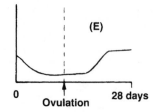

a. A
b. B
c. C
d. D
e. E

**441.** An 18-year-old emaciated woman who has been on a strict diet regimen and training for a marathon presents with amenorrhea. Exogenous pulsatile administration of GnRH restores ovulation and menses. Ovulation is caused by a sudden increase in the secretion of which of the following hormones?

a. LH
b. FSH
c. GnRH
d. Estrogen
e. Progesterone

**442.** In the following graph of changes in endometrial thickness during a normal 28-day menstrual cycle, the event designated A corresponds most closely to which of the following phases?

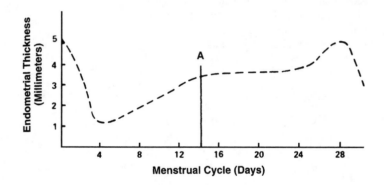

a. The menstrual phase
b. The maturation of the corpus luteum
c. The early proliferative phase
d. The secretory phase
e. Ovulation

**443.** A couple presents at the fertility center concerned that they have not been able to conceive a child. The reproductive endocrinologist evaluates the wife to be certain that she is ovulating. Which of the following is an indication that ovulation has taken place?

a. An increase in serum FSH levels
b. A drop in body temperature
c. An increase in serum LH levels
d. An increase in serum progesterone levels
e. An increase in serum estrogen levels

**444.** A 26-year-old man with Klinefelter syndrome has seminiferous tubule dysgenesis. Which of the following is a function of Sertoli cells in the seminiferous tubules?

a. Secretion of FSH into the tubular lumen
b. Secretion of testosterone into the tubular lumen
c. Maintenance of the blood-testis barrier
d. Synthesis of estrogen after puberty
e. Expression of surface LH receptors

**445.** A 34-year-old woman discovers that she is pregnant using a home pregnancy test that detects the presence of human chorionic gonadotropin (hCG). In a normal pregnancy, hCG prevents the involution of the corpus luteum that normally occurs at the end of the menstrual cycle. Which of the curves shown below approximates the level of this hormone during pregnancy?

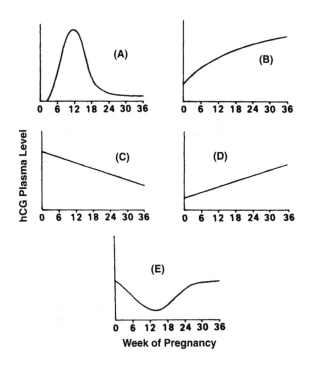

a.  A
b.  B
c.  C
d.  D
e.  E

**446.** A woman presents to her obstetrician with concerns that she has had trouble breast feeding. She reports that her mother-in-law told her that alcohol would relax her and allow her milk to flow more readily, but it has not helped, even with drinking up to a bottle of wine a day. Which of the following hormones is involved in the ejection of milk from a lactating mammary gland?

a. Growth hormone
b. FSH
c. LH
d. Prolactin
e. Oxytocin

**447.** A 26-year-old woman purchases an ovulation predictor kit at her local pharmacy. Assuming a regular menstrual cycle of 28 to 30 days, ovulation would be expected to occur between which of the following days?

a. Days 6 and 8
b. Days 10 and 12
c. Days 14 and 16
d. Days 18 and 20
e. Days 22 and 24

**448.** An 18-year-old college woman is brought to the emergency department by her roommate after she was raped walking back to the dorm from the library at night. She requests the "morning after pill" she has heard about to prevent pregnancy from the violation. She is given a postcoital contraceptive to prevent implantation and induce regression of the corpus luteum. Which of the following best describes the implantation of the zygote in the uterine wall?

a. Precedes formation of the zona pellucida
b. Involves infiltration of the endometrium by the syncytiotrophoblast
c. Occurs 3 to 5 days after fertilization
d. Occurs when the embryo consists of approximately 128 cells
e. Is inhibited by secretion of progesterone from the corpus luteum

**449.** A 22-year-old woman presents to the obstetrician-gynecologist's office with complaints of painful menstruation accompanied by profuse menstrual flow. The doctor prescribes a low-dose oral contraceptive for the menorrhagia and ibuprofen for the dysmenorrhea. Biological actions of estrogens include a decrease in which of the following?

a. Ovarian follicular growth
b. Duct growth in the breasts
c. Uterine smooth muscle motility
d. Serum cholesterol levels
e. Libido

**450.** A 23-year-old woman presents to her primary care physician with significant weight loss and amenorrhea. She has a high-intensity exercise regimen and seems preoccupied with food. She is diagnosed with anorexia nervosa. With respect to menstrual cycles in normal individuals, which of the following hormones is primarily responsible for development of ovarian follicles prior to ovulation?

a. Chorionic gonadotropin
b. Estradiol
c. Follicle-stimulating hormone
d. Luteinizing hormone
e. Progesterone

## Questions 451 and 452

**451.** A 30-year-old woman with polycystic ovarian syndrome (PCOS) uses an estrogen/progesterone combination for androgen excess and endometrial protection. Which of the following is most likely regarding progesterone?

a. Progesterone is secreted by the corpus luteum.
b. Progesterone secretion by the placenta increases at week 6 of gestation.
c. Plasma levels of progesterone increase during menses.
d. Plasma levels of progesterone remain constant after implantation.
e. Plasma levels of progesterone decrease after ovulation.

**452.** In regards to estrogen, administration of estrogens in women will do which of the following?

a. Limit the growth of ovarian follicles
b. Produce cyclic changes in the vagina and endometrium
c. Cause cervical mucus to become thicker and more acidic
d. Retard ductal proliferation in the breast
e. Decrease bone density

**453.** A young couple presents with concerns that they have not been able to conceive a child. Physical examination of the 22-year-old husband reveals mild obesity, gynecomastia, and decreased facial and axillary hair. He has male genitalia, but penile length is decreased and the testes are small. Chromosomal analysis reveals the XXY pattern of Klinefelter syndrome. Which of the following is the principal androgen responsible for transforming undifferentiated external genitalia in the fetus into male external genitalia?

a. Testosterone
b. Androstenedione
c. Androsterone
d. Dihydrotestosterone
e. Müllerian-inhibiting substance

**454.** A 12-year-old girl presents to her pediatrician's office because she has not yet begun her menstrual periods and she lacks breast development. After evaluation, she is found to have Turner syndrome. Which of the following best describes a patient with Turner syndrome?

a. The most common karyotype is 45, X/46, XX mosaicism.
b. Tall stature is common.
c. It is not associated with renal abnormalities.
d. Ovarian dysgenesis (streak ovary) is characteristic.
e. It is not associated with hypothyroidism.

**455.** A 55-year-old woman is experiencing the signs and symptoms of menopause. Her gynecologist discusses with her the possibility of hormone replacement therapy, which has which of the following effects?

a. Returns the menstrual cycle pattern to normal
b. Reduces the incidence of hot flashes
c. Reduces the risk of coronary artery disease and stroke
d. Reduces the risk of breast cancer
e. Increases the risk of osteoporosis

**456.** A couple has been having difficulty conceiving a child. The woman is evaluated at a fertility clinic and her examination and other investigations are unremarkable. The husband is asked to give a sample of ejaculate for analysis. Which of the following is most accurate regarding semen?

a.  The bulk of semen volume is contributed by the prostate gland.
b.  Semen prevents sperm capacitation.
c.  Semen is propelled out of the urethra by contraction of the smooth muscle comprising the bulbocavernosus muscle.
d.  Semen activates sperm motility in the male reproductive tract.
e.  In the population, sperm counts in semen have increased over the last 20 years.

**457.** A 29-year-old woman delivers a 7-lb 6-oz baby girl without complication. She begins to produce and eject breast milk (via prolactin and oxytocin) a few days later. Prolactin secretion is tonically suppressed in nonpregnant women by which of the following hormones?

a.  Estrogen
b.  Progesterone
c.  Dopamine
d.  FSH
e.  LH

**458.** A young couple has been trying to conceive a baby. The medical director of the fertility center has advised the woman to take her basal temperature readings on a daily basis and for them to have intercourse at the time the woman appears to be ovulating. Once conception takes place, which of the following must occur in order for the pregnancy to proceed uneventfully?

a.  The corpus luteum must secrete progesterone to sustain the endometrium.
b.  The pituitary must secrete hCG to maintain the corpus luteum.
c.  The pituitary must secrete prolactin to sustain the placenta.
d.  The placenta must secrete FSH to maintain ovarian function.
e.  The placenta must secrete LH to maintain ovarian function.

**459.** A 32-year-old woman presents at her physician's office complaining of nausea and vomiting. The history reveals that her symptoms have been present for over a month and that they seem to be worse in the morning. A urine sample is taken and shows that the woman is pregnant. Physiological changes that occur during pregnancy include which of the following?

a. Decreased production of cortisol and corticosterone
b. Increased conversion of glucose to glycogen
c. Hypercapnia
d. Increased hematocrit
e. Reduced circulating gonadotropin levels

**460.** A 35-year-old woman presents to her obstetrician/gynecologist's office for her annual well-woman examination. She reports that she may have "a touch of the flu" because she has been tired and nauseated the past week and also has had fleeting episodes of lower abdominal pain. She wasn't sure when her last menstrual period started but after looking at a calendar, realized that it had been 38 days. A right adnexal mass was palpated on routine pelvic examination and subsequently observed on ultrasound. Urinalysis confirmed that the woman was pregnant and serum levels of the tumor marker CA-125 were elevated. The gynecologist informed the woman that she may have an ovarian cancer and may need her ovary removed, but that they need to wait another week or two to do the laparotomy in order to protect her fetus. Ovariectomy before the sixth week of pregnancy leads to abortion, but thereafter has no effect on pregnancy because the placenta secretes adequate amounts of which of the following hormones?

a. Estrogens and progesterone
b. Estrogen and relaxin
c. Progesterone and human chorionic gonadotropin (hCG)
d. Human chorionic somatomammotropin (hCS) and hCG
e. Growth hormone releasing hormone (GnRH) and corticotropin releasing hormone (CRH)

# Reproductive Physiology

## Answers

**435. The answer is b.** *(Fauci, pp 601, 2317, 2345. Ganong, pp 425-427, 433.)* The temperature of the testes must be considerably below that of the internal body temperature for spermatogenesis to occur. The testes are normally maintained at a temperature of about 89.6°F (32°C), and are kept cool by a countercurrent heat exchange between the spermatic arteries and veins and by air circulating around the scrotum. The testes develop in the abdomen but normally descend into the scrotum during fetal development. In approximately 10% of newborn infants, one or, less commonly, both testes remain in the abdominal cavity or inguinal canal. Although most (98%) of undescended testes (cryptorchidism) spontaneously descend by 1 year, and all but 0.3% spontaneously descend by puberty, early surgical treatment is recommended because abdominal temperatures can cause irreversible damage to the spermatogenic epithelium and the incidence of malignant tumors is higher in undescended than in scrotal testes. Maturation of spermatogonia, the primitive germ cells, into primary spermatocytes does not begin until adolescence. Throughout the reproductive life of the human male, 100 to 200 million sperm are produced daily. Of critical importance to the hormonal regulation of spermatogenesis is the pulsatile release of GnRH and the subsequent involvement of FSH and LH at their target cells. FSH acts directly on the Sertoli cells of the seminiferous tubules to initiate mitotic and meiotic activity of germ cells. LH effects are thought to be mediated via stimulation of testosterone secretion by the Leydig cells.

**436. The answer is d.** *(Fauci, pp 2195, 2204-2205. Ganong, pp 236, 248-249, 421-424, 450-452.)* Prolactin is a single-chain protein structurally homologous to growth hormone, which is secreted by the anterior pituitary and has the principal physiologic effects of lactation (ie, milk production), decreased reproductive function, and suppressed sexual drive. Normal adult serum levels of prolactin are about the same or only slightly higher in females compared to males. Consistent with its role in lactogenesis, prolactin secretion increases during pregnancy. Suckling increases prolactin secretion, but milk ejection during suckling is due to oxytocin release. Prolactin inhibits reproductive function by inhibiting hypothalamic GnRH release and pituitary gonadotropin secretion. Hyper prolactinemia is the most common pituitary hormone hypersecretion syndrome in both males and females. Pregnancy and lactation are the most important physiological causes of hyperprolactinemia. Prolactin-secreting pituitary adenomas, hypothyroidism, and drug-induced inhibition or disruption of dopaminergic receptor function are other common causes of hyperprolactinemia.

**437 and 438. The answers are c. and b.** (*Ganong, pp 448-451. Widmaier, pp 632-633.*) During the first 2 months of pregnancy, estrogen and progesterone production is primarily the responsibility of the corpus luteum. The placenta serves as the source of the hormones during the remainder of pregnancy. Progesterone is essential to maintain placental implantation, inhibit uterine contractions, and suppress the maternal immune system response to fetal antigens. Estrogens serve to increase the size of the uterus, induce progesterone and oxytocin receptors, stimulate maternal hepatic protein secretion, and promote breast development. Estriol is the major estrogen produced during pregnancy. The production of estrogen and progesterone during gestation requires cooperation between the maternal, placental, and fetal compartments—the fetoplacental unit.

**439. The answer is c.** (*Ganong, pp 438-439. Widmaier, pp 619-622.*) Ovulation takes place just after the peak of the LH and estrogen curves, which occurs on approximately the 14th day of the menstrual cycle. Although FSH is primarily responsible for follicular maturation within the ovary, LH is necessary for final follicular maturation; without it, ovulation cannot take place. Both estrogen, following a sharp preovulatory rise in plasma concentration, and progesterone are secreted in abundance by the postovulatory corpus luteum.

**440. The answer is d.** (*Ganong, pp 438-439. Widmaier, pp 619-622.*) There is a marked increase in progesterone secretion following ovulation. Almost all the progesterone secreted in nonpregnant women is secreted by the corpus luteum. Secretion of both progesterone and estrogen is controlled by LH released by the adenohypophysis, and LH release itself is under the direction of a hypothalamic releasing factor.

**441. The answer is a.** (*Fauci, pp 2327-2328. Ganong, pp 434, 438-439.*) Ovulation is caused by a sudden increase in LH secretion. Both LH and FSH blood levels increase during the follicular phase of the menstrual cycle and reach peak blood levels prior to ovulation. Estrogen levels follow a similar pattern during the follicular phase. The physiological signal for ovulation is a surge in LH blood levels. Under the influence of LH, thecal and granulosa cells become the luteal cells of the corpus luteum. Progesterone production by the corpus luteum increases significantly. Estrogen levels also increase, but do not reach the levels achieved during the follicular phase. In anorexia nervosa, the regulation of virtually every endocrine system is altered, but the most striking changes occur in the reproductive system. Amenorrhea in anorexia nervosa is hypothalamic in origin and reflects decreased production of GnRH (with low levels of LH and FSH) that may be due to a marked reduction in leptin associated with the decreased mass of adipose tissue. In up to 25% of patients, however, amenorrhea precedes significant weight loss.

**442. The answer is e.** (*Fauci, pp 2327-2328. Ganong, pp 433-437.*) Ovulation occurs at point A on the graph. In response to estrogen secretion by the ovary, the endometrial lining of the uterus undergoes proliferation of both glandular epithelium and supporting stroma during the first 10 to 14 days of the menstrual cycle. Following ovulation, the glands begin to secrete mucus and the stroma undergoes pseudodecidual reaction in preparation for potential pregnancy. When ovulation is not followed by implantation of a fertilized ovum, progesterone secretion declines as the corpus luteum involutes, and the endometrial lining is almost completely shed during menses.

**443. The answer is d.** (*Fauci, pp 2324-2328. Ganong, pp 438-440. Le, pp 442-443. Widmaier, 619-623.*) Progesterone production by the corpus luteum increases significantly at the time of ovulation. Progesterone affects the set point for thermoregulation and increases body temperature approximately 0.58°F. Both LH and FSH blood levels increase during the follicular phase of the menstrual cycle and reach peak blood levels prior to ovulation. Estrogen levels follow a similar pattern during the follicular phase. The physiologic signal for ovulation is a surge in LH blood levels. Under the influence of LH, thecal and granulosa cells become the luteal cells of the corpus luteum. Estrogen levels also increase, but do not reach the levels achieved during the follicular phase.

**444. The answer is c.** (*Ganong, pp 424-427. Widmaier, p 608.*) The Sertoli cells rest on a basal lamina and form a layer around the periphery of the seminiferous tubules. They are attached to each other by specialized junctional complexes that limit the movement of fluid and solute molecules from the interstitial space and blood to the tubular lumen, and thus form a blood-testis barrier that provides an immunologically privileged environment for sperm maturation. Sertoli cells are intimately associated with developing spermatozoa and play a major role in germ-cell maturation. They secrete a variety of serum proteins and an androgen-binding protein into the tubular fluid in response to FSH and testosterone stimulation. Testosterone is synthesized and secreted by the interstitial Leydig cells. Estrogen is produced in small amounts by the Sertoli cells before puberty.

**445. The answer is a.** (*Ganong, p 449. Widmaier, p 632.*) Human chorionic gonadotropin (hCG) begins to appear in the maternal blood approximately 6 to 8 days following ovulation, upon implantation of the fertilized ovum in the endometrium. The secretion of hCG is essential to prevent involution of the corpus luteum and to stimulate secretion of progesterone and estrogens, which continues until the placenta becomes large enough to secrete sufficient quantities of those hormones. Following a peak at 7 to 9 weeks, hCG secretion gradually declines to a low level by 20 weeks' gestation.

**446. The answer is e.** (*Fauci, p 2218. Ganong, pp 236, 247-248, 451-452.*) A combined neurogenic and hormonal reflex involving oxytocin, a posterior pituitary hormone, causes the actual ejection ("let-down") of milk from breast tissue. Although estrogen and progesterone are essential for the physical development of breast tissue during pregnancy, both hormones inhibit milk secretion. Milk secretion is regulated by prolactin, a pituitary hormone secreted throughout pregnancy and after parturition. Adequate amounts of growth hormone are required to provide the nutrients that are essential for milk production by breast tissue. Suckling on breast tissue is the stimulus that leads to milk secretion. The secretion of oxytocin is increased by stressful stimuli, and inhibited by alcohol. Furthermore, alcohol is transferred from the mother's bloodstream into her breast milk and to the nursing infant, where it can have many deleterious effects.

**447. The answer is c.** (*Fauci, pp 2327-2328. Ganong, pp 433-438. Widmaier, pp 621-622.*) In a woman with a menstrual cycle of 28 to 30 days, ovulation generally occurs between days 14 and 16. The menstrual cycle is divided physiologically into three phases. The follicular phase begins with the onset of menses and lasts 9 to 13 days. The ovulatory phase lasts 1 to 3 days and culminates in ovulation. The luteal phase, the most constant phase of the cycle, lasts about 14 days and ends with the onset of menstrual bleeding.

**448. The answer is b.** (*Ganong, pp 448-450. Widmaier, pp 638-639.*) Implantation of a zygote into the uterine wall involves infiltration of the endometrium by the syncytiotrophoblast. Fertilization and early cleavage of the zygote occur in the fallopian tube in the human female. After approximately 3 days, the zygote enters the uterine cavity, where it undergoes additional divisions over a period of 3 to 4 days to form a morula of approximately 60 cells that is transformed into a blastocyst consisting of the yolk sac and embryo. Enzymatic digestion of the zona pellucida and infiltration of the endometrium by the syncytiotrophoblast, which forms the outer layer of the blastocyst, result in implantation of the blastocyst within the endometrium, where it erodes into maternal vessels. During these early stages of embryogenesis, the endometrium is primed by progesterone secreted by the corpus luteum in the ovary in response to pituitary gonadotropin secretion. After 10 to 15 days, placental gonadotropins maintain the corpus luteum until placental synthesis of progesterone is established at 6 to 8 weeks of gestation. Large-dose estrogens, diethystilbesterol, and mifepristone (RU486) are examples of postcoital contraceptives.

**449. The answer is d.** (*Ganong, pp 306, 441-443. Le, p 442.*) Estrogens have a significant plasma cholesterol-lowering action. Estrogens stimulate the growth and development of the female reproductive tract, including the ovarian follicles, duct growth and enlargement of the breasts, and uterine smooth muscle and its motility, as well as its blood flow. Estrogen increases libido in humans and has a protective effect against osteoporosis.

**450. The answer is c.** (*Fauci, pp 474-475. Ganong, pp 248, 444-448. Widmaier, pp 620-621.*) Preparation of primordial ovarian follicles for ovulation is the primary function of FSH. FSH stimulates development of the theca and granulosa cells of the follicles and promotes the synthesis of estrogens, including estradiol. LH promotes luteinization of the postovulatory follicle and stimulates progesterone secretion by the corpus luteum. During pregnancy, hCG is secreted by the placenta and continues progesterone production. Amenorrhea is seen in patients with anorexia nervosa due to decreased production of GnRH in the hypothalamus and subsequent low levels of FSH and LH.

**451 and 452. The answers are a. and b.** *(Fauci, pp 306, 2195. Ganong, pp 438-444. Widmaier, p 640.)* Progesterone is secreted by the corpus luteum. The plasma level of progesterone is low during the menses and remains low until just prior to ovulation. It rises substantially after ovulation, owing to secretion by the corpus luteum. If fertilization occurs, the corpus luteum continues to secrete progesterone until the placenta develops and begins to produce large amounts of the hormone. The plasma level of progesterone rises steadily throughout pregnancy after the placenta takes over production at about 12 weeks of gestation. Estrogens cause the mucus secreted by the cervix to become thinner and more alkaline and to exhibit a fernlike pattern upon drying. Estrogens can stimulate growth of ovarian follicles even in hypophysectomized women and also stimulate growth of the glandular epithelium of the endometrium, the smooth muscle of the uterus, and the uterine vascular system. Growth of the glandular elements of the breast is stimulated by progesterone; growth of the ductal elements is stimulated by estrogen. Estrogen helps maintain bone density.

**453. The answer is d.** *(Fauci, p 2340. Ganong, pp 413-417, 433. Widmaier, p 613.)* The testosterone metabolite dihydrotestosterone (DHT) induces the formation of the male external genitalia and male secondary sex characteristics. The fetus develops with bipotential internal and external genitalia that can develop (at about 40 days gestation) into either a testis or ovary, depending upon which genes are expressed. When the embryo has functional testes, male internal and external genitalia develop. The Leydig cells of the fetal testis secrete testosterone and the Sertoli cells secrete Müllerian-inhibiting substance (MIS), also known as antimüllerian hormone (AMH), a member of the TGF-$\beta$ growth factor family. The development of male internal genitalia depends upon testosterone, which stimulates growth and development of the Wolffian ducts and MIS, which stimulates Müllerian duct regression. Individuals with Klinefelter syndrome have an XXY chromosomal pattern, which is the most common sex chromosome disorder. These individuals have internal and external male genitalia, and testosterone secretion at puberty is often great enough for the development of male characteristics. However, the testes are small and the seminiferous tubules are abnormal, leading to infertility, eunuchoid proportions, gynecomastia, and poor virilization in phenotypic males. Mental retardation, developmental delay, or learning disabilities may be present. Patients with mosaic forms of Klinefelter syndrome have less severe clinical features, larger testes, and may achieve fertility.

**454. The answer is d.** *(Fauci, pp 2341-2342. Ganong, pp 407, 414. Le, p 445.)* Gonadal dysgenesis is characteristic of Turner syndrome. Most females have primary amenorrhea and lack pubertal development. The 45, X karyotype is most common and short stature is also typically seen. Renal manifestations, such as horseshoe kidney, are also frequently observed. In addition, other abnormalities include bicuspid aortic valve, coarctation of the aorta, hypertension, and hypothyrodism.

**455. The answer is b.** *(Fauci, pp 2404-2405, 2334-2335. Widmaier, pp 639-640.)* Because of the challenge of weighing the benefits versus risks for each individual, whether or not to use postmenopausal hormone therapy is one of the most complex health-care decisions facing women. In both observational studies and randomized trials, hormone therapy (either estrogen alone or estrogen/progestin) shows definite improvement in vasomotor symptoms (ie, hot flashes and night sweats) and vaginal dryness, and in increasing bone density and reducing the risk of fractures. However, observational studies promoting the use of hormone therapy as a strategy to delay the postmenopausal onset of cardiovascular disease have recently been refuted by randomized trials showing an increased risk of coronary artery disease in stroke with hormone replacement therapy. Hormone therapy also increases the risk of endometrial cancer, breast cancer (with long-term use), venous thromboembolism, and gallbladder disease. Estrogen therapy does not restore a woman's ability to have children.

**456. The answer is b.** *(Ganong, pp 424-428. Widmaier, p 606.)* Semen contains chemicals that prevent sperm capacitation, thereby prolonging the viability of the sperm. Semen is secreted primarily by the seminiferous tubules and the alkaline nature of the secretion buffers the acidity of the vagina. In recent years, the average sperm count has decreased from approximately 100 M/mL of semen to 60 to 70 M/mL of semen. The bulbocavernosus muscle is a skeletal muscle.

**457. The answer is c.** *(Fauci, pp 2204, 2195. Ganong, pp 421-424. Widmaier, pp 332, 637.)* In nonpregnant women, the secretion of prolactin is kept tonically suppressed by secretion of dopamine from the hypothalamus. Prolactin is the main hormone of lactation. Hormone levels increase early in pregnancy due to the influence of estrogens. However, lactation does not occur early in pregnancy because estrogens and progesterone inhibit the interaction of prolactin with receptors located on the alveolar cell membranes. At term, estrogen and progesterone levels decrease and milk production begins usually within 3 days of delivery.

**458. The answer is a.** *(Fauci, pp 2327-2328. Ganong, pp 448-451. Le, p 444. Widmaier, p 632.)* The corpus luteum in the ovary at the time of fertilization fails to regress and instead enlarges in response to stimulation by hCG secreted by the placenta. During the first trimester, placental production of hCG sustains the corpus luteum and ensures continued progesterone secretion by the corpus luteum, which is essential for development of the fetus.

**459. The answer is e.** *(Ganong, pp 448-451. Widmaier, pp 632-634.)* During pregnancy, the maternal hypothalamic-pituitary axis is suppressed due to high circulating levels of sex hormones. This leads to reduced gonadotropin levels, and, thus, ovulation does not occur. Additionally, hyperventilation leads to decreased arterial carbon dioxide levels. Increased water retention leads to decreased hematocrit. Maternal use of glucose declines and, as a result, gluconeogenesis increases. Plasma cortisol levels increase as the result of progesterone-mediated displacement from transcortin and its subsequent binding to globulin.

**460. The answer is a.** *(Fauci, pp 604-607. Ganong, pp 448-451. Le, pp 448-449.)* The placenta produces all of the hormones listed in the five answers at various times during pregnancy but it is the production of progesterone and estrogens (estradiol and estriol) from maternal and fetal precursors, which take over the function of the corpus luteum after the sixth week of pregnancy.

# Endocrine Physiology

## Questions

**461.** A 43-year-old man develops a brain tumor that impinges on the supraoptic nucleus in the hypothalamus. As a result, the secretion of which of the following hormones is affected?

a. Adrenocorticotropic hormone (ACTH)
b. Antidiuretic hormone (ADH)
c. Follicle-stimulating hormone (FSH)
d. Growth hormone (GH)
e. Prolactin

**462.** Following neck surgery, a patient develops circumoral paresthesia and a long QT interval on the electrocardiogram consistent with hypocalcemia resulting from injury to the parathyroid glands. Which of the following best describes parathyroid hormone (PTH)?

a. It is synthesized and secreted from the oxyphil cells in the parathyroid glands.
b. Secretion is increased in response to an increase in plasma-free $Ca^{2+}$ concentration.
c. It acts directly on bone cells to increase $Ca^{2+}$ resorption and mobilize $Ca^{2+}$.
d. It acts directly on intestinal cells to increase $Ca^{2+}$ absorption.
e. It increases phosphate reabsorption in the renal proximal tubular cells.

**463.** A 39-year-old man with an enlarged head, hands, and feet, osteoarthritic vertebral changes and hirsutism presents with a complaint of gynecomastia and lactation. The patient is most likely suffering from a tumor in which of the following locations?

a. Hypothalamus
b. Anterior pituitary
c. Posterior pituitary
d. Adrenal cortex
e. Breast

**464.** A 33-year-old major league baseball player takes human growth hormone to increase his performance. Which of the following best describes human growth hormone?

a. Secretion is stimulated by somatostatin and inhibited by ghrelin.
b. It has a long half-life.
c. It inhibits protein synthesis.
d. It decreases lipolysis.
e. It stimulates production of somatomedins (insulin-like growth factors I and II) by the liver, cartilage, and other tissues.

**465.** A 28-year-old woman develops a posterior pituitary tumor. Which of the following hormones is secreted by the posterior pituitary gland?

a. α-Melanocyte-stimulating hormone (α-MSH)
b. β-Lipotropin (β-LPH)
c. Leutinizing hormone (LH)
d. Oxytocin
e. Thyroid-stimulating hormone (TSH)

**466.** A 36-week pregnant mother has a decrease in urinary estriol excretion, indicating a decline in fetal adrenal cortical activity. Which of the following is the principal steroid secreted by the fetal adrenal cortex?

a. Cortisol
b. Corticosterone
c. Dehydroepiandrosterone
d. Progesterone
e. Pregnenolone

**467.** A 22-year-old woman presents with a recurrent vaginal candidiasis that is refractory to nystatin treatment. Diabetes screening shows elevated fasting blood glucose, and the patient is started on 25 U of insulin per day. Which aspect of glucose transport is enhanced by insulin?

a. Transport into adipocytes
b. Transport across the tubular epithelium of the kidney
c. Transport into the brain
d. Transport through the intestinal mucosa
e. Transport against a concentration gradient

**468.** A 52-year-old woman with a chief complaint of snoring is referred for a sleep study. As shown in the graph below, the concentration of a hormone varied over the 24-hour period of study. This diurnal variation in plasma level results from the secretion of which of the following hormones?

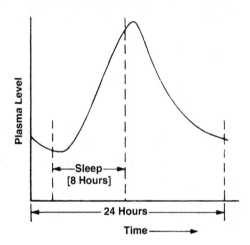

a. Thyroxine
b. Insulin
c. Parathyroid hormone
d. Cortisol
e. Estrogen

**469.** A 24-year-old pregnant woman and her 3-year-old child are seen in a medical mission clinic in Sudan. The child is short in stature, has a potbelly and enlarged protruding tongue, and is developmentally delayed. Iodine is prescribed for mother and child, with the hope of preventing mental retardation in the developing fetus. Iodides are stored in the thyroid follicles mainly in the form of which of the following?

a. Thyroxine
b. Triiodothyronine
c. Thyroglobulin
d. Monoiodotyrosine
e. Thyroid peroxidase

**470.** A 15-year-old girl presents with loss of the outer one-third of her eyebrows. Physical examination demonstrates slight enlargement of the thyroid gland and delayed relaxation phase of deep tendon reflexes. Blood work shows an elevation in creatine phosphokinase (CPK) and thyroid-stimulating hormone (TSH). Thyroid hormone therapy is ordered. Physiologically active thyroxine exists in which of the following forms?

a. Bound to albumin
b. Bound to prealbumin
c. Bound to globulin
d. As a glucuronide
e. Unbound

**471.** A 47-year-old man with uncontrolled diabetes has an increase in the plasma concentration of free fatty acids that parallels his increase in plasma glucose. Which of the following is most likely regarding activation of hormone-sensitive lipase in adipocytes?

a. It causes increased hydrolysis of cholesterol esters.
b. It is mediated by a cyclic AMP-dependent protein kinase.
c. It is prevented by cortisol.
d. It is stimulated by insulin.
e. It results in accumulation of monoglycerides and diglycerides in adipocytes.

**472.** A 3-year-old patient with DiGeorge congenital thymic aplasia presents with a seizure. An elevated serum phosphorus and low serum calcium confirm a hypoparathyroid state. Plasma levels of calcium can be increased most rapidly by the direct action of PTH on which of the following?

a. Kidney
b. Intestine
c. Thyroid gland
d. Bones
e. Skeletal musculature

**473.** A 20-year-old man presents with increasing daytime somnolence. A 24-hour sleep study showing a sudden onset of rapid eye movement (REM) sleep without previous slow-wave sleep confirms a diagnosis of narcolepsy. REM sleep decreases the secretion of growth hormone. The physiological secretion of growth hormone is increased by which of the following?

a. Hypoglycemia
b. Hyperglycemia
c. Free fatty acids
d. Somatostatin
e. Growth hormone

**474.** A 50-year-old male alcoholic presents with cirrhotic liver disease and chronic pancreatitis. He has been nauseated for the past several days, and not eating. Blood glucagon levels are elevated with which of the following results?

a. Stimulation of glycogenolysis in muscle
b. Inhibition of insulin secretion
c. Stimulation of gluconeogenesis in the liver
d. Inhibition of adenylate cyclase
e. Inhibition of phospholipase C

**475.** A patient in hyperkalemic renal failure is given an infusion of glucose and insulin. The actions of insulin include which of the following?

a. Converting glycogen to glucose
b. Stimulating gluconeogenesis
c. Increasing plasma amino acid concentration
d. Enhancing potassium entry into cells
e. Reducing urine formation

**476.** A 47-year-old woman with an anterior pituitary tumor presents with poor wound healing and hypertension. The endogenous secretion of ACTH is correctly described in which of the following statements?

a. It shows a circadian rhythm in humans.
b. It is decreased during periods of stress.
c. It is inhibited by aldosterone.
d. It is stimulated by glucocorticoids.
e. It is stimulated by epinephrine.

**477.** A patient with tuberculosis becomes confused and complains of muscle cramps and nausea. Lab results show a plasma sodium concentration of 125 mEq/L, serum osmolarity of 200 mOsm/kg, urine osmolarity of 1500 mOsm/kg, urine sodium of 400 mEq/d, and a normal blood volume. These clinical findings are consistent with which of the following?

a. Increased secretion of atrial natriuetic peptide
b. Decreased secretion of aldosterone
c. Increased secretion of aldosterone
d. Decreased secretion of antidiuretic hormone
e. Increased secretion of antidiuretic hormone

**478.** A 29-year-old man recovering from a viral upper respiratory tract infection develops a tender, enlarged thyroid gland and subacute thyroiditis, requiring hormone therapy. Injection of thyroid hormone into a human subject will result in which of the following?

a. Decrease the rate of oxygen consumption
b. Increase muscle protein synthesis
c. Decrease the need for vitamins
d. Increase the plasma concentration of cholesterol
e. Decrease the rate of lipolysis

**479.** An abdominal computed tomography (CT) in a 50-year-old patient with Conn syndrome (primary hyperaldosteronism) shows multiple small adrenocortical masses. Which of the following clinical findings are most likely present?

a. Hypertension
b. Hyperkalemia
c. Decreased extracellular fluid volume
d. Increased concentrating ability of the kidney
e. Increased hematocrit

**480.** A 75-year-old woman with primary hyperparathyroidism presents at her physician's office with dehydration and malaise. Which of the following plasma levels are most likely to be decreased?

a. Phosphate
b. Sodium
c. Calcium
d. Potassium
e. Calcitonin

**481.** A 65-year-old woman with metastatic small cell lung cancer presents to the ER with nausea, vomiting, and tachycardia. She is diagnosed as having Addison disease. Which of the following is most consistent with a patient in this condition?

| | Serum Na | Serum K | Blood glucose | Blood pressure |
|---|---|---|---|---|
| a. | Increased | increased | decreased | decreased |
| b. | Decreased | increased | increased | decreased |
| c. | Decreased | increased | decreased | decreased |
| d. | Increased | decreased | increased | decreased |
| e. | Decreased | decreased | increased | increased |

**482.** A 37-year-old woman presents with exophthalmus and an enlarged thyroid gland. The levels of free thyroxine in her blood are elevated. Other clinical findings of Graves disease include which of the following?

a. Anorexia
b. Increased basal metabolic rate
c. Bradycardia
d. Increased weight gain
e. Decreased sweating

**483.** A 20-year-old diabetic man forgets to take his insulin prior to the start of the National Collegiate Athletic Association (NCAA) swimming championships. Insulin-independent glucose uptake occurs in which of the following sites?

a. Adipose tissue
b. Cardiac muscle
c. Skeletal muscle
d. The brain
e. The uterus

**484.** A 46-year-old woman on lithium therapy for her bipolar disorder presents with complaints of weakness, arthralgia, and constipation. Blood work reveals hypercholesterolemia, increased levels of TSH, and decreased free $T_4$ levels. Which of the following is also likely to be associated with her hypothyroid state?

a. Tachycardia
b. Increased metabolic rate
c. Heat intolerance
d. Sleepiness
e. Decreased body mass index

**485.** A multisystem trauma patient develops hyperpyrexia, severe tachycardia, and high-output congestive heart failure with volume depletion, consistent with thyroid storm. Which of the following is the most appropriate treatment for the exaggerated hyperthyroidism?

a. $T_3$ administration to induce negative feedback inhibition of $T_4$
b. Aspirin to treat the fever
c. Propylthiouracil to block synthesis of new thyroid hormone
d. $\beta_2$-Adrenergic agents to mediate vasodilation and bronchodilation
e. Iodine followed by propylthiouracil to block release and synthesis of thyroid hormone

**486.** A 5-year-old boy presents with sexual precocity. Twenty-four hour melatonin concentrations are found to be lower than normal. Which of the following best describes melatonin?

a. It is synthesized in the anterior pituitary gland.
b. It regulates skin pigmentation in humans.
c. Its secretion is increased by darkness.
d. Its secretion is inhibited by norepinephrine from the sympathetic nervous system.
e. It is synthesized from the amino acid L-arginine.

**487.** A patient presents with Whipple triad, including plasma glucose < 60 mg/dL, symptomatic hypoglycemia, and improvement of symptoms with administration of glucose. CT of the abdomen is suggestive of islet cell carcinoma. Which of the following best describes the islets of Langerhans?

a. They are found primarily in the head of the pancreas.
b. They constitute approximately 30% of the pancreatic weight.
c. They contain six distinct endocrine cell types.
d. They have a meager blood supply.
e. They secrete insulin and glucagon.

**488.** A 59-year-old man is brought to his physician's office by his wife. She reports that he has been weak, nauseated, and urinates frequently. She has also noticed a fruity odor on her husband's breath. A urine sample is strongly positive for ketones and the finger-stick glucose is high, leading to a presumptive diagnosis of diabetes. As a result of insulin deficiency, which of the following will most likely occur?

a. Increased cellular uptake of glucose
b. Decreased intracellular α-glycerophosphate in liver and fat cells
c. Enhanced glucose uptake and use except by brain tissue
d. Decreased fatty acid release from adipose tissue
e. Indirect depression of glucose utilization due to excess fatty acids in the blood

**489.** A 24-year-old woman presents with a slightly elevated blood pressure. She has high plasma levels of total $T_4$, cortisol, and renin activity, but no symptoms or signs of thyrotoxicosis or Cushing syndrome. Which of the following is the most likely explanation?

a. She has been treated with ACTH and TSH.
b. She has been treated with $T_3$ and cortisol.
c. She has an adrenocortical tumor.
d. She is in the third trimester of pregnancy.
e. She has been subjected to chronic stress.

**490.** A 57-year-old postmenopausal woman takes calcium and vitamin D supplements daily to prevent osteoporosis. Which of the following best describes vitamin D?

a. It is a water-soluble vitamin.
b. Deficiency is seen in areas with high sun exposure.
c. 1,25 (OH)2-vitamin D is the physiologically active form of vitamin D.
d. It is converted to 1,25 (OH)2-vitamin D in the liver.
e. 1,25 (OH)2-vitamin D production increases when PTH secretion decreases.

**491.** A 13-year-old girl presents for her annual sports physical. Her height is measured at 50 in (> 3 SD below the mean for her age), and the history suggests that the girl may be suffering from anorexia nervosa. Which of the following about growth and development is most likely?

a. Growth hormone activates the JAK2-STAT pathway.
b. Linear growth ceases earlier in boys than in girls.
c. Serum IGF-I levels decrease throughout childhood.
d. Growth hormone is essential for prenatal linear growth.
e. Normal growth during puberty is independent of thyroid function.

**492.** A 22-year-old woman with insulin-dependent diabetes mellitus presents to the ER with nausea, vomiting, and a blood glucose of 600. She is found to be in diabetic ketoacidosis (DKA). Which of the following is true regarding patients in DKA?

a. Respiratory rate decreases.
b. Serum potassium levels are increased.
c. Serum potassium levels are decreased.
d. Intracellular potassium levels are increased
e. IV fluids correct the acidosis.

**493.** A 34-year-old patient with chronic asthma is started on glucocorticoid therapy. The treatment may result in bone loss because glucocorticoids do which of the following?

a. Inhibit bone formation
b. Increase calcium absorption from the GI tract
c. Increase osteoblast growth
d. Inhibit bone resorption
e. Suppress vitamin D activation

**494.** A 29-year-old woman presents with paroxysmal episodes of headaches, anxiety, and palpitations. The physician suspects an anxiety disorder, but orders laboratory studies to rule out underlying disease. The lab findings of hypercalcemia and elevated urinary catecholamines suggest the possibility of type II multiple endocrine neoplasia (MEN II). Which of the following is the hallmark of pheochromocytoma?

a. Hypoglycemia
b. Weight gain
c. Dry skin
d. Lethargy
e. Hypertension

**495.** A 36-year-old male computer programmer works for a company that has just been acquired in a corporate takeover. He experiences symptoms of tachycardia, palpitations, and an irregular heart beat, particularly at night. His plasma catecholamine levels are found to be increased, which may result from which of the following?

a. An increase in blood pressure
b. An increase in blood volume
c. An increase in plasma cortisol
d. An increase in blood glucose
e. Changing from the standing to the supine position

**496.** An 18-year-old man with hemophilia A suffered multiple internal injuries from a motorcycle accident. He is now presenting with dizziness, abdominal pain, dark patches on his elbows and knees, and cravings for chips and french fries. He is referred to an endocrinologist who makes the diagnosis of Addison disease, and prescribes cortisol. Cortisol administration to a patient with adrenal insufficiency will result in which of the following?

a. Increased insulin sensitivity in muscle
b. Enhanced wound healing
c. Increased corticotropin-releasing hormone secretion
d. Increased ACTH secretion
e. Increased gluconeogenesis

**497.** An 80-year-old man reports increasing dyspnea, which worsens with exertion. The cardiologist orders an echocardiogram, brain natriuretic peptide (BNP), and atrial natriuretic peptide (ANP) to evaluate possible congestive heart failure. Which of the following is most likely with atrial natriuretic peptide?

a. ANP enhances antidiuretic hormone (ADH) secretion.
b. ANP constricts afferent renal arterioles.
c. ANP acts only on the distal nephron to increase urine flow.
d. ANP secretion increases when central venous pressure increases.
e. ANP secretion is stimulated by hyponatremia.

**498.** A patient with multiple endocrine neoplasia type I (MEN I) and acromegaly is found to have a deletion of the 11q13 region of chromosome 11, a suppressor gene for growth hormone. Growth hormone excess results in which of the following?

a. Decreased gluconeogenesis
b. Hypoglycemia
c. Insulin resistance
d. Decreased protein synthesis
e. Decreased lipolysis

**499.** Sulfonylurea treatment in a 53-year-old type 2 diabetic patient causes a fall in the patient's plasma glucose concentration to 45 mg/dL. Which of the following is a sign and symptom of hypoglycemia?

a. Dry skin
b. Bradycardia
c. Insomnia
d. Loss of fine motor skills
e. Satiety

**500.** Radiation treatment for a pituitary tumor in an 8-year-old boy results in the complete loss of pituitary function. As a result, the child is likely to experience which of the following symptoms?

a. Absent sexual maturation
b. Accelerated growth spurts
c. Increased ACTH
d. Increased TSH levels

**501.** A 49-year-old male patient with AIDS and declining CD4 counts has an increased frequency of systemic infections and develops sick euthyroid syndrome. Which of the following would be expected with normal thyroid function?

a. TSH initiates thyroid hormone secretion via activation of nuclear receptors in thyroid gland cells.
b. Secretion of TSH is regulated primarily by the pituitary level of $T_3$.
c. TSH is secreted from the posterior pituitary.
d. $T_4$ is the physiologically active hormone.
e. $T_4$ is formed from $T_3$ by the process of monodeiodination.

**502.** The second-year medical students started a hunger strike to protest the reduction in library hours. After 3 days of fasting, the students will most likely manifest which of the following?

a. Decreased lipolysis
b. Increased urinary excretion of nitrogen
c. Decreased gluconeogenesis
d. Increased glucose utilization by the brain
e. Increased secretion of insulin

# Endocrine Physiology

## Answers

**461. The answer is b.** (*Ganong, pp 234-236, 242-250. Widmaier, pp 330-334.*) Antidiuretic hormone (ADH), also called arginine vasopressin (AVP), is secreted from the posterior lobe of the pituitary gland (neurohypophysis) into the general circulation from the endings of supraoptic neurons in the hypothalamus. ACTH, FSH, GH, and prolactin are all secreted by the anterior pituitary gland (adenohypophysis) into the portal hypophyseal circulation from the endings of arcuate and other hypothalamic neurons.

**462. The answer is c.** (*Ganong, pp 390-392. Stead, pp 88-89, 232-233.*) Parathyroid hormone (PTH), secreted by the chief cells of the parathyroid gland, is essential for life. PTH has a direct effect on bone to increase bone resorption and mobilize $Ca^{2+}$; this effect is mediated by increasing intracellular cAMP levels in osteoblasts. PTH also increases calcium absorption from the gut, although that effect is the result of PTH-mediated increases in renal 1,25-dihydroxy-cholecalciferol. PTH has a phosphaturic action due to a decrease in phosphate reabsorption in the proximal tubules. The secretion

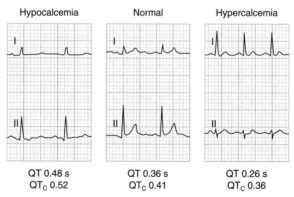

| Hypocalcemia | Normal | Hypercalcemia |
|---|---|---|
| QT 0.48 s | QT 0.36 s | QT 0.26 s |
| QT$_C$ 0.52 | QT$_C$ 0.41 | QT$_C$ 0.36 |

(Reproduced, with permission, from Fauci AS, Braunwald E, Kasper DL, et al. Harrison's Principles of Internal Medicine, 17th ed. New York: McGraw-Hill, 2008:1396.)

of PTH is inversely related to the circulating levels of ionized calcium. A prolonged QT interval is typical in hypocalcemia whereas a shortened QT interval is seen with hypercalcemia.

**463. The answer is b.** (*Ganong, pp 399-402, 409. Stead, pp 74-75, 233.*) Tumors of the somatotropes of the anterior pituitary gland secrete large amounts of growth hormone, leading to acromegaly in adults. When the epiphyses have not yet fused to the long bones, growth is stimulated by excess growth hormone leading to gigantism in children. Once the epiphyses have closed, linear growth is no longer possible, and growth hormone produces the pattern of bone and soft tissue abnormalities typical of acromegaly. Hypersecretion of growth hormone is accompanied by hypersecretion of prolactin in up to 40% of patients with acromegaly. Human growth hormone also has intrinsic lactogenic activity. Acromegaly can be caused by hypothalamic tumors that secrete growth hormone-releasing hormone (GHRH), but these are rare.

**464. The answer is e.** (*Ganong, pp 248, 305, 352, 398-406. Widmaier, pp 347-349, 576.*) Growth hormone (GH) exerts many of its effects on growth and metabolism by stimulating the production and release of polypeptide growth factors called somatomedins from the liver, cartilage, and other tissues. In humans, the principal circulating somatomedins are insulin-like growth factor I (IGF-I, somatomedin C) and IGF-II. GH release is stimulated by growth hormone-releasing hormone (GHRH) and ghrelin and inhibited by somatostatin. All of these peptides are synthesized and released by the hypothalamus, though the main site of ghrelin synthesis and secretion is the stomach. GH increases lipolysis; the resultant increase in free fatty acids, which takes several hours to develop, provides a ready source of energy for the tissues during hypoglycemia, fasting, and stressful stimuli. GH also has a protein anabolic effect. GH is metabolized rapidly; the half-life of circulating GH in humans is 6 to 20 minutes.

**465. The answer is d.** (*Ganong, pp 242, 396-397. Widmaier, pp 330-331.*) Oxytocin is secreted from the posterior lobe of the pituitary gland (neurohypophysis) into the general circulation from the endings of paraventricular neurons in the hypothalamus. LH, TSH, and β-lipotropin are all secreted by the anterior pituitary gland (adenohypophysis). α-MSH is released from the intermediate lobe of the pituitary.

**466. The answer is c.** (*Ganong, pp 356, 361-366, 450.*) Because it lacks 3β-hydroxysteroid dehydrogenase, the enzyme that converts pregnenolone to progesterone (the initial step in both glucocorticoid and mineralocorticoid synthesis), the fetal cortex synthesizes primarily dehydroepiandrosterone. This steroid is metabolized further to estrogen and androgen by the placenta. During fetal life, the adrenal cortex consists of a thin subcapsular rim, which eventually gives rise to the adult cortex, and a thick inner fetal cortex, which constitutes 80% of the gland. This zone undergoes rapid involution after birth.

**467. The answer is a.** (*Fauci, pp 2275-2283. Ganong, pp 336-338. Stead, pp 63-65.*) Insulin increases glucose uptake by adipocytes. Transport of glucose into cells is by facilitated diffusion. Insulin increases the number of transporters available for glucose uptake in many cells, including adipocytes, skeletal and cardiac muscle, and some smooth muscle. Insulin does not enhance glucose transport into brain cells, intestinal mucosal cells, or renal tubular epithelial cells. Diabetics have increased susceptibility to infections due to decreased efficacy of granulocytes despite a normal number. Type 1 diabetes mellitus patients must use insulin. They cannot use oral hypoglycemic agents because they do not have any functional pancreatic β cells.

**468. The answer is d.** (*Fauci, pp 2192-2193. Ganong, pp 372-374.*) Cortisol is a hormone that has a diurnal variation, as shown in the graph accompanying the question. Plasma cortisol levels rise sharply during sleep, peaking soon after awakening, and sinking to a low level approximately 12 hours later. This pattern is intimately related to the secretory rhythm of ACTH, which governs, and in turn is partly governed by, plasma concentration of cortisol.

**469. The answer is c.** (*Fauci, pp 2224-2226. Ganong, pp 317-322, 328-329.*) The thyroid gland stores iodide primarily as thyroglobulin. The thyroid gland has a specialized active transport system that very efficiently traps iodide from circulating blood and can accumulate iodide against a large concentration gradient. Within the thyroid, the iodide rapidly undergoes organification by which it is oxidized and covalently linked to tyrosine residues in thyroglobulin. The iodinated tyrosine residues gradually become coupled to form thyroxine, the major secretion product of the thyroid. Children who are hypothyroid from birth or before are sometimes referred to as cretins. Worldwide, congenital hypothyroidism is one of the most common causes of preventable mental retardation. Outside of the United States and most other developed countries, maternal iodine deficiency is a major cause of congenital hypothyroidism.

**470. The answer is e.** *(Ganong, pp 321-323. Stead, pp 81-83.)* Only the free unbound form of thyroxine is physiologically active. Circulating thyroxine can be bound to albumin, thyroxine-binding prealbumin (TBPA), or thyroxine-binding globulin (TBG). Most thyroxine is bound, and, despite the large available pool of albumin, most of it is bound to TBG. This reflects the relatively greater affinity of TBG for thyroxine.

**471. The answer is b.** *(Ganong, pp 305, 342.)* Hormone-sensitive lipase is a cytoplasmic enzyme in adipocytes that catalyzes the complete hydrolysis of triglyceride to fatty acids and glycerol. It is activated by a cyclic AMP-dependent protein kinase that phosphorylates the enzyme, converting it to its active form. Because no accumulation of monoglycerides or diglycerides is detected in adipocytes following the action of hormone-sensitive lipase, it is the initial hydrolysis of triglyceride to fatty acid and diglyceride that is the rate-limiting step. Hormone-sensitive lipase is sensitive to several hormones in vitro, but it appears to be regulated in vivo primarily by epinephrine and glucagon, which activate it by increasing cyclic AMP, and insulin, which inhibits it by preventing cyclic AMP-dependent phosphorylation. Cortisol enhances lipolysis indirectly by promoting increased enzyme synthesis.

**472. The answer is d.** *(Fauci, pp 413, 2057. Ganong, pp 390-392.)* PTH increases plasma calcium levels primarily by mobilizing bone calcium. The main function of the parathyroid gland is to maintain a constant ionized calcium level in the extracellular fluid. To do this, PTH stimulates increased plasma calcium levels, chiefly by mobilizing calcium from bones. Although PTH can also increase renal tubular reabsorption of calcium and intestinal absorption of calcium, these effects depend on adequate dietary ingestion of calcium and thus occur more slowly.

**473. The answer is a.** *(Ganong, pp 201, 400-406. Stead, p 71.)* Synthesis and secretion of growth hormone (GH) by the anterior pituitary is regulated by a variety of metabolic factors, many of which act to alter the balance between release of growth hormone-releasing hormone (GHRH) and somatostatin (SS) from the hypothalamus. Among the stimuli that increase

GH secretion are: (1) conditions in which there is a deficiency of energy substrate (eg, hypoglycemia, exercise, and fasting); (2) stressful stimuli (eg, fever, various psychological stresses); (3) an increase in arginine and some other amino acids (eg, protein meal); (4) glucagon; (5) L-dopa and dopamine receptor agonists; (6) estrogens and androgens; and (7) going to sleep. Stimuli that decrease GH secretion include somatostatin, REM sleep, glucose, cortisol, free fatty acids, and GH itself.

**474. The answer is c.** *(Fauci, pp 1969-1973. Ganong, pp 348-350. Stead, pp 114-117.)* The primary action of glucagon is to increase blood glucose concentration, which it accomplishes by promoting gluconeogenesis and glycogenolysis in the liver but not in muscle. These effects are mediated by cyclic AMP, which is produced by hepatic adenylate cyclase following interaction of glucagon with its plasma membrane receptor. Interaction of glucagon with different hepatic plasma membrane receptors activates phospholipase C, which results in a rise in concentration of intra-cellular $Ca^{2+}$, which further stimulates glycogenolysis. Although glucagon opposes the action of insulin, it does not directly affect insulin secretion.

**475. The answer is d.** *(Ganong, pp 336-338.)* One of insulin's major effects is the stimulation of the $Na^+$-$K^+$ pump, which increases potassium entry into cells, with a resultant lowering of the extracellular $K^+$ concentration. Insulin given along with glucose, to prevent hypoglycemia, is often used as a treatment for hyperkalemia. Insulin's major effect on metabolism is the synthesis of proteins and lipids and the storage of glucose as glycogen. Insulin stimulates the uptake of amino acids and glucose by most cells of the body and decreases the rate of gluconeogenesis. Insulin has no effect on urine formation, but in diabetes, when glucose levels increase to a level at which the kidney can no longer reabsorb the filtered glucose, glucose acts as an osmotic diuretic and increases the formation of urine.

**476. The answer is a.** *(Fauci, p 2212. Ganong, pp 372-375.)* The secretion of ACTH occurs in several irregular bursts during the day; the peak occurs early in the morning prior to awakening and thus is not due to the stress of arising. This circadian rhythm, maximum secretion in early morning and minimum secretion in the evening, is regulated by the hypothalamus through the secretion of corticotropin-releasing hormone (CRH) into the hypothalamic-hypophyseal portal capillary system. In addition to the basal rhythm, physical or mental stress will lead to increased ACTH secretion within minutes. ACTH is also regulated as a result of feedback inhibition by the hormones whose synthesis it stimulates, such as glucocorticoids. Aldosterone is a mineralocorticoid and is not controlled by ACTH. Epinephrine does not appear to have any effect on ACTH secretion.

**477. The answer is e.** (*Ganong, pp 246-247, 378-379, 729-730. Stead, pp 77-78, 226-228. Widmaier, pp 502-503.*) An increase in antidiuretic hormone is associated with isovolemic, hypotonic hyponatremia, and an increase in both urine osmolarity and urine sodium. The etiology of syndrome of inappropriate antidiuretic hormone secretion (SIADH) includes idiopathic overproduction of ADH that is often associated with disorders of the CNS (encephalitis, stroke, head trauma) and pulmonary disease (TB, pneumonia). Hyperaldosteronism leads to decreased sodium (and water) excretion and thus hypernatremia and an increase in extracellular fluid volume. A decrease in aldosterone would be associated with hypovolemic hyponatremia. A decrease in ANP would lead to decreased sodium and water excretion.

**478. The answer is b.** (*Ganong, pp 323-326. Stead, pp 85-86.*) Thyroid hormone affects all aspects of metabolism; it increases calorigenesis in every tissue in the body. The hormone stimulates protein synthesis, which may be directly responsible for a portion of its calorigenic effect. Thyroid hormone affects both synthesis and degradation of lipids; the net effect is a decrease in lipid stores. By increasing the mechanisms by which cholesterol is eliminated from the body, thyroid hormone decreases plasma cholesterol levels. Because of its stimulatory effect on metabolic processes, thyroid hormone increases the demand for coenzymes and vitamins.

**479. The answer is a.** (*Fauci, pp 281, 2693. Ganong, pp 375-381. Stead, pp 93-94.*) The symptoms of primary hyperaldosteronism (Conn syndrome) develop from chronic excess secretion of aldosterone from the zona glomerulosa of the adrenal cortex. Patients are hypertensive and have an expanded blood volume with a decreased hematocrit. They are not markedly hypernatremic because of a renal escape phenomenon. Patients are severely depleted of potassium and, as a consequence, suffer kidney damage, with a resulting loss in concentrating ability.

**480. The answer is a.** (*Ganong, pp 390-393. Stead, pp 87-88, 233-234.*)
PTH is essential for maintaining plasma calcium and phosphate levels. It is
released in response to decreased plasma calcium and acts to increase
calcium reabsorption and phosphate excretion. Thus, hyperparathyroidism
is characterized by hypophosphatemia and hypercalcemia.

**481. The answer is c.** (*Ganong, p 381. Stead, pp 89-91. Widmaier, p 344.*)
This patient has primary adrenal insufficiency due to bilateral adrenal
destruction from a metastatic lung cancer. The deficiency of cortisol results
in hypoglycemia. The deficiency of the mineralocorticoids (aldosterone)
results in hyponatremia and hyperkalemia from the loss of aldosterone's
affect on the distal tubules of the kidney and subsequent volume depletion
that takes place.

**482. The answer is b.** (*Fauci, pp 2233-2237. Ganong, pp 329-330. Stead,
pp 78-81.*) Hyperthyroidism can increase the basal metabolic rate 60% to
100% above normal. Thyroid hormone causes nuclear transcription of
large numbers of genes in virtually all cells of the body. The result is a generalized increase in functional cell activity and metabolism. The increased
metabolic activity of patients with hyperthyroidism is accompanied by
increased food intake. Nevertheless, their body weight decreases. The generalized increase in cellular activity results in increased sweat production
and increased heart rate.

**483. The answer is d.** (*Ganong, pp 336-338. Widmaier, p 572.*) Insulin
does not promote glucose uptake by most brain cells. Insulin does increase
glucose uptake in skeletal muscle, cardiac muscle, smooth muscle, adipose
tissue, leukocytes, and the liver. In most insulin-sensitive tissues, insulin
acts to promote glucose transport by enhancing facilitated diffusion of glucose down a concentration gradient. In the liver, where glucose freely per-
meates the cell membrane, glucose uptake is increased as a result of its
phosphorylation by glucokinase. Formation of glucose-6-phosphate reduces
the intra cellular concentration of free glucose and maintains the concentration gradient favoring movement of glucose into the cell.

**484. The answer is d.** (*Ganong, pp 323-326. Stead, pp 81-83.*) Sleepiness is
common in patients with hypothyroidism. Hypothyroidism is a condition
usually characterized by low levels of $T_3$ and $T_4$, owing to atrophy of the

thyroid gland. In very rare cases there is resistance to the effects of thyroid hormones. A deficiency of thyroid hormones or their effects results in bradycardia, which is due to decreased sympathetic activity, and a decreased metabolic rate with its associated sleepiness, weight gain, and cold intolerance. Excess thyroid hormone increases metabolic rate, which increases heat production, stimulates the appetite, and causes weight loss even in the face of increased intake of food. Heat intolerance is characteristic of hyperthyroidism.

**485. The answer is c.** (*Ganong, pp 321-326. Stead, pp 79-80.*) Thyroid storm is an exaggerated manifestation of hyperthyroidism. Thyroid storm is a medical emergency and mortality is high (20%-50%) even with the correct treatment. After primary stabilization of the airway, breathing and oxygenation, circulation, and fluid balance, treatment includes propylthiouracil (PTU) or methimazole to block the synthesis of new thyroid hormone and β-blockers to block adrenergic effects. Iodine should not be given until after PTU has taken effect or more thyroid hormone will be produced. Aspirin displaces $T_4$ from thyroid binding protein, and therefore should not be used to treat fever. $T_3$ and $T_4$ inhibit the release of thyrotropin-releasing hormone (TRH) from the hypothalamus, which regulates thyroid-stimulating hormone (TSH) secretion from the anterior pituitary gland.

**486. The answer is c.** (*Ganong, pp 420, 462-465.*) Synthesis and secretion of melatonin are increased in the dark via input from norepinephrine secreted by postganglionic sympathetic neurons. Melatonin is synthesized in the pineal gland from the amino acid tryptophan. Pinealomas (tumors of the pineal gland) that destroy the pineal gland and reduce secretion of melatonin and cause hypothalamic damage may cause precocious puberty by removing the inhibitory effect of melatonin on the pituitary response to gonadotropin-releasing hormone. Melatonin causes amphibian skin to become lighter in color but has no role in the regulation of skin color in humans.

**487. The answer is e.** (*Ganong, pp 333-334. Stead, pp 69-70.*) The islets of Langerhans, which constitute 1% to 2% of the pancreatic weight, secrete insulin, glucagon, somatostatin, and pancreatic polypeptide. Each is secreted from a distinct cell type, A, B, D, and F, respectively. The islets are scattered throughout the pancreas, but are more plentiful in the tail than in the body or head.

**488. The answer is b.** (*Ganong, pp 340-343. Stead, pp 63-68. Widmaier, pp 578-580.*) α-Glycerophosphate is produced in the course of normal use of glucose. In the absence of adequate quantities of α-glycerophosphate, a normal acceptor of free fatty acids in triglyceride synthesis, lipolysis will be the predominant process in adipose tissue. As a result, fatty acids will be released into the blood. The prevailing insulin level is decisive in the selection of substrate by a tissue for the production of energy. Insulin promotes use of carbohydrate, and a lack of the hormone causes use of fat mainly to the exclusion of uptake and use of glucose, except by brain tissue. Indirect depression of glucose utilization due to excess fatty acids is a result, and not a contributing cause, of increased use of fat.

**489. The answer is d.** (*Ganong, pp 322, 449-450, 456.*) Thyroxin-binding globulin (TBG) is increased in estrogen-treated patients and during pregnancy, increasing the total plasma levels of $T_3$ and $T_4$, but with a normal level of the free thyroid hormones, such that the clinical state is euthyroid. Cortisol levels also increase during pregnancy and parturition due to increased production of corticotropin-releasing hormone (CRH) by the placenta (as well as the fetal hypothalamus). Although tissue renin contributes little to the circulating renin pool, pregnancy is associated with increased renin levels that may arise from components of the tissue renin-angiotensin system found in the uterus, the placenta, and the fetal membranes. Amniotic fluid contains large amounts of prorenin.

**490. The answer is c.** (*Ganong, pp 387-389. Widmaier, pp 354-355.*) 1,25 (OH)2-vitamin D is the physiologically active form of vitamin D and the conversion to this form occurs in the kidney, not the liver. It is a fat soluble vitamin with metabolism occurring in the skin with exposure to sunlight. When PTH secretion increases, so does the production of 1,25 (OH)2-vitamin D.

**491. The answer is a.** (*Ganong, pp 44-47, 326, 400-407.*) Growth hormone activates many different intracellular enzyme cascades, including the JAK2-STAT pathway, which also mediates the effects of various growth factors and prolactin. Secretion of insulin-like growth factor I (IGF-I) increases throughout childhood and stimulates cell proliferation and growth in many different cell types, including chondrocytes within growth plates. Linear growth ends earlier in girls than in boys. IGF-II is largely independent of growth hormone and plays a role in the growth of the fetus before birth. Thyroid hormones are essential for normal linear growth and skeletal development. The growth-promoting effects of thyroid hormones occur via a synergistic effect with growth hormone.

**492. The answer is b.** *(Fauci, pp 2282-2284. Ganong, pp 340-343.)* Patients in diabetic ketoacidosis have an increased serum potassium at presentation. This is not due to an excess of potassium stores, but is the result of the shift of potassium out of the cells because of the acidosis. Thus, intracellular potassium is actually low and needs to be replaced as the acidosis resolves. Kussmaul respirations (rapid, deep breathing) occur as carbon dioxide is exhaled. While IV fluids help with the intravascular volume depletion that occurs with DKA (due to glucosuria), only insulin therapy can correct the acidosis.

**493. The answer is a.** *(Fauci, pp 1641, 2365-2367. Ganong, p 395.)* Glucocorticoids lower plasma $Ca^{2+}$ levels by inhibiting osteoclast formation and activity. Over long periods of time, glucocorticoids cause osteoporosis by decreasing bone formation and increasing bone resorption. They decrease bone formation by inhibiting protein synthesis in osteoblasts. Glucocorticoids also decrease the absorption of $Ca^{2+}$ and $PO_4^{3-}$ from the intestine and increase the renal excretion of these ions. Vitamin D formation is facilitated when plasma $Ca^{2+}$ levels are low.

**494. The answer is e.** *(Fauci, pp 2269-2273. Ganong, pp 360, 642. Stead, pp 94-95.)* The hallmark of pheochromocytoma is either sustained or paroxysmal hypertension. Pheochromocytoma is a rare catecholamine-secreting tumor of the adrenal chromaffin cells. Patients with the disease often have associated episodes of sweating, anxiety or nervousness, palpitations, headache, diaphoresis, and hyperglycemia. In adults, approximately 80% of pheochromocytomas are unilateral and solitary. The 10% rule applies to pheochromocytomas as follows: 10% in adults are bilateral, 10% are extra-adrenal, 10% are malignant, and 10% are familial, inherited as an autosomal dominant trait either alone or in combination with MEN 2.

**495. The answer is c.** (*Ganong, pp 358-359.*) Phenylethanolamine-*N*-methyltransferase (PNMT), the enzyme that catalyzes the formation of epinephrine from norepinephrine, is found in appreciable quantities only in the brain and the adrenal medulla. Adrenal medullary PNMT is induced by glucocorticoiods and glucocorticoids are necessary for the normal development of the adrenal medulla. Circumstances that increase sympathetic nerve input to the adrenal medulla increase catecholamine secretion. Major stressors include decreased intravascular volume or pressure, fear or rage, a change in posture from supine to standing, and hypoglycemia.

**496. The answer is e.** (*Ganong, pp 366-372. Stead, pp 89-91. Widmaier, p 344.*) Cortisol is defined as a glucocorticoid because it promotes the conversion of amino acids to glucose (gluconeogenesis). It also decreases glucose uptake by muscle and adipocytes by decreasing the sensitivity of the cells to insulin. The net result is to provide more glucose to non-insulin-requiring cells. Cortisol retards wound healing. It also decreases CRH and ACTH secretion by feedback inhibition.

**497. The answer is d.** (*Ganong, pp 460-462, 723. Widmaier, pp 509-510.*) Atrial natriuretic peptide (ANP) is synthesized, stored, and secreted by cardiac atrial muscle, the latter in response to increased central venous pressure or increased plasma sodium concentrations. ANP increases glomerular filtration by simultaneous dilation of afferent and constriction of efferent renal arterioles. It decreases salt and water reabsorption along the entire length of the kidney. The excretion of water is enhanced by inhibition of ADH.

**498. The answer is c.** (*Ganong, pp 400-404. Stead, pp 74-75.*) Patients with acromegaly have insulin resistance. In addition, they manifest increased lipolysis and increased gluconeogenesis due to their high growth hormone levels. The combination of enhanced glucose production and insulin resistance can produce hyperglycemia and diabetes mellitus. Protein synthesis increases to support tissue growth and proliferation.

**499. The answer is d.** (*Ganong, pp 344-346, 353-354. Stead, pp 69-70. Widmaier, p 580.*) Hypoglycemia can lead to loss of fine motor skills. Hypoglycemia refers to abnormally low blood glucose levels and is dangerous because glucose is the primary energy source for brain cells. Dysfunction of the nervous system can lead to dizziness, headache, mental confusion, convulsion, and loss of consciousness. Increased sympathetic activity can produce sweating, tachycardia, hunger, and anxiety.

**500. The answer is a.** *(Ganong, pp 396-397, 404-409. Stead, pp 72-76.)* Radiation treatment likely produced panhypopituitarism in the young child. Sexual maturation and growth during development will not occur because of low levels of GH, FSH, LH, ILGF1, TSH and thyroid hormones, and gonadal hormones. The cortisol response to stress is decreased due to low ACTH levels.

**501. The answer is b.** *(Fauci, pp 2225-2227. Ganong, pp 317-324.)* Secretion of TSH is regulated primarily by the pituitary levels of $T_3$. As plasma thyroid hormone levels increase, pituitary $T_3$ levels rise and lead to inhibition of TSH synthesis and secretion. TSH stimulates thyroid gland function by binding to specific cell membrane receptors and increasing the intracellular levels of cAMP. The thyroid gland secretes thyroxine ($T_4$) and triiodothyronine ($T_3$); the latter is the physiologically active hormone. The majority of $T_3$ is formed in the peripheral tissues by deiodination of $T_4$.

**502. The answer is c.** *(Ganong, pp 290-291, 298.)* With prolonged fasting of 3 days or more, gluconeogenesis is decreased partly due to increased ketogenesis and lipolysis. The increased availability of ketones and fatty acids as a source of fuel for brain cells decreases the demand by the brain for glucose. The decreased gluconeogenesis is reflected in a nitrogen excretion level at or below normal values. Insulin levels would decrease in this situation.

# Bibliography

Fauci AS, Braunwald E, Kasper DL, et al. *Harrison's Principles of Internal Medicine.* 17th ed. New York, NY: McGraw-Hill; 2008.

Ganong WF. *Review of Medical Physiology.* 22nd ed. New York, NY: The McGraw-Hill Companies, Inc.; 2005.

Guyton AC, Hall MN. *Textbook of Medical Physiology.* 10th ed. Philadelphia, PA:WB Saunders; 2000.

Le T, Bhushan V, Rao D. *First Aid for the USMLE Step 1.* 20th ed. New York, NY: McGraw-Hill; 2008.

Levitzky MG. *Pulmonary Physiology.* 7th ed. New York, NY: The McGraw-Hill Companies, Inc.; 2008.

McPhee SJ, Lingappa V, Ganong WF. *Pathophysiology of Disease: An Introduction to Clinical Medicine.* 5th ed. New York, NY: The McGraw-Hill Companies, Inc.; 2006.

Stead LG, Stead SM, Kaufman MS, et al. *First Aid for the Medicine Clerkship.* 2nd ed. New York, NY: McGraw-Hill; 2006.

Widmaier E, Hershel R, Strang K. *Vander's Human Physiology.* 11th ed. New York, NY: McGraw-Hill; 2008.

# Index

Note: Page numbers followed by "*t*" indicate table and page numbers followed by "*f*" indicate figure.

Second messengers, 7, 55, 62
Secondary active transport, 1-2
Secondary hyperaldosteronism, 164
Secondary hypoaldosteronism, 14
Second-degree heart block, 236, 267
Secretin, 48, 318
Segmentation, 47
Seizures, 57, 65
Semen, 385, 393
Seminiferous tubules, 380
Semipermeable membrane, 4, 56
Senses
    hearing, 25-27, 129, 134, 151-152, 155
    sight, 27-29, 133, 154-155
Sensory neurons, 23-24
Sensory receptors, 23
Serotonin, 143, 165
Sertoli cells, 380, 389-390
SGLT, 302, 320
Short-chain fatty acids (SCFAs), 66, 303, 320
Shunt percentage fraction, 203, 227
Sickle cell anemia, 114, 121
Sickle cell crisis, 114, 121
Sickle cell trait, 111, 119
Sight, 27-29
Signal transduction pathways, 63
Sildenafil, 55, 62
Simple diffusion, 1, 3
Sinoatrial nodal cells, 245
Skeletal muscle
    action potential of, 172, 179
    calcium release, 29
    characteristics of, 31
    contractile responses of, 171-172, 178-179
    contraction of, 29, 126, 149, 170, 176-177
    end-plate potential in, 171, 177
    excitation-contraction coupling of, 178
    fibers of, 29-30, 64, 167, 174
    glucose transport into, 65
    ryanodine receptor in, 169, 175
Skeletal muscle cells, 23
Sleep apnea, 197, 224
Slow-oxidative muscle fibers, 30
Small intestine, 49
    inflammation of, 316
    motility in, 291, 309
    removal of proximal segments,
        294, 312
    sodium absorption from, 308, 325
    vitamin absorption in, 291, 310
Smooth muscle
    bronchial, 206, 230
    contraction of, 59, 129, 151, 171, 178,
        264, 289, 291, 309
    excitation-contraction coupling of, 178
    gastrointestinal, 301, 321
Smooth muscle autoantibodies, 67

Sodium
    absorption of, 308, 325
    equilibrium potential, 144, 165-166
    fractional excretion of, 330, 353, 371
    gastrointestinal absorption of, 47
    membrane potential affected by, 163
    reabsorption of, 14, 51, 292, 311,
        328-329, 339, 343-347, 351-352,
        362, 365-369
    regulation of, 11
    transference, 164
    transport of, 66
Sodium channels, 28, 38, 175
Somatomedins, 396, 409
Somatostatin, 143, 165, 321, 399, 411
Spasticity, 126, 149
Spermatogenesis, 375, 387
Sphingomyelin, 55, 103-104
Spike potential, 22
Spirometer, 209, 232-233
Splitting of heart sound, 246, 276
ST segment, 39, 277, 284
Stagnant hypoxia, 188, 216
Stapes, 26
Starling curve, 42, 252, 280
Starling forces, 225, 271
Starling law, 46, 220
Steady-state volume of cell, 5-6
Steatorrhea, 296, 298-299, 314, 316-317
Stereocilia, 26
Stokes-Adam syndrome, 267
Stomach, 49
Stress incontinence, 368
Stress test, 244, 274
Stroke, 71, 90
Stroke volume, 41-42, 246-248, 269, 271,
        276-278
Stroke work, 42, 265, 290
Subatmospheric intraalveolar pressure, 34
Subatmospheric intrapleural pressure, 36
Substance P, 143, 165
Subthalamus, 128, 151
Succinylcholine, 140, 162
Surfactant, 187, 193, 215-216, 219
Swallowing, 46
Swan-Ganz catheter, 220
Synapse, 23
Syncope, 235, 266-267
Syndrome of inappropriate antidiuretic
        hormone (SIADH), 102, 342, 364, 413
Systemic circulation, 265, 290
Systolic murmurs, 45, 243-244, 246, 273, 277

**T**
T wave, 39, 279
Tardive dyskinesia, 25
Terminal bronchioles, 33